MW01106634

# Substance Use Disorders, Part I

*Editors*

RAY CHIH-JUI HSIAO
LESLIE RENEE WALKER

# CHILD AND ADOLESCENT PSYCHIATRIC CLINICS OF NORTH AMERICA

www.childpsych.theclinics.com

*Consulting Editor*
HARSH K. TRIVEDI

July 2016 • Volume 25 • Number 3

**ELSEVIER**

1600 John F. Kennedy Boulevard • Suite 1800 • Philadelphia, Pennsylvania, 19103-2899

http://www.theclinics.com

CHILD AND ADOLESCENT PSYCHIATRIC CLINICS OF NORTH AMERICA Volume 25, Number 3
July 2016 ISSN 1056-4993, ISBN-13: 978-0-323-44841-3

Editor: Lauren Boyle
Developmental Editor: Kristen Helm

*Child and Adolescent Psychiatric Clinics of North America* (ISSN 1056-4993) is published quarterly by Elsevier Inc., 360 Park Avenue South, New York, NY 10010-1710. Months of issue are January, April, July, and October. Business and Editorial Offices: 1600 John F. Kennedy Boulevard, Suite 1800, Philadelphia, PA 19103-2899. Periodicals postage paid at New York, NY and additional mailing offices. Subscription prices are $310.00 per year (US individuals), $544.00 per year (US institutions), $100.00 per year (US students), $360.00 per year (Canadian individuals), $662.00 per year (Canadian institutions), $200.00 per year (Canadian students), $430.00 per year (international individuals), $662.00 per year (international institutions), and $200.00 per year (international students). International air speed delivery is included in all *Clinics* subscription prices. All prices are subject to change without notice. **POSTMASTER:** Send address changes to *Child and Adolescent Psychiatric Clinics of North America*, Elsevier Health Sciences Division, Subscription Customer Service, 3251 Riverport Lane, Maryland Heights, MO 63043. **Customer Service: 1-800-654-2452 (U.S. and Canada); 314-447-8871 (outside U.S. and Canada). Fax: 314-447-8029. E-mail:** JournalsCustomer Service-usa@elsevier.com **(for print support) or** journalsonlinesupport-usa@elsevier.com **(for online support).**

*Reprints.* For copies of 100 or more of articles in this publication, please contact the Commercial Reprints Department, Elsevier Inc., 360 Park Avenue South, New York, New York 10010-1710 Tel.: 212-633-3874; Fax: 212-633-3820, E-mail: reprints@elsevier.com.

*Child and Adolescent Psychiatric Clinics of North America* is covered in *MEDLINE/PubMed (Index Medicus), ISI, SSCI, Research Alert, Social Search, Current Contents,* and *EMBASE/Excerpta Medica.*

Printed in the United States of America.

# Contributors

## CONSULTING EDITOR

**HARSH K. TRIVEDI, MD, MBA**
Executive Director and Chief Medical Officer; Behavioral Health Vice Chair for Clinical Affairs; Associate Professor of Psychiatry, Vanderbilt University School of Medicine, Nashville, Tennessee

## CONSULTING EDITOR EMERITUS

**ANDRÉS MARTIN, MD, MPH**

## FOUNDING CONSULTING EDITOR

**MELVIN LEWIS, MBBS, FRCPSYCH, DCH**

## EDITORS

**RAY CHIH-JUI HSIAO, MD**
Associate Professor, Department of Psychiatry and Behavioral Sciences, University of Washington School of Medicine; Co-Director, Adolescent Substance Abuse Program, Seattle Children's Hospital, Seattle, Washington

**LESLIE RENEE WALKER, MD**
Professor and Vice-Chair of Faculty Affairs, Department of Pediatrics, University of Washington School of Medicine; Co-Director, Adolescent Substance Abuse Program, Seattle Children's Hospital, Seattle, Washington

## AUTHORS

**ALEXIS APLASCA, MD**
Assistant Professor, Departments of Psychiatry and Pediatrics, Director of Psychiatric Services for Pediatrics, Children's Hospital of Richmond, Virginia Commonwealth University, Richmond, Virginia

**GABRIELLE BARNETT, MA**
Mountain Manor Treatment Center, Baltimore, Maryland

**LAURA BLACK, MD**
Resident, Department of Psychiatry, New York University, New York, New York

**ANN BRUNER, MD**
Mountain Manor Treatment Center; Department of Pediatrics, Johns Hopkins University, Baltimore, Maryland

**DEEPA R. CAMENGA, MD, MHS**
Assistant Professor of Emergency Medicine, Yale School of Medicine, New Haven, Connecticut

**RICHARD F. CATALANO, PhD**
Social Development Research Group, University of Washington School of Social Work, Seattle, Washington

**TAMERA COYNE-BEASLEY, MD, MPH, FAAP, FSAHM**
Division of General Pediatrics and Adolescent Medicine, Department of Pediatrics, University of North Carolina, Chapel Hill, North Carolina

**MARC FISHMAN, MD**
Mountain Manor Treatment Center; Department of Psychiatry, Johns Hopkins University, Baltimore, Maryland

**SCOTT E. HADLAND, MD, MPH**
Division of Adolescent/Young Adult Medicine, Department of Medicine, Boston Children's Hospital; Department of Health Policy and Management, Harvard T. H. Chan School of Public Health; Instructor, Department of Pediatrics, Harvard Medical School, Boston, Massachusetts

**WILLIAM F. HANING III, MD, DFASAM, DFAPA**
Department of Psychiatry, John A. Burns School of Medicine, University of Hawaii, Honolulu, Hawaii

**RASHAD HARDAWAY, MD**
Child and Adolescent Psychiatry Fellow, University of Washington, Seattle Children's Hospital, Seattle, Washington

**ERIN HARROP, MSW**
University of Washington School of Social Work, Seattle, Washington

**BRIDGET HOCHWALT, BA**
MPH Candidate 2017, Division of General Pediatrics and Adolescent Medicine, Department of Pediatrics, University of North Carolina, Chapel Hill, North Carolina

**RAY CHIH-JUI HSIAO, MD**
Associate Professor, Department of Psychiatry and Behavioral Sciences, University of Washington School of Medicine; Co-Director, Adolescent Substance Abuse Program, Seattle Children's Hospital, Seattle, Washington

**ALICIA GRATTAN JORGENSON, MD**
Acting Assistant Professor, Seattle Children's Hospital, Seattle, Washington

**JONATHAN D. KLEIN, MD, MPH**
Associate Executive Director, Director, Julius B. Richmond Center, American Academy of Pediatrics, Elk Grove Village, Illinois

**SHARON LEVY, MD, MPH**
Associate Professor, Department of Pediatrics, Harvard Medical School; Division of Developmental Medicine, Department of Medicine, Boston Children's Hospital, Boston, Massachusetts

**MORGAN LIDDELL, MD**
Fellow in Child and Adolescent Psychiatry, Department of Child Psychiatry, Seattle Children's Hospital, Seattle, Washington

**JULIE LINKER, PhD**
Assistant Professor, Division of Child and Adolescent Psychiatry, Department of Psychiatry, Virginia Commonwealth University, Richmond, Virginia

**VIKTORIYA MAGID, PhD**
Assistant Professor, Department of Psychiatry and Behavioral Services, Medical University of South Carolina, Charleston, South Carolina

**CECILIA PATRICA MARGRET, MD, PhD, MPH**
Child and Adolescent Psychiatrist, Acting Assistant Professor, Department of Psychiatry and Behavioral Sciences, University of Washington, Seattle Children's Hospital, Seattle, Washington

**MICHAEL J. MASON, PhD**
Associate Professor, Director, Commonwealth Institute for Child and Family Studies, Division of Child and Adolescent Psychiatry, Department of Psychiatry, Virginia Commonwealth University, Richmond, Virginia

**JON McCLELLAN, MD**
Professor, Department of Psychiatry, University of Washington, Seattle, Washington

**ROSA MORALES-THEODORE, MD**
Assistant Professor, Division of Child and Adolescent Psychiatry, Department of Psychiatry, Virginia Commonwealth University, Richmond, Virginia

**JONATHAN D. MORROW, MD, PhD**
Assistant Professor, Department of Psychiatry, University of Michigan Addiction Treatment Services, University of Michigan, Ann Arbor, Michigan

**TARYN M. PARK, MD**
Department of Psychiatry, John A. Burns School of Medicine, University of Hawaii, Honolulu, Hawaii

**NICHOLAS C. PEIPER, PhD, MPH**
RTI International, Behavioral and Urban Health Program, Research Triangle Park, North Carolina

**TY A. RIDENOUR, PhD, MPE**
RTI International, Behavioral and Urban Health Program, Research Triangle Park, North Carolina

**RICHARD K. RIES, MD**
Professor of Psychiatry, Director of Addictions Division, Department of Psychiatry and Behavioral Sciences, Harborview Medical Center, University of Washington, Seattle, Washington

**JASON SCHWEITZER, MD**
Child and Adolescent Psychiatry Fellow, University of California-San Diego, Rady Children's Hospital, San Diego, California

**ADITI SHARMA, MD**
Department of Psychiatry and Behavioral Sciences, University of Washington School of Medicine, Seattle, Washington

**BIKASH SHARMA, MD**
Mountain Manor Treatment Center, Baltimore, Maryland

**ANNABELLE K. SIMPSON, MD**
Child and Adolescent Psychiatry Fellow, University of Washington, Seattle Children's Hospital, Seattle, Washington

**MICHAEL STORCK, MD**
Associate Professor of Psychiatry and Behavioral Sciences, Department of Child Psychiatry, Seattle Children's Hospital, Seattle, Washington

**JOJI SUZUKI, MD**
Department of Psychiatry, Brigham and Women's Hospital, Boston, Massachusetts

**LESLIE RENEE WALKER, MD**
Professor and Vice-Chair of Faculty Affairs, Department of Pediatrics, University of Washington School of Medicine; Co-Director, Adolescent Substance Abuse Program, Seattle Children's Hospital, Seattle, Washington

**CHENG-FANG YEN, MD, PhD**
Professor, Department of Psychiatry, Kaohsiung Medical University Hospital, School of Medicine, College of Medicine, Kaohsiung Medical University, Kaohsiung, Taiwan, China

**CASSIE YU, MD**
Acting Assistant Professor, Department of Psychiatry, University of Washington, Seattle, Washington

**NIKOLA ZAHARAKIS, PhD**
Senior Project Manager, Commonwealth Institute for Child and Family Studies, Division of Child and Adolescent Psychiatry, Department of Psychiatry, Virginia Commonwealth University, Richmond, Virginia

# Contents

Substance use and consequent disorders have burdened US health care, criminal justice, and society at large for centuries. Pathological substance use almost invariably begins before 25 years of age, demonstrating how critical adolescence is within the etiology, prevention, and treatment of substance use disorder. This article provides a high-level overview of the prevalence of substance use disorders to provide a context within which the remaining issue provides in-depth descriptions of the evidence on specific topics. Described herein are trends in substance use, substance use disorder, and demographic comparisons.

There are many facets of the neurobiology of substance use that are distinct in adolescence as compared with adulthood. The adolescent brain is subject to intense subcortical reward processes, but is left with an immature prefrontal control system that is often unable to resist the pull of potentially exciting activities like substance use, even when fully aware of the dangers involved. Peer influences serve only to magnify these effects and foster more sensation-seeking, risky behavior. The unique aspects of neurobiology should be taken into consideration when designing prevention programs and clinical interventions for adolescent substance use disorders.

Substance abuse disorders have a strong genetic component. Genetic risk factors associated with alcohol abuse include common variants in genes coding for alcohol-metabolizing enzymes and gamma-aminobutyric acid A receptors. Functional missense mutations in *ADH1B* and *ALDH2* are protective against alcohol dependence. Nicotine use disorders are associated with polymorphisms in a cluster of nicotinic acetylcholine receptors on chromosome 15q24, and mutations that reduce the enzymatic activity of *CYP2A6*. Genetic risk factors for other illicit drug use have not been well-studied. Most genetic vulnerability toward substance use disorders remains unexplained. Future research will benefit from advanced whole-genome sequencing technologies.

Due to the significant consequences of adolescent substance use behaviors, researchers have increasingly focused on prevention approaches. The field of prevention science is based on the identification of predictors of problem behaviors, and the development and testing of prevention programs that seek to change these predictors. As the field of prevention science moves forward, there are many opportunities for growth, including the integration of prevention programs into service systems and primary care, an expansion of program adaptations to fit the needs of local populations, and a greater emphasis on the development of programs targeted at young adult populations.

Alcohol drinking in childhood and adolescence is a serious public health concern. Adolescence is a vulnerable period for risk-taking tendencies. Understanding the influences of problematic alcohol use is important for evolving interventions. Alcohol use in early years foreshadows a lifetime risk for psychiatric and substance use disorders. Early screening and assessment can alter tragic sequelae. We discuss clinical aspects such as confidentiality, differential levels of care, and criteria for best fitting treatments. Given the prevalence of drinking and its impact on psychiatric and substance use disorders, the need for further study and prevention are emphasized.

Cannabis use in the adolescent population poses a significant threat of addiction potential resulting in altered neurodevelopment. There are multiple mechanisms of treatment of cannabis use disorder including behavioral therapy management and emerging data on treatment via pharmacotherapy. Recognizing the diagnostic criteria for cannabis use disorder, cannabis withdrawal syndrome, and mitigating factors that influence adolescent engagement in cannabis use allows for comprehensive assessment and management in the adolescent population.

Tobacco use is a pervasive public health problem and the leading cause of preventable morbidity and mortality in the United States. This article reviews the epidemiology of tobacco use in youth, with a description of cigarettes, alternative tobacco product, and polytobacco use patterns among the general population and among adolescents with psychiatric and/or substance use disorders. The article also provides an update on the diagnosis and assessment of tobacco use disorder in adolescents, with a particular focus on the clinical management of tobacco use in adolescents with co-occurring disorders.

> Compared with other illicit substances, stimulants are not commonly used by adolescents; however, they represent a serious concern regarding substance use among youths. This article uses methamphetamine as a model for stimulant use in adolescents; cocaine and prescription stimulants are also mentioned. Methamphetamine use among adolescents and young adults is a serious health concern with potentially long-term physical, cognitive, and psychiatric consequences. Brain development and the effects of misusing stimulants align such that usage in adolescents can be more dangerous than during adulthood. It seems helpful to keep in mind the differences between adolescents and young adults when implementing interventions.

> Opioid use and addiction in adolescents and young adults is a health problem of epidemic proportions, with devastating consequences for youth and their families. Opioid overdose is a life-threatening emergency that should be treated with naloxone, and respiratory support if necessary. Overdose should always be an opportunity to initiate addiction treatment. Detoxification is often a necessary, but never sufficient, component of treatment for OUDs. Treatment for OUDs is effective but treatment capacity is alarmingly limited and under-developed. Emerging consensus supports the incorporation of relapse prevention medications such as buprenorphine and extended release naltrexone into comprehensive psychosocial treatment including counseling and family involvement.

> Use of hallucinogenic substances as a public health concern has increased over the past decade. Among adolescents, there are increasing emergency department presentations for intoxication with these drugs, contrary to decreasing reported use of classical hallucinogens such as LSD (lysergic acid diethylamide). Academic and governmental groups have monitored use of hallucinogens, highlighting a notable change in perceptions about use among adolescents thought to contribute to these trends. Special populations and religious groups, though, have been granted governmental permission to use hallucinogens for their cultural practices. Novel designer hallucinogens have gained popularity and may have serious medical and psychological side effects from use.

> Inhalant abuse is the intentional inhalation of a volatile substance for the purpose of achieving an altered mental state. As an important, yet under-recognized form of substance abuse, inhalant abuse crosses all demographic, ethnic, and socioeconomic boundaries, causing significant morbidity and mortality in school-aged and older children. This review

presents current perspectives on epidemiology, detection, and clinical challenges of inhalant abuse and offers advice regarding the medical and mental health providers' roles in the prevention and management of this substance abuse problem. Also discussed is the misuse of a specific "over-the-counter" dissociative, dextromethorphan.

because test results can be misleading if not interpreted in the correct clinical context, clinicians should always conduct a careful interview with adolescent patients to understand what testing is likely to show and then use testing to validate or refute their expectations. Because of the ease with which samples can be tampered, providers should also carefully reflect on their own collection protocols and sample validation procedures to ensure optimal accuracy.

# CHILD AND ADOLESCENT PSYCHIATRIC CLINICS

AACAP Members: Please go to www.jaacap.org for information on access to the Child and Adolescent Psychiatric Clinics. *Resident* Members of AACAP: Special access information is available at www.childpsych.theclinics.com.

**THE CLINICS ARE AVAILABLE ONLINE!**
Access your subscription at:
www.theclinics.com

# Preface

# Understanding Adolescent Substance Use Disorders in the Era of Marijuana Legalization, Opioid Epidemic, and Social Media

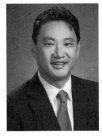 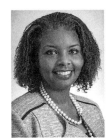

Ray Chih-Jui Hsiao, MD    Leslie Renee Walker, MD
*Editors*

With the prescription opioid abuse and heroin epidemic claiming the lives of tens of thousands of Americans each year, President Barack Obama recently announced new initiatives to combat the epidemic, including several measures targeting vulnerable adolescents and young adults, as a priority of his administration. The President's call to action draws renewed attention to the perils of substance use and untreated substance use disorders in adolescents. In addition, the ongoing public debate about efforts to legalize marijuana in specific states and federally challenges clinicians caring for adolescents with requiring an increasingly broad scope of clinical knowledge in their daily practice. Therefore, many clinicians in the trenches are desiring additional educational resources that can augment their understanding of adolescent substance use disorders and enhance their clinical skills to keep up with constant changes such as the emerging popularity of novel illicit substances of abuse or new routes of abuse for existing illicit substances and the proliferation of social media and its impact on substance use patterns and perception. In response to this demand, the editorial team of the *Child and Adolescent Psychiatric Clinics of North America* has decided to devote the July and October 2016 issues to adolescent substance use disorders. For the purpose of these two issues, the age range for adolescents is defined as 12 to 21. The July issue focuses on the prevalence of substance use in adolescents and the clinical presentation of various substance use and co-occurring disorders with an emphasis on assessment. The October issue will focus on the latest advances

Child Adolesc Psychiatric Clin N Am 25 (2016) xiii–xiv
http://dx.doi.org/10.1016/j.chc.2016.04.001
1056-4993/16/$ – see front matter © 2016 Published by Elsevier Inc.

childpsych.theclinics.com

in treatment and management approaches for substance use and co-occurring disorders.

In the July issue, readers start out with an overview of the prevalence and patterns of substance use in adolescents and develop an appreciation for substance use as a common occurrence rather than an exception in teenagers. By the time that adolescents reach the twelfth grade, almost 70% will have tried alcohol; half will have experimented with an illegal drug; about 40% will have smoked a cigarette, and over 20% will have used a prescription drug for nonmedical purposes. Despite the high rate of lifetime use, most adolescents do not develop full-blown substance use disorders, and there are various current theories on why selected individuals are more prone to develop a disorder. We highlight the current theories on neurobiological mechanisms of addiction in the article by Sharma and Morrow and review the latest genetic findings in the article by Yu and McClellan. The article by Harrop and Catalano provides an in-depth discussion of leading evidence-based prevention programs for adolescent substance use and their underlying theoretical background. The next 7 articles cover the most common substances of abuse and their implications in clinical practice through focused discussions on clinical presentation and assessment. With the evolution of DSM-5 to include behavioral addictions, the article by Jorgenson and colleagues provides a brief discussion on the best established behavioral addiction, pathologic gambling, and devotes significant attention to the most prominent behavioral addiction in adolescents, Internet addiction. This issue concludes with articles on psychiatric and medical comorbidities of substance use disorders and a review of available objective testing methods for assessment purposes.

We would like to thank our contributors for sharing their expertise on this very important topic, and we would be remiss if we didn't acknowledge our wonderful editorial and publishing teams at Elsevier, especially Lauren Boyle and Kristen Helm, for their amazing support throughout the planning and publishing process. We hope our fellow clinicians will appreciate our efforts to target the contents of this issue with a clinical focus that's geared toward frontline health care providers who are working with adolescents.

Ray Chih-Jui Hsiao, MD
Seattle Children's Hospital
M/S OA.5.154, PO Box 5371
Seattle, WA 98145-5005, USA

Leslie Renee Walker, MD
Seattle Children's Hospital
M/S CSB-200, PO Box 5371
Seattle, WA 98145-5005, USA

E-mail addresses:
rhsiao@uw.edu (R.C.-J. Hsiao)
leslie.walker@seattlechildrens.org (L.R. Walker)

# Overview on Prevalence and Recent Trends in Adolescent Substance Use and Abuse

CrossMark

Nicholas C. Peiper, PhD, MPH[a], Ty A. Ridenour, PhD, MPE[a],
Bridget Hochwalt, BA[b], Tamera Coyne-Beasley, MD, MPH[b],*

## KEYWORDS

- Adolescent • Substance use • Epidemiology

## KEY POINTS

- Several large national surveillance surveys have documented significant trends in adolescent substance use over the past 25 years.
- The prevalence of cigarette smoking has significantly decreased, but electronic cigarette and hookah use have emerged as common forms of nicotine and tobacco use among adolescents.
- From 1991 to 2015, the prevalence of lifetime, 12-month, and 30-day use of marijuana all increased among adolescents.
- Between 2002 and 2014, male and female adolescents aged 12 to 17 years had similar 12-month prevalence rates of substance use disorders as well as slightly decreasing trends that were nearly identical.
- Compared with any other age group, the highest 12-month prevalence of substance use disorder occurs in 18 to 25 year olds; they had the steepest decline in prevalence between 2002 and 2014.

Disclosure Statement: The authors have no commercial or financial conflicts of interest associated with this article.

The project described was supported by the National Institute on Drug Abuse (grant award number R42 DA02212) and the National Center for Advancing Translational Sciences, National Institutes of Health (grant award number UL1TR001111). The content is solely the responsibility of the authors and does not necessarily represent the official views of National Institute on Drug Abuse or the National Institutes of Health.

[a] RTI International, Behavioral and Urban Health Program, Research Triangle Park, NC 27709-2194, USA; [b] Department of Pediatrics, Division of General Pediatrics and Adolescent Medicine, University of North Carolina, CB # 7225, 231 MacNider, Chapel Hill, NC 27599, USA
* Corresponding author.
E-mail address: tamera_coyne-beasley@med.unc.edu

Substance use (SU) and SU disorder (SUD) exact monumental tolls on individuals, health care systems, and societies. SU consequences cost the United States more than $600 billion annually (eg, due to SUD treatment, crime, medical and psychiatric disorders, and sexually transmitted infection).[1] Globally, the 4th, 5th, and 15th leading contributors to disease burden are smoking, alcoholism, and illegal drug use, respectively.[2] They additionally contribute to the propensity for other illnesses, both physical and mental. To illustrate, smoking leads to the first, second, fifth, and seventh leading causes of disease burden (eg, cardiovascular disease, lung cancer, chronic obstructive pulmonary disease).[2]

Understanding the epidemiology of SU and SUD requires evidence from adolescents. Virtually all individuals who consume an addictive substance initiate some form of SU before adulthood. Moreover, except for recent increases in misuse of prescription opiate medications among the elderly, SUD almost invariably onsets before 25 years of age.[3,4] Moreover, earlier onset of SU contributes to the risk for SUD.[5,6] For space efficiency, herein the term *substance* refers to any substance with addictive potential and *drug* refers to any illicit substance (including marijuana and inhalants).

## PREVALENCE OF ADOLESCENT SUBSTANCE USE

In the United States, the National Institutes of Health, Substance Abuse and Mental Health Services Administration, and Centers for Disease Control and Prevention have devoted substantial resources to ongoing surveillance of adolescent SU and its consequences for several decades.[7] In particular, data from the National Survey on Drug Use and Health (NSDUH), Monitoring the Future (MTF) study, and Youth Risk Behavior Survey (YRBS) all show that SU, as well as accepting attitudes and beliefs toward use, increases throughout middle and high school.[7,8] This increase is especially notable with regard to the approximate doubling of 30-day alcohol, cigarette, and marijuana use prevalence that occurs between grade 8 and 10 (**Table 1**).[9]

## ALCOHOL USE

Alcohol is the substance most frequently used by adolescents.[10] As part of a downward trend since the 1990s, the lifetime, annual, and 30-day measures of alcohol use were at historic lows in the 2015 MTF. Data from the 1991 to 2015 MTF highlight these trends (**Fig. 1**)[11]:

- In 2015, 10% of 8th graders, 22% of 10th graders, and 35% of 12th graders reported 30-day alcohol use for an overall rate of 22%.
- One-fourth of students (26%) have consumed any alcohol by 8th grade, 47% by 10th grade, and 64% by 12th grade.
- For binge drinking (ie, 5 or more drinks in a row at one occasion), the 2-week prevalence rate of 22% among students peaked in 1997 and then decreased to 11% in 2015.
- The rate of 30-day alcohol intoxication reached a high of 21% in 1997 and progressively declined to 11% in 2015.

## TOBACCO USE

Like alcohol, trends in cigarette smoking and smokeless tobacco on the MTF have also significantly decreased over the past 25 years[11,12]:

- In 2015, the 30-day prevalence of cigarette smoking was 3.6% for 8th graders, 6.3% for 10th graders, and 11.4% for 12th graders.

**Table 1**
**Estimates of substance use in US adolescents**

| | | Grade 8 | | | Grade 10 | | | Grade 12 | | |
|---|---|---|---|---|---|---|---|---|---|---|
| | Time | 1991 | 2015 | Difference | 1991 | 2015 | Difference | 1991 | 2015 | Difference |
| Alcohol | Lifetime | 70.1 | 26.1 | −44.0 | 83.8 | 47.1 | −36.7 | 88.0 | 64.0 | −24.0 |
| | 12-mo | 54.0 | 21.0 | −33.0 | 72.3 | 41.9 | −30.4 | 77.7 | 58.2 | −19.5 |
| | 30-d | 25.1 | 9.7 | −15.4 | 42.8 | 21.5 | −21.3 | 54.0 | 35.3 | −18.7 |
| Intoxication | Lifetime | 26.7 | 10.9 | −15.8 | 50.0 | 28.6 | −21.4 | 65.4 | 46.7 | −18.7 |
| | 12-mo | 17.5 | 7.7 | −7.8 | 40.1 | 23.4 | −16.7 | 52.7 | 37.7 | −15.0 |
| | 30-d | 7.6 | 3.1 | −4.5 | 20.5 | 10.3 | −10.2 | 31.6 | 20.6 | −11.0 |
| Cigarettes | Lifetime | 44.0 | 13.3 | −30.7 | 55.1 | 19.9 | −35.2 | 63.1 | 31.1 | −32.0 |
| | 12-mo | — | — | — | — | — | — | — | — | — |
| | 30-d | 14.3 | 3.6 | −10.7 | 20.8 | 6.3 | −14.5 | 28.3 | 11.4 | −16.9 |
| Smokeless tobacco | Lifetime | 20.7 | 8.6 | 12.1 | 26.6 | 12.3 | 14.3 | 32.4 | 13.2 | 19.2 |
| | 12-mo | — | — | — | — | — | — | — | — | — |
| | 30-d | 7 | 3.2 | −3.8 | 9.6 | 4.9 | −4.7 | 11.4 | 6.1 | −5.3 |
| Marijuana | Lifetime | 10.2 | 15.5 | +5.3 | 23.4 | 31.1 | +7.7 | 36.7 | 44.7 | +8.0 |
| | 12-mo | 6.2 | 11.8 | +5.6 | 16.5 | 25.4 | +8.9 | 23.9 | 34.9 | +11.0 |
| | 30-d | 3.2 | 6.5 | +3.3 | 8.7 | 14.8 | +6.1 | 13.8 | 21.3 | +7.5 |
| Any illicit drug | Lifetime | 14.3 | 10.3 | −4.0 | 19.1 | 14.6 | −4.5 | 26.9 | 21.1 | −5.8 |
| | 12-mo | 8.4 | 6.3 | −2.1 | 12.2 | 10.5 | −1.7 | 16.2 | 15.2 | −1.0 |
| | 30-d | 3.8 | 3.1 | −0.7 | 5.5 | 4.9 | −0.6 | 7.1 | 7.6 | +0.5 |

Note: Estimates of 12-month use of cigarettes and smokeless tobacco were not available. Difference represents percentage point difference. Any illicit drug refers to any use of drugs other than marijuana: hallucinogens, crack, cocaine, heroin, and prescription drugs.
*Data from* Johnston LD, O'Malley PM, Miech RA, et al. Monitoring the future national survey results on drug use, 1975-2015: overview, key findings on adolescent drug use. Ann Arbor (MI): Institute for Social Research; University of Michigan; 2015.

- In 1996 and 1997, the 30-day prevalence among US students reached a high of 28.3% before decreasing to 7.0% in 2015.
- The prevalence of 30-day smokeless tobacco use increased from 4.9% in 2007% to 6.5% in 2010, before steadily decreasing to 4.7% in 2015.

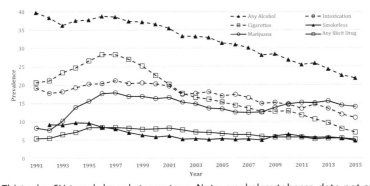

**Fig. 1.** Thirty-day SU trends by substance type. Note: smokeless tobacco data not available for 1991. Any illicit drug refers to any use of drugs other than marijuana: hallucinogens, crack, cocaine, heroin, and prescription drugs. (*Data from* Johnston LD, O'Malley PM, Miech RA, et al. Monitoring the future national survey results on drug use, 1975-2015: overview, key findings on adolescent drug use. Ann Arbor (MI): Institute for Social Research; University of Michigan; 2015.)

Data from the YRBS and National Youth Tobacco Survey (NYTS) also reveal several trends in frequent cigarette smoking (ie, 20 or more days in the past 30 days) and alternative tobacco use like electronic cigarettes (e-cigarettes) and hookah[12–14]:

- Between 1991 and 1997, the prevalence of frequent cigarette smoking increased from 13% to 17% before decreasing to 6% in 2013.
- The 30-day prevalence of e-cigarette use among US high schoolers vastly increased from 1.5% to 13.4% between 2011 and 2014 and from 4.1% to 9.4% for 30-day hookah use.
- In 2015, the 30-day prevalence of e-cigarette use surpassed every other tobacco product on both the MTF and NYTS.

## MARIJUANA USE

Marijuana remains the most widely consumed illicit drug in the United States:

- In the MTF, the 30-day prevalence increased from 8.3% in 1991 to a high of 17.9% in 1997 before declining to 14.0% in 2015.
- By grade in the MTF, the prevalence of 30-day use among 8th graders decreased from 10.4% in 2008[8] to 9.3% in 2015 but increased from 13.8% to 14.8% for 10th graders and 19.4% to 21.3% for 12th graders.
- In a 2013 study using 2002 to 2011 NSDUH data, 12 to 17 year olds composed 13% of frequent marijuana users (ie, 21 or more days in the past month) in 2002 compared with 7% in 2011.[15]

## ILLICIT DRUG USE

As marijuana increases the overall prevalence of illicit drug use, the use of other drugs is lower. Overall, drug use other than marijuana remains common and typically increases from adolescence to emerging adulthood:

- In the 2014 NSDUH, 13.4% of individuals 12 to 17 years old tried a drug other than marijuana in their lifetime, 8.5% in the past 12 months, and 3.6% in the past 30 days.[16]
- The 2015 MTF found that 10.3% of 8th graders, 14.6% of 10th graders, and 21.1% of 12th graders tried a drug other than marijuana.[11]
- Between 1991 and 2015, the 30-day prevalence of illicit drug use other than marijuana increased from 5.4% in 1991 to a high of 8.4% in 1997 before declining to 5.1% in 2015.

## NONMEDICAL PRESCRIPTION DRUG USE

One type of illicit drug use that has received considerable attention over the past 15 years is nonmedical prescription drug (NMPD) use. Compared with the substances that peaked in the late 1990s, nonmedical use of amphetamines, opioids, and tranquilizers all peaked around the early 2000s[17,18]:

- Between 2005 and 2015, the 12-month rate of any prescription drug use decreased from 17.1% to 12.9% in the MTF.
- On the 2015 MTF, the 12-month rate of 12.9% among 12th graders was the second highest illicit drug after marijuana use at 34.9%.[11]

## SOCIAL AND DEMOGRAPHIC DIFFERENCES IN SUBSTANCE USE

There are several subgroup differences in SU that merit discussion. In terms of sex, males have historically been shown to have higher rates of illicit drug use than females, including higher rates of frequent use.[19–21] One notable exception is with higher nonmedical use of amphetamines, sedatives, and tranquilizers among female adolescents.[22,23] NMPD use among female adolescents tends to be associated with self-medication of negative affect and stress, whereas male use tends to involve experimentation and antisocial behavior.[24–30] For most substances, however, the sex differences are small and have recently narrowed for alcohol and binge drinking, 2 indicators whereby males had higher rates of use during the 1990s and 2000s.[11]

Several notable differences have been shown among the 3 largest racial and ethnic groups in the United States: Caucasians, African Americans, and Hispanics. Historically, higher rates of illicit drug use have been found among Caucasians; but disparities have recently narrowed because of changes in marijuana use.[31–34] In the NSDUH, the proportion of Caucasians composing frequent marijuana users decreased from 75% in 2002% to 66% in 2011, whereas the rates increased from 14% to 16% for African Americans and 8% to 14% for Hispanics.[15] Among 18 to 25 year olds in the 2005 to 2012 NSDUH, 26.6% of African American youths used marijuana before tobacco compared with 14.3% among their Caucasian counterparts; by 2012, these rates increased to 41.5% and 24.0%, respectively.[35] For Hispanic youths on the 2015 MTF, overall SU rates decreased between Caucasians and African Americans, whereas 8th and 12th grade Hispanic students had the highest rates for inhalants, cocaine, crack, methamphetamine, and crystal methamphetamine.[36]

In terms of geographic differences over the past 15 years, the South and Midwest have demonstrated higher rates of cigarette smoking, underage binge drinking, NMPD use, and their associations with treatment admissions and preventable morbidity and mortality.[37–39] Although the United States as a whole has demonstrated increases in prescription opioid use and its consequences since the early 2000s, the highest rates of use have been found among rural populations in Appalachia and the Midwest, areas with concentrated socioeconomic deprivation and impoverishment.[37–41]

There have also been differences in adolescent SU in states with medical marijuana laws.[42,43] In a recent study with the 1991 to 2014 MTF, 30-day marijuana use was more prevalent in states with a medical marijuana law (15.9%) any time up to 2014 compared with other states (13.3%).[43] However, marijuana use in states before passing a medical marijuana law (16.3%) did not significantly differ from states after passing a law (15.5%). As states in the Midwest and South tend to fully prohibit cannabis or only allow nonpsychoactive forms, the significantly lower rates of cigarette smoking, other tobacco use, and NMPD use found in states with medical marijuana laws suggests other social and demographic factors may influence adolescent marijuana use.[37–44]

Taken together, large shifts in adolescent SU have taken place over the past 25 years. Such changes emphasize the heterogeneity of birth cohorts with multiple levels of risk and resiliency that vary over time. As cohort effects have been shown to be more predictive of marijuana and alcohol use than period effects in the 1976 to 2007 MTF, peer group norms may exert greater influence on adolescent SU than individual-level perceptions and attitudes that are broadly influenced by larger sociopolitical forces.[45,46] Moreover, the collective emergence of birth cohort differences in the initiation and use of tobacco, alcohol, marijuana, prescription drugs, and heroin illustrates the continued need to monitor adolescent SU with federally funded epidemiological surveys.[35,45–50] Moving forward, there remain great opportunities to more thoroughly investigate adolescent SU through data harmonization across surveys and reconcile ongoing discrepancies in SU estimates from differences in survey methodologies.[49–53]

## PREVALENCE OF ADOLESCENT SUBSTANCE USE DISORDERS
### Methodological Considerations

Trends in prevalence rates of SUD cannot be entirely disentangled from the evolving nomenclatures on which the diagnoses are based as well as the instrumentation that is used to collect data.[52,54,55] Thus, differences between recent iterations of SUD no-menclatures are briefly discussed before presenting trends. Because the *International Classification of Diseases* is generally not used in the United States, data herein are from the American Psychiatric Association's *Diagnostic and Statistical Manual of Mental Disorders* (*DSM*) nomenclature.

Ongoing efforts to better epitomize SUD have resulted in several iterations to *DSM* classifications since the first SUD taxonomy was presented in the *DSM-III*.[56,57] The *DSM-III* was criticized for emphasizing physiological criteria and social impairment, lack of a specific theoretical underpinning, and inclusion of 2 SUDs, abuse and dependence.[58–61] The Edwards and Gross Alcohol Dependence Syndrome[62,63] served as the theoretical basis for subsequent *DSM-III-R*, *DSM-IV* and *DSM-5* nomenclatures, whereas abuse and dependence diagnoses were not aggregated into a single disorder until the *DSM-5*. The *DSM-IV* nomenclature differed from *DSM-III-R* in several ways,[64,65] including (1) abuse and dependence diagnoses were made to be distinct; (2) abuse diagnosis criteria were expanded from 2 to 4; (3) the clustering criterion was more specific (at least 3 dependence criteria were required to occur during a 12-month period); and (4) dependence diagnoses were further specified as either physiological (ie, tolerance or withdrawal was experienced) or nonphysiological. Changes from the *DSM-IV* to the *DSM-5* included:

- Dependence and abuse diagnoses being combined into a single disorder that is graded in terms of severity;
- Elimination of the criterion of SU causing legal problems;
- Addition of a craving criterion.[66]

Assessment instruments also differ among the epidemiological studies that have been conducted to estimate SUD prevalence. For adults, the most commonly used in-struments have been the Composite International Diagnostic Interview and its Sub-stance Abuse Module,[67–69] the Alcohol Use Disorder and Associated Disabilities Interview Schedule–*DSM-IV* Version (Grant and colleagues,[70] 2001), the NSDUH (Center for Behavioral Health Statistics and Quality, 2015),[16] and the Schedules for Clinical Assessment in Neuropsychiatry.[71] These instruments generally offer acceptable to excellent psychometrics, but they also have been shown to generate discordance in terms of who meets the criteria for specific diagnoses.[72] Large epide-miological studies of adolescents have derived diagnoses based on the NIMH Diag-nostic Interview Schedule for Children, the Alcohol Use Disorder and Associated Disabilities Interview Schedule,[73] the Composite International Diagnostic Interview,[74] and the NSDUH.[16] These instruments also have adequate to excellent psychometrics but also likely generate discordance among them.

## PREVALENCE OF ADOLESCENT SUBSTANCE USE DISORDERS
### Developmental Considerations

Further complicating prevalence estimates is that existing classification systems of SUD have been developed using theory about, and data collected from, adults rather than adolescents. Shortcomings of the nomenclatures for adults also pertain to ado-lescents, but additional uncertainties exist regarding classification of adolescents' SUD because of the developmental differences between adolescents and adults.[75–79]

To illustrate, duration and regularity of SU (eg, at least once per month over a 6-month period) are associated with the development of diagnostic criteria.[76,80] On average, adolescent regular SU has been over a far shorter time period than adults who consume the same substances. Even so, adolescents with SUDs generally consume the substance regularly over much shorter time periods than adults with the same SUDs.[76,81,82] Hence, psychotropic effects of a substance may affect adolescents differently than adults because of biological, social, or cognitive reasons.[76,77,83,84]

Although developmental differences have critical implications for how to classify adolescents' SUDs, understanding their cause, and intervention strategy, much remains unknown regarding nomenclature differences between adolescents and adults. Two examples, from mild and severe forms of pathological SU, illustrate well the clinical implications that arise from applying to adolescents a nomenclature that is designed for adults. Physiological dependence characterizes a severe form of SUD[85–87] as indicated by changes in metabolism of a substance and altered biological functioning that results from physiological adjustments to attempt to normalize functioning during long-term and heavy SU.[86] It is diagnosed by the presence of either or both of tolerance (needing more of a substance to attain the same subjective experience) or withdrawal (either experiencing substance-specific symptoms that occur when discontinuing use or continued use to avoid these symptoms). Some have suggested that physiological dependence is necessary and sufficient to diagnose SUD at least for certain substances.[86] However, this classification scheme fails to distinguish persons who are ill from those who are well, particularly among adolescents.[86] Proportions of adolescents in SUD treatment who experience withdrawal are usually less than 33%.[80,86,88,89] The clinical implication of using the physiological dependence criterion in place of the broader dependence diagnosis (specifically for the *DSM-IV*) is that in regions where substance abuse is not considered to be severe enough to fund treatment, treatment would be withheld from more than two-thirds of the adolescents in need of treatment.

On the other extreme is mild pathological SU in the form of diagnostic orphans who meet diagnostic criteria but not full diagnoses.[90–93] Compared with persons who report no criteria, diagnostic orphans experience more SU-related severe problems (eg, extent of SU, number of psychiatric disorders, earlier age of SU onset, proportion meeting criteria for substance dependence at a 1-year follow-up). Within the *DSM-IV* nomenclature, adult and adolescent diagnostic orphans closely resemble persons meeting the criteria for abuse in severity of substance involvement.[92,93] However, among adolescent regular drinkers, nearly one-third fit the diagnostic orphan description in contrast to only 20% of adult regular drinkers.[91,93] Consistent with recommendations for adolescents,[92,93] the *DSM-5* simplifies the qualification for a diagnosis. Even so, substantial proportions of young adults and adolescents remain diagnostic orphans because they meet only one SUD criterion (2 or more are required for diagnosis).[69,94]

## PREVALENCE OF UNITED STATES ADULT SUBSTANCE USE DISORDERS

Compared with adolescents, SUD in adults has garnered much greater focus in epidemiology research. Lifetime prevalence of alcohol abuse or dependence and drug abuse or dependence, respectively, was estimated at 13.8% and 6.2% from the Epidemiologic Catchment Area (ECA) study of the early 1980s.[95,96] Lifetime prevalence of alcohol abuse and drug abuse was 23.5% and 11.9%, respectively, from the National Comorbidity Study (NCS) of the early 1990s.[97] The National Longitudinal Alcohol Epidemiologic Survey (NLAES) of the early 1990s estimated the lifetime prevalence of alcohol dependence at 13.3% and any drug use disorder at 6.2%.[98,99] Finally, the prevalence of any alcohol disorder was 30.3% and any drug use disorder was 10.3% in the National Epidemiologic Survey on Alcohol and Related Conditions (NESARC) of the early 2000s.[100,101] Effects of nomenclature, instrumentation, and survey methodologies notwithstanding, lifetime prevalence of SUDs in US adults seems to have increased since the 1980s.

However, to estimate trends in adult SUDs, 12-month prevalence estimates of dependence may provide a better gauge because of potential recall bias in study participants due to reporting experiences from years and sometime decades earlier that may affect lifetime estimates[102] and dependence diagnostic criteria were more consistent among nomenclatures compared with abuse (described later). Alcohol and drug dependence 12-month prevalence rates were 5.9% and 2.5% from the ECA study,[103] 4.4% and 0.8% from the NLAES, 1.3% and 0.4% from the NCS Replication,[104] and 3.8% and 0.6% from the NESARC. In contrast to lifetime prevalence estimates, 12-month prevalence rates of dependence suggest little to no change in US adults' alcohol or drug use disorder prevalence since 1980.

The methodological similarities between the 2001 to 2002 NESARC and the 1991 to 1992 NLAES provided an opportunity to directly compare 12-month prevalence in alcohol abuse and dependence between the two time periods.[4] Prevalence of 12-month alcohol abuse and dependence was 4.7% and 3.8% in 2001 to 2002 compared with 3.0% and 4.4% in 1991 to 1992. Thus, it seems that after accounting for nosology and instrumentation differences among studies, relatively little change in prevalence of alcohol use disorders occurred among US adults over the 10-year span ending the twentieth century.

## PREVALENCE OF UNITED STATES ADOLESCENT SUBSTANCE USE DISORDERS

As mentioned, compared with epidemiological studies of adults, less evidence is available regarding US adolescents. Aside from the NSDUH (which is described later), 3 studies conducted during approximately the same time span as those described earlier provided data for general population prevalence estimates. The Great Smoky Mountain Study (1997–1998) of western North Carolina estimated lifetime SUD of any kind to be 12.2% by 16 years of age (*DSM-IV*).[105] The Center for Antisocial Drug Dependence of Colorado aggregated 3 large samples of 12 to 18 year olds to estimate the prevalence of lifetime abuse and dependence (*DSM-III-R*) as 10.0% and 8.5% for alcohol and 13.9% and 11.5% for any illicit drug.[106] The NCS Replication (2001–2004) included 13- to 18-year-old participants, but participants were required to qualify for abuse before they were asked about dependence; thus, only abuse prevalence could be estimated from their data.[55,69] Within this US epidemiological sample, lifetime and 12-month prevalence was, respectively, 6.5% and 4.7% for alcohol abuse and 8.9% and 5.7% for abuse of any illegal drug.[107,108]

Methodological considerations notwithstanding, prevalence of SUDs seems to have declined since the early 1990s in contrast to the implied trends from adult epidemiological studies. Additional confounds to making direct comparisons among the samples include some consisting of local populations (eg, North Carolina and Colorado populations) and not reporting the same diagnoses.

As with adult abuse and dependence diagnoses, one study has used the same methods and diagnoses over time, thereby, providing data to directly investigate trends in adolescent SUD over time. NSDUH has monitored rates of any alcohol use disorder and any drug use disorder since 2002.[16] For comparison, similar data have been collected for adults during that time span.

Trends in 12-month prevalence of any alcohol use disorder as well as any drug use disorder since 2002 appear in **Fig. 2** for adolescents and adults. Solid-lined trends depict prevalence of drug use disorder, whereas dashed-lined trends depict prevalence of alcohol use disorder. Shapes of data points correspond to age groups. Adolescents aged 12 to 17 years are the only age group whose 12-month prevalence rates and trends are nearly identical between drugs and alcohol. Perhaps the most parsimonious explanation is that many of same individuals who experience drug use disorder also experience alcohol use disorder. Greater 12-month prevalence of SUDs occurs in 18 to 25 year olds compared with any other age group. In both of these age groups, SUD prevalence has declined slightly in recent years, whereas prevalence of alcohol and drug use disorders have increased slightly in adults aged 26 years and older. Regardless of the direction of recent trends, the largest change has been a reduction in 18 to 25 year olds' alcohol use disorders (from nearly 18% in 2002 to slightly more than 12% in 2014). Otherwise, changes in trends have been generally negligible.

## PREVALENCE OF UNITED STATES ADOLESCENT SUBSTANCE USE DISORDERS
### Sex Differences

Historically, SU and SUD have been far more prevalent across all age groups in males than females.[109] For certain substances, this sex difference remains in contemporary trends.[110] However, in the 2013 NSDUH participants aged 12 to 17 years, the 30-day prevalence of alcohol use was 11.2% for boys and 11.9% for girls, continuing a trend of younger girls' prevalence of alcohol involvement becoming more similar to boys' in recent cohorts.[111] Marijuana use (by far the most commonly used illegal drug in 12–17 year olds in NSDUH) 30-day prevalence was lower in NSDUH compared with MTF (**Fig. 3**; likely because of differences between sampling designs), whereas prevalence rates were only slightly greater in boys than girls with the difference being negligible in certain years.[110]

Prevalence of past-year substance dependence or abuse of any substance among 12 to 17 year olds in the 2013 NSDUH was 5.3% in boys and 5.2% in girls.[109] The corresponding prevalence from the 2006 NSDUH was 8.0% for boys and 8.1% for girls.[111] Thus, whereas a greater prevalence of boys may initiate use of particular

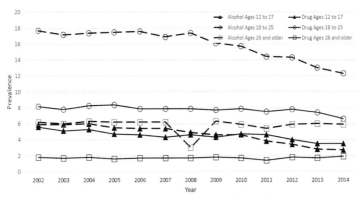

**Fig. 2.** SUD trends by age group and substance type. (*Data from* Center for Behavioral Health Statistics and Quality. Behavioral health trends in the United States: results from the 2014 National Survey on Drug Use and Health. In HHS publication No. SMA 15-4927, NSDUH series H-50. 2015. Available at: http://www.samhsa.gov/data/. Accessed February 12, 2016.)

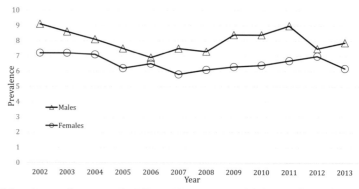

**Fig. 3.** Thirty-day marijuana use in NSDUH 12 to 17 year olds by sex. (*Data from* Substance Abuse and Mental Health Services Administration. Results from the 2013 National Survey on Drug Use and Health: summary of national findings, NSDUH series H-48, HHS publication No. (SMA) 14-4863. Rockville (MD): Substance Abuse and Mental Health Services Administration; 2014.)

substances during adolescence, overall rates of recent and pathological SU in contemporary populations have been nearly equal in adolescents.

## SUMMARY

In sum, to understand the cause and SU and consequential SUD requires understanding them in adolescence. By young adulthood, nearly all persons who will experience lifetime SU or SUD have initiated, and spent years engaging in, these experiences. Given SUD's chronicity, heavy burden on health care, cost to society, and tragic effects on the individuals and their families, understanding its cause in adolescence is an important investment and critical to reducing its prevalence via evidence-based prevention and treatment.

## REFERENCES

1. National Drug Intelligence Center. The economic impact of illicit drug use on American Society. In: U.S. department of justice. 2011. Available at: www.justice.gov/archive/ndic/pubs44/44731/44731p.pdf. Accessed September 7, 2013.
2. Lopez AD, Mathers CD, Ezzati M, et al. Global and regional burden of disease and risk factors, 2001: systematic analysis of population health data. Lancet 2006;367:1747–57.
3. Chen CY, O'Brien MS, Anthony JC. Who becomes cannabis dependent soon after onset of use? Epidemiological evidence from the United States: 2000-2001. Drug Alcohol Depend 2005;79(1):11–22.
4. Grant BF, Dawson DA, Stinson FS, et al. The 12-month prevalence and trends in DSM-IV alcohol abuse and dependence: United States, 1991–1992 and 2001–2002. Drug Alcohol Depend 2004;74(3):223–34.
5. Grant BF, Stinson FS, Harford TC. Age at onset of alcohol use and *DSM-IV* alcohol abuse and dependence: a 12-year follow-up. J Subst Abuse 2001; 13(4):493–504.
6. Jackson KM, Barnett NP, Colby SM, et al. The prospective association between sipping alcohol by the sixth grade and later substance use. J Stud Alcohol Drugs 2015;76(2):212–21.

7. Schulden JD, Thomas YF, Compton WM. Substance abuse in the United States: findings from recent epidemiologic studies. Curr Psychiatry Rep 2009;11(5): 353–9.
8. Merikangas KR, McClair VL. Epidemiology of substance use disorders. Hum Genet 2012;131(6):779–89. Available at: http://dx.doi.org/10.1007/s00439-012-1168-0.
9. Miech RA, Johnston LD, O'Malley PM, et al. Monitoring the future national survey results on drug use, 1975-2014: Volume I, Secondary school students. Ann Arbor (MI): Institute for Social Research; University of Michigan; 2015.
10. Lanza ST, Vasilenko SA, Dziak JJ, et al. Trends among U.S. high school seniors in recent marijuana use and associations with other substances: 1976-2013. J Adolesc Health 2015;57(2):198–204. Available at: http://dx.doi.org/10.1016/j.jadohealth.2015.04.006.
11. Johnston LD, O'Malley PM, Miech RA, et al. Monitoring the future national survey results on drug use, 1975-2015: overview, key findings on adolescent drug use. Ann Arbor (MI): Institute for Social Research; University of Michigan; 2015.
12. Creamer MR, Perry CL, Harrell MB, et al. Trends in multiple tobacco product use, among high school students. Tob Regul Sci 2015;1(3):204–14.
13. Kann L, Kinchen S, Shanklin SL, et al. Youth risk behavior surveillance–United States, 2013. MMWR Suppl 2014;63(Suppl 4):1–168.
14. Arrazola RA, Singh T, Corey CG, et al. Tobacco use among middle and high school students - United States, 2011-2014. MMWR Morb Mortal Wkly Rep 2015;64(14):381–5.
15. Burns RM, Caulkins JP, Everingham SS, et al. Statistics on cannabis users skew perceptions of cannabis use. Front Psychiatry 2013;4:138. Available at: http://dx.doi.org/10.3389/fpsyt.2013.00138.
16. Center for Behavioral Health Statistics and Quality. Behavioral health trends in the United States: results from the 2014 National Survey on Drug Use and Health. In HHS publication No. SMA 15-4927, NSDUH series H-50. 2015. Available at: http://www.samhsa.gov/data/. Accessed February 12, 2016.
17. Young AM, Glover N, Havens JR. Nonmedical use of prescription medications among adolescents in the United States: a systematic review. J Adolesc Health 2012;51(1):6–17. Available at: http://dx.doi.org/10.1016/j.jadohealth.2012.01.011.
18. Schepis TS, West BT, Teter CJ, et al. Prevalence and correlates of co-ingestion of prescription tranquilizers and other psychoactive substances by U.S. high school seniors: results from a national survey. Addict Behav 2016;52:8–12. Available at: http://dx.doi.org/10.1016/j.addbeh.2015.08.002.
19. Schepis TS, Desai RA, Cavallo DA, et al. Gender differences in adolescent marijuana use and associated psychosocial characteristics. J Addict Med 2011; 5(1):65–73. Available at: http://dx.doi.org/10.1097/ADM.0b013e3181d8dc62.
20. Lee YO, Hebert CJ, Nonnemaker JM, et al. Youth tobacco product use in the United States. Pediatrics 2015;135(3):409–15. Available at: http://dx.doi.org/10.1542/peds.2014-3202.
21. Mistry R, Heinze JE, Cordova D, et al. Transitions in current substance use from adolescence to early-adulthood. J Youth Adolesc 2015;44(10):1871–83. Available at: http://dx.doi.org/10.1007/s10964-015-0309-x.
22. Cotto JH, Davis E, Dowling GJ, et al. Gender effects on drug use, abuse, and dependence: a special analysis of results from the national survey on drug use and health. Gend Med 2010;7(5):402–13. Available at: http://dx.doi.org/10.1016/j.genm.2010.09.004.

23. McCabe SE, West BT, Teter CJ, et al. Co-ingestion of prescription opioids and other drugs among high school seniors: results from a national study. Drug Alcohol Depend 2012;126(1–2):65–70. Available at: http://dx.doi.org/10.1016/j.drugalcdep.2012.04.017.

24. McCabe SE, Cranford JA, West BT. Trends in prescription drug abuse and dependence, co-occurrence with other substance use disorders, and treatment utilization: results from two national surveys. Addict Behav 2008;33(10):1297–305. Available at: http://dx.doi.org/10.1016/j.addbeh.2008.06.005.

25. McCabe SE, Cranford JA, Boyd CJ, et al. Motives, diversion and routes of administration associated with nonmedical use of prescription opioids. Addict Behav 2007;32(3):562–75. Available at: http://dx.doi.org/10.1016/j.addbeh.2006.05.022.

26. McCabe SE, Boyd CJ, Young A. Medical and nonmedical use of prescription drugs among secondary school students. J Adolesc Health 2007;40(1):76–83. Available at: http://dx.doi.org/10.1016/j.jadohealth.2006.07.016.

27. McCabe SE, West BT, Teter CJ, et al. Medical and nonmedical use of prescription opioids among high school seniors in the United States. Arch Pediatr Adolesc Med 2012;166(9):797–802. Available at: http://dx.doi.org/10.1001/archpediatrics.2012.85.

28. Lasopa SO, Cottler L, Vaddiparti K, et al. Gender differences in risk factors for nonmedical use of prescription stimulants among youth 10 to 18 years in the US. Drug Alcohol Depend 2015;146:e169. Available at: http://dx.doi.org/10.1016/j.drugalcdep.2014.09.376.

29. King KA, Vidourek RA, Merianos AL. Sex and grade level differences in lifetime nonmedical prescription drug use among youth. J Prim Prev 2013;34(4):237–49. Available at: http://dx.doi.org/10.1007/s10935-013-0308-1.

30. Wu L-T, Pilowsky DJ, Patkar AA. Non-prescribed use of pain relievers among adolescents in the United States. Drug Alcohol Depend 2008;94(1–3):1–11. Available at: http://dx.doi.org/10.1016/j.drugalcdep.2007.09.023.

31. Brook JS, Adams RE, Balka EB, et al. Early adolescent marijuana use: risks for the transition to young adulthood. Psychol Med 2002;32(1):79–91.

32. Zapolski TCB, Pedersen SL, McCarthy DM, et al. Less drinking, yet more problems: understanding African American drinking and related problems. Psychol Bull 2014;140(1):188–223. Available at: http://dx.doi.org/10.1037/a0032113.

33. Chen P, Jacobson KC. Developmental trajectories of substance use from early adolescence to young adulthood: gender and racial/ethnic differences. J Adolesc Health 2012;50(2):154–63. Available at: http://dx.doi.org/10.1016/j.jadohealth.2011.05.013.

34. Keyes KM, Vo T, Wall MM, et al. Racial/ethnic differences in use of alcohol, tobacco, and marijuana: is there a cross-over from adolescence to adulthood? Soc Sci Med 2015;124:132–41. Available at: http://dx.doi.org/10.1016/j.socscimed.2014.11.035.

35. Kennedy SM, Patel RP, Cheh P, et al. Tobacco and marijuana initiation among African American and white young adults. Nicotine Tob Res 2016;18(Suppl 1):S57–64. Available at: http://dx.doi.org/10.1093/ntr/ntv194.

36. Johnston LD, O'Malley PM, Bachman JG, et al. Demographic subgroup trends among adolescents in the use of various licit and illicit drugs: 1975-2014. Ann Arbor (MI): Institute for Social Research; 2015.

37. Young AM, Havens JR, Leukefeld CG. A comparison of rural and urban nonmedical prescription opioid users' lifetime and recent drug use. Am J Drug Alcohol Abuse 2012;38(3):220–7.

38. Gfroerer JC, Larson SL, Colliver JD. Drug use patterns and trends in rural communities. J Rural Health 2007;23(Suppl:10–15). http://dx.doi.org/10.1111/j.1748-0361.2007.00118.x.

39. Eberhardt MS, Pamuk ER. The importance of place of residence: examining health in rural and nonrural areas. Am J Public Health 2004;94(10):1682–6.

40. Keyes KM, Cerdá M, Brady JE, et al. Understanding the rural–urban differences in nonmedical prescription opioid use and abuse in the United States. Am J Public Health 2014;104(2):e52–9.

41. Bachhuber MA, Saloner B, Cunningham CO, et al. Medical cannabis laws and opioid analgesic overdose mortality in the United States, 1999-2010. JAMA Intern Med 2014;174(10):1668–73.

42. Wall MM, Poh E, Cerdá M, et al. Adolescent marijuana use from 2002 to 2008: higher in states with medical marijuana laws, cause still unclear. Ann Epidemiol 2011;21(9):714–6.

43. Hasin DS, Melanie W, Keyes KM, et al. Medical marijuana laws and adolescent marijuana use in the USA from 1991 to 2014: results from annual, repeated cross-sectional surveys. Lancet Psychiatry 2015;2(7):601–8.

44. Cicero TJ, Ellis MS, Surratt HL, et al. The changing face of heroin use in the United States: a retrospective analysis of the past 50 years. JAMA Psychiatry 2014;71(7):821–6.

45. Keyes KM, Schulenberg JE, O'Malley PM, et al. The social norms of birth cohorts and adolescent marijuana use in the United States, 1976-2007. Addiction 2011;106(10):1790–800.

46. Keyes KM, Schulenberg JE, O'Malley PM, et al. Birth cohort effects on adolescent alcohol use: the influence of social norms from 1976 to 2007. Arch Gen Psychiatry 2012;69(12):1304–13.

47. Novak SP, Bluthenthal R, Wenger L, et al. Initiation of heroin and prescription opioid pain relievers by birth cohort. Am J Public Health 2016;106(2):298–300.

48. Novak SP, Peiper NC, Zarkin GA. Nonmedical prescription pain reliever and alcohol consumption among cannabis users. Drug Alcohol Depend 2016;106: 298–300.

49. Peiper NC, Clayton R, Wilson R, et al. The performance of the K6 Scale in a large school sample. Psychol Assess 2015;27(1):228–38. Available at: http://psycnet.apa.org/journals/pas/27/1/228/.

50. Peiper NC, Lee A, Lindsay S, et al. The performance of the K6 Scale in a large school sample: a follow-up study evaluating measurement invariance on the Idaho Youth Prevention Survey. Psychol Assess 2015. http://dx.doi.org/10.1037/pas0000188.

51. Biondo G, Chilcoat HD. Discrepancies in prevalence estimates in two national surveys for nonmedical use of a specific opioid product versus any prescription pain reliever. Drug Alcohol Depend 2014;134:396–400.

52. Grucza RA, Abbacchi AM, Przybeck TR, et al. Discrepancies in estimates of prevalence and correlates of substance use and disorders between two national surveys. Addiction 2007;102(4):623–9.

53. Miller JW, Gfroerer JC, Brewer RD, et al. Prevalence of adult binge drinking: a comparison of two national surveys. Am J Prev Med 2004;27(3):197–204.

54. Ridenour TA, Fazzone T, Cottler LB. Classification and assessment of adolescent substance use - related disorders. In: Essau CA, editor. Substance abuse and dependence in adolescence. New York: Taylor & Francis; 2002. p. 21–62.

55. Ridenour TA, Bray BC, Scott HS, et al. Classification and assessment of substance use disorders in adolescents. In: Essau CA, editor. Adolescent

addiction: epidemiology, assessment, and treatment. Burlington, MA: Elsevier; 2008. p. 17–57.

56. American Psychiatric Association. Diagnostic and statistical manual of mental disorders 3rd edition (DSM-III). Washington, DC: American Psychiatric Association; 1980.

57. Robins LN, Helzer JE. Diagnosis and clinical assessment: the current state of psychiatric diagnosis. Annu Rev Psychol 1986;37:409–32.

58. Caetano R. A commentary on the proposed changes in DSM-III concept of alcohol dependence. Drug Alcohol Depend 1987;19:345–55.

59. Nathan PE. Psychoactive substance dependence. In: Widiger T, Frances A, Pincus H, et al, editors. The DSM-IV source book, vol. 1. Washington, DC: American Psychiatric Association Press; 1994. p. 33–43.

60. Rounsaville BJ. An evaluation of the DSM-III substance use disorders. In: Tischler G, editor. Diagnosis and classification in psychiatry. New York: Cambridge University Press; 1987. p. 175–94.

61. Schuckit MA. Keeping current with the DSMs and substance use disorders. In: Dunner D, editor. Current psychiatric therapy. Philadelphia: W.B. Saunders Co; 1993. p. 89–91.

62. Edwards G, Gross GG. Alcohol dependence: provisional description of a clinical syndrome. Br Med J 1976;1:1058–61.

63. Edwards G. The alcohol dependence syndrome: a concept as stimulus to enquiry. Br J Addict 1986;8:171–83.

64. American Psychiatric Association. Diagnostic and statistical manual of mental disorders. 4th edition. Washington, DC: American Psychiatric Association; 1994.

65. Cottler LB, Schuckit MA, Helzer JE, et al. The DSM-IV field trial for substance use disorders: major results. Drug Alcohol Depend 1995;38:59–69.

66. American Psychiatric Association. American Psychiatric Association: diagnostic and statistical manual of mental disorders, 5th edition (DSM-5). Washington, DC: American Psychiatric Association; 2013.

67. Cottler LB, Compton WM. Advantages of the CIDI family of instruments in epidemiological research of substance use disorders. Int J Methods Psychiatr Res 1993;3:109–19.

68. Kessler RC, Ustun TB. The World Mental Health (WMH) survey initiative version of the World Health Organization (WHO) composite international diagnostic interview (CIDI). Int J Methods Psychiatr Res 2004;13:93–121.

69. Ridenour TA, Bray BC, Cottler LB. Reliability of use, abuse, and dependence of four types of inhalants in adolescents and young adults. Drug Alcohol Depend 2007;91:40–9.

70. Grant BF, Dawson DA, Hasin DS. The alcohol use disorder and associated disabilities interview schedule–DSM-IV version (AUDADIS-IV). Bethesda (MD): National Institute on Alcohol Abuse and Alcoholism; 2001.

71. Wing JK, Babor T, Brugha T, et al. SCAN: schedules for clinical assessment in neuropsychiatry. Arch Gen Psychiatry 1990;47:589–93.

72. Cottler LB, Grant BF, Blaine J, et al. Concordance of DSM-IV alcohol and drug use disorder criteria and diagnoses as measured by AUDADIS-ADR, CIDI and SCAN. Drug Alcohol Depend 1997;47(3):195–205.

73. Grant BF, Dawson DA, Hasin DS. The alcohol use disorder and associated disabilities interview schedule. Rockville (MD): National Institute on Alcohol Abuse and Alcoholism; 1992.

74. Merikangas K, Avenevoli S, Costello J, et al. National comorbidity survey replication adolescent supplement (NCS-A), I: background and measures. J Am Acad Child Adolesc Psychiatry 2009;48(4):367–9.

75. Dawes MA, Antelman SM, Vanyukov MM, et al. Developmental sources of variation in liability to adolescent substance use disorders. Drug Alcohol Depend 2000;61:3–14.

76. Deas D, Riggs P, Langenbucher J, et al. Adolescents are not adults: developmental considerations in alcohol users. Alcohol Clin Exp Res 2000;24:232–7.

77. Lamminpaa A. Alcohol intoxication in childhood and adolescence. Alcohol Alcohol 1995;30:5–12.

78. Meyers K, Hagan TA, Zanis D, et al. Critical issues in adolescent substance use assessment. Drug Alcohol Depend 1999;55:235–46.

79. Weinberg NZ, Rahdert E, Colliver JD, et al. Adolescent substance abuse: a review of the past 10 years. J Am Acad Child Adolesc Psychiatry 1998;37:252–61.

80. Mikulich SK, Hall SK, Whitmore EA, et al. Concordance between DSM-III-R and DSM-IV diagnoses of substance use disorders in adolescents. Drug Alcohol Depend 2001;61:237–48.

81. Brown SA, Mott MA, Myers MG. Adolescent alcohol and drug treatment outcome. In: Watson RR, editor. Drug and alcohol abuse prevention, drug and alcohol abuse review. Clifton (NJ): Humana; 1990. p. 373–403.

82. Brown SA, Mott MA, Stewart MA. Adolescent alcohol and drug abuse. In: Walker CE, Roberts MC, editors. Handbook of clinical child psychology. 2nd edition. Oxford (United Kingdom): John Wiley & Sons; 1992. p. 677–93.

83. Dunn ME, Goldman MS. Age and drinking-related differences in the memory organization of alcohol expectancies in 3rd-, 6th-, 9th-, and 12th-grade children. J Consult Clin Psychol 1998;66:579–85.

84. Lamminpaa A. Acute alcohol intoxication among children and adolescents. Eur J Pediatr 1994;153:868–72.

85. Langenbucher JW, Morgenstern J, Miller KJ. DSM-III, DSM-IV and ICD-10 as severity scales for drug dependence. Drug Alcohol Depend 1995;39:139–50.

86. Langenbucher J, Martin CS, Labouvie E, et al. Toward the DSM-IV: the withdrawal-gate model versus the DSM-IV in the diagnosis of alcohol abuse and dependence. J Consult Clin Psychol 2000;68:799–809.

87. Woody GE, Cottler LB, Cacciola J. Severity of dependence: data from the DSM-IV field trials. Addiction 1993;88:1573–9.

88. Stewart MA, Brown SA. Withdrawal and dependency symptoms among adolescent alcohol and drug abusers. Addiction 1995;90:627–35.

89. Winters KC, Stinchfield RD. Current issues and future needs in the assessment of adolescent drug abuse. In: Rahdert E, Czechowicz D, editors. Adolescent drug abuse: clinical assessment and therapeutic interventions (NIDA research monograph 156). Rockville (MD): US Dept. of Health and Human Services; 1995. p. 146–71.

90. Hasin D, Paykin A. Dependence symptoms but no diagnosis: diagnostic 'orphans' in a community sample. Drug Alcohol Depend 1998;50:19–26.

91. Hasin D, Paykin A. Dependence symptoms but no diagnosis: diagnostic 'orphans' in a 1992 national sample. Drug Alcohol Depend 1999;53:215–22.

92. Pollock NK, Martin CS. Diagnostic orphans: adolescents with alcohol symptoms who do not qualify for DSM-IV abuse or dependence diagnoses. Am J Psychiatry 1999;156:897–901.

93. Sarr M, Bucholz KK, Phelps DL. Using cluster analysis of alcohol use disorders to investigate 'diagnostic orphans': subjects with alcohol dependence symptoms but no diagnosis. Drug Alcohol Depend 2000;60:295–302.

94. Hagman BT, Cohn AM, Schonfeld L, et al. College students who endorse a subthreshold number of DSM-5 alcohol use disorder criteria: alcohol, tobacco, and illicit drug use in DSM-5 diagnostic orphans. Am J Addict 2014;23(4):378–85.

95. Anthony JC, Helzer JE. Syndromes of drug abuse and dependence. In: Robins LN, Regier DA, editors. Psychiatric disorders in America: the epidemiologic catchment area study. New York: Free Press; 1991. p. 116–54.

96. Helzer JE, Burnam A, McEvoy LT. Alcohol abuse and dependence. In: Robins LN, Regier DA, editors. Psychiatric disorders in America: the epidemiologic catchment area study. New York: Free Press; 1991. p. 81–115.

97. Kessler RC, McGonagle KA, Zhao S, et al. Lifetime and 12-month prevalence of DSM-III-R psychiatric disorders in the United States: results from the National Comorbidity Survey. Arch Gen Psychiatry 1994;51(1):8–19.

98. Grant BF. Prevalence and correlates of drug use and *DSM-IV* drug dependence in the United States: results of the National Longitudinal Alcohol Epidemiologic Survey. J Subst Abuse 1996;8:195–210.

99. Grant BF, Dawson DA. Age of onset of drug use and its association with *DSM-IV* drug abuse and dependence: results from the National Longitudinal Alcohol Epidemiologic Survey. J Subst Abuse 1998;10:163–73.

100. Compton WM, Thomas YF, Stinson FS, et al. Prevalence, correlates, disability, and comorbidity of DSM-IV drug abuse and dependence in the United States: results from the national epidemiologic survey on alcohol and related conditions. Arch Gen Psychiatry 2007;64(5):566–76.

101. Hasin DS, Stinson FS, Ogburn E, et al. Prevalence, correlates, disability, and co-morbidity of DSM-IV alcohol abuse and dependence in the United States: results from the National Epidemiologic Survey on Alcohol and Related Conditions. Arch Gen Psychiatry 2007;64(7):830–42.

102. Simon GE, VonKorff M. Recall of psychiatric history in cross-sectional surveys: implications for epidemiologic research. Epidemiol Rev 1994;17(1):221–7.

103. Bourdon KH, Rae DS, Locke BZ, et al. Estimating the prevalence of mental disorders in US adults from the epidemiologic catchment area survey. Public Health Rep 1992;107(6):663.

104. Kessler RC, Chiu WT, Demler O, et al. Prevalence, severity, and comorbidity of 12-month DSM-IV disorders in the national comorbidity survey replication. Arch Gen Psychiatry 2005;62(6):617–27.

105. Costello EJ, Mustillo S, Erkanli A, et al. Prevalence and development of psychiatric disorders in childhood and adolescence. Arch Gen Psychiatry 2003;60(8):837–44.

106. Young SE, Corley RP, Stallings MC, et al. Substance use, abuse and dependence in adolescence: prevalence, symptom profiles and correlates. Drug Alcohol Depend 2002;68(3):309–22.

107. Swendsen J, Conway KP, Degenhardt L, et al. Mental disorders as risk factors for substance use, abuse and dependence: results from the 10-year follow-up of the National Comorbidity Survey. Addiction 2010;105(6):1117–28.

108. Merikangas KR, He JP, Burstein M, et al. Lifetime prevalence of mental disorders in US adolescents: results from the national comorbidity survey replication–adolescent supplement (NCS-A). J Am Acad Child Adolesc Psychiatry 2010; 49(10):980–9.

109. National Institute on Drug Abuse. Sex and gender differences in substance use. 2015. Available at: https://www.drugabuse.gov/publications/research-reports/substance-use-in-women/sex-gender-differences-in-substance-use. Accessed February 12, 2016.
110. Substance Abuse and Mental Health Services Administration. Results from the 2013 National Survey on Drug Use and Health: summary of national findings, NSDUH series H-48, HHS publication No. (SMA) 14–4863. Rockville (MD): Substance Abuse and Mental Health Services Administration; 2014.
111. Substance Abuse and Mental Health Services Administration. Results from the 2006 National Survey on Drug Use and Health: national findings (office of applied studies, NSDUH series H-32, DHHS publication No. SMA 07–4293). Rockville (MD): 2007.

# Neurobiology of Adolescent Substance Use Disorders

Aditi Sharma, MD[a], Jonathan D. Morrow, MD, PhD[b,*]

**KEYWORDS**

- Adolescence • Addiction • Neurobiology • Development • Substance use

**KEY POINTS**

- Subcortical reward processes are stronger in adolescents than adults, but prefrontal cortical executive control systems are weaker.
- Peer influences enhance reward-related neural responses of adolescents and increase sensation-seeking, risky behavior.
- Adolescents are more susceptible to stress, and some turn to substance use as a coping strategy.
- Adolescents are less sensitive to some of the acute negative consequences of substance use that can serve as a signal to limit intake, but more sensitive to long-term problems such as neurodegeneration and cognitive deficits.

## INTRODUCTION

Developmental tasks of adolescence include emotional maturation, individuation, establishment of meaningful relationships outside the family, and progress toward independence from the family of origin. In this context, typical adolescent characteristics, including increased appetitive drives, sensory-seeking behavior, and experimentation, likely serve an adaptive function. These tendencies lead to increased risk-taking behaviors, including experimentation with substance use, as a common part of the adolescent experience. In fact, experimentation with drugs and alcohol can be considered a normative behavior, and only a fraction of those who experiment with drugs and alcohol go on to develop substance use disorders. In a longitudinal study of 101 subjects, it was found that those who experimented with drug use during adolescence had better "psychological health" than adolescents who either abstained completely or used substances frequently.[1]

[a] Department of Psychiatry and Behavioral Sciences, University of Washington School of Medicine, 4800 Sand Point Way NE, Mailstop OA.5.154, PO Box 5371, Seattle, WA 98105-0371, USA; [b] Department of Psychiatry, University of Michigan Addiction Treatment Services, University of Michigan, 4250 Plymouth Road, Ann Arbor, MI 48109, USA
* Corresponding author.
*E-mail address:* jonmorro@med.umich.edu

Child Adolesc Psychiatric Clin N Am 25 (2016) 367–375
http://dx.doi.org/10.1016/j.chc.2016.02.001
1056-4993/16/$ – see front matter © 2016 Elsevier Inc. All rights reserved.
childpsych.theclinics.com

For numerous reasons, adolescence is a remarkably vulnerable time, characterized by changes in physiology, cognition, environmental influence, and social dynamics. Biological changes, mostly hormonally mediated, include physical growth, development of secondary sex characteristics, and alterations in neurobiology. Physiologic vulnerability to stress increases.[2,3] Some aspects of cognition begin to mature, whereas other aspects, particularly executive functioning, lag behind. External demands begin to exert more influence, including academic pressures, employment, and generally increased levels of responsibility. Peer influence and approval become more important, and social focus shifts away from the family of origin. Many psychiatric disorders have their onset in adolescence, including depression, anxiety, and substance use disorders. For adolescents who do engage in substance use, it is known that earlier onset of use is a significant predictor of development of a substance or alcohol use disorder over the lifetime, as well as predicting greater addiction severity.[4,5]

## REVIEW OF NEUROBIOLOGY OF SUBSTANCE USE

Of all psychiatric disorders, the pathophysiology of addiction is perhaps the best understood. Only a small fraction of the millions of known chemical compounds support addictive behavior, and yet drugs of abuse have a startling diversity of chemical structures, including, for example, complex aromatic cannabinoids, opioid peptides, modified catecholamines, and even extremely simple molecules such as ethanol and nitrous oxide. The one property all these compounds share is that they cause dramatic increases in dopamine release within the nucleus accumbens.[6] Other salient rewards, such as food, sex, and other pleasurable activities, also cause dopamine release in the nucleus accumbens; indeed this dopaminergic activity is likely necessary for instigating and supporting all motivated behaviors that are aimed at repeating pleasurable experiences. The critical difference from these other rewards is that drugs of abuse stimulate accumbal dopamine release through *pharmacological*, as well as psychological, mechanisms.

## ROLE OF NUCLEUS ACCUMBENS

The nucleus accumbens is the major component of the ventral striatum. It is a part of the basal ganglia, which is a set of subcortical structures that serve as a critical interface between limbic and motor circuitry, essentially allowing emotional responses to be translated into motor activity. Nucleus accumbens projection neurons send information through iterative cortico-striatal-thalamic loops, where neural activity is repeatedly modulated by afferents from multiple brain areas before ultimately exiting into the motor system to produce motivated behavior.[7] Glutamatergic projections carry information from a number of different structures to the nucleus accumbens, including processed multimodal sensory information from the amygdala, and contextual memory information from the hippocampus. Importantly, the prefrontal cortex provides executive control and decision-making information to the nucleus accumbens, and these prefrontal cortical afferents serve as a major source of inhibitory control over subcortical impulses, including urges to use drugs.[8] A relatively small group of brainstem neurons known as the ventral tegmental area provides dopaminergic input to the nucleus accumbens. Dopamine does not directly influence action potentials. Rather, it modifies neuronal responses to specific glutamatergic inputs. One long-lasting consequence of drug-induced spikes in accumbal dopamine is an alteration of synaptic density within this structure, such that specific circuits associated with drug-seeking behaviors become strengthened at the expense of synapses involved in other goal-directed behaviors.[9]

## BRAIN CHANGES OCCURRING IN ADOLESCENCE

During brain development from childhood through adolescence and to adulthood, various changes occur, many of which affect the functioning of the reward circuitry outlined previously. Maturation does not occur simultaneously across the entire brain; rather, various areas of the brain mature at different rates during development. Among the first areas to mature are subcortical structures, including the nucleus accumbens and other parts of the striatum.[10,11] Cortical white matter is shown to increase linearly, due to increased myelination. In contrast, human brain imaging studies have shown that there is an increase in cortical gray matter during childhood, followed by a sustained decrease starting around puberty, which reflects a refinement of neuronal connections known as "synaptic pruning." This decrease in gray matter occurs at different times throughout the cortex, according to a consistent sequence across individuals.[12] Gogtay and colleagues,[13] in studying brain maturation from childhood through adulthood via MRI, found that higher-order association cortices matured later than primary sensorimotor cortices. Among the last regions of the brain to mature is the prefrontal cortex.

Rodent studies have shown increases in dopaminergic activity across the brain during adolescence, particularly in limbic areas.[14,15] Stanwood and colleagues[16] found that D1 and D2 receptor density increased in the nucleus accumbens, the striatum, and the prefrontal cortex until the age of 40 days, followed by a progressive decline.[17] Although baseline dopamine levels may be lower in adolescents compared with adults, rewarding stimuli tend to evoke higher levels of dopamine release in adolescents.[18] At the same time, glutamatergic projections from the prefrontal cortex to subcortical structures including amygdala and nucleus accumbens are underdeveloped in adolescence as compared with adulthood.

## FUNCTIONAL IMPLICATIONS OF MATURATION PATTERN

The changes to the limbic system outlined previously seem almost designed to make adolescents more vulnerable to substance use disorders. Galvan and colleagues[19] found that when comparing children, adolescents, and adults in a reward-based task, nucleus accumbens activity in adolescents most closely resembled that of adults, but the activity of the orbitofrontal cortex was more similar to that of children. Thus, during adolescence, areas of the limbic system associated with primary urges and cravings are functioning at peak performance, whereas areas that provide control and context to those primary motivations remain immature.[19] Numerous studies support this basic finding, which has clear functional consequences. For example, adolescents perform poorly compared with adults on tasks that test inhibitory control, such as anti-saccade tasks that involve suppressing an eye-gaze response.[20] This type of behavioral disinhibition, also described as impulsivity, is well-known to predispose individuals to substance use disorders.[21,22] For example, Mahmood and colleagues[23] examined activation of the ventromedial prefrontal cortex and other brain regions of interest during a go/no-go task (to assess activation of various brain regions during a response-inhibition task) in 39 adolescents who were high-frequency substance users and 41 adolescents who were low-frequency substance users. They found that increased engagement of the prefrontal/executive control circuitry during a response-inhibition task predicted better outcomes 18 months later, as evidenced by fewer symptoms of drug and alcohol dependence in both groups.[23] Other aspects of executive function also improve over the course of adolescence, including working memory, problem-solving, and selective attention, all of which may also contribute to substance use disorders.[24]

In addition to impulsivity resulting from a lack of prefrontal cortical control over subcortical urges, there is evidence that subcortical incentive processes themselves are more powerful in adolescents. As mentioned in the previous section, reward-related dopaminergic activity in the nucleus accumbens and other regions is enhanced in adolescence, even compared with adulthood.[25] This increased dopamine response may underlie increased sensation seeking and risk taking among adolescents.[26,27] Risky behavior can be defined as the pursuit of rewards despite the possibility of danger, failure, or loss. By 15 years of age, teens are as capable as adults of logically assessing risk and probabilities of success.[28] However, if novelty and rewards are simply more salient for them, adolescents may be more inclined to engage in risky behaviors, including drug and alcohol use, despite a roughly equal assessment of the potential dangers involved.

## NEUROBIOLOGY OF PEER INFLUENCE

During adolescence, the social environment can have a profound influence over risky behaviors, such as substance use. Social cues activate limbic circuitry more strongly in adolescents than adults.[29,30] Adolescents spend more time with peers,[31] and begin to place increasing value on peer relationships and approval. Peer influence is a known factor contributing to adolescent substance use,[32] as well as other risky behaviors.[33] In fact, even the mere presence of peers has been shown to increase risk-taking behavior in adolescents.[34] For example, one study of adolescents and adults performing a task alone and in the presence of peers, showed that when performing a task while being observed by peers, adolescents engaged in riskier behavior and showed more activation in the ventral striatum and orbitofrontal cortex, than compared with when they were not being observed by peers. Adults performing the same task did not exhibit riskier behavior when in the presence of peers, and also did not show significant differences in ventral striatum and orbitofrontal cortex activity. Among adolescents, but not adults, increased activity in the ventral striatum and orbitofrontal cortex was also associated with risky decision-making.[35] This does not necessarily mean that the presence of peers has direct influences on neurobiology, as the presence of peers could also be influencing cognitions and behavior, which in turn could account for the functional MRI changes seen. However, the finding is consistent with the concept that peer influence can enhance the salience of rewards and thereby increase the likelihood of high-risk substance use behaviors.

## UNIQUE VULNERABILITY TO STRESS

Stress is a known risk factor for initiation of substance use and relapse to substance use.[36] For numerous reasons, adolescence is a time of increasing stress. Increasing academic demands, social changes, emphasis on peer acceptance, changing family dynamics, and emergence of psychiatric disorders, are some, but not all of the factors implicated. In addition to being a time of increased exposure to stress, adolescence is also a time of increased physiologic vulnerability to stress. Baseline salivary levels of the stress hormone cortisol have been shown to increase as pubertal status progresses in humans.[37] Rodent studies reveal increased behavioral responses, sympathetic activation, and hypothalamic-pituitary axis activity in responses to stressors during adolescence.[38] Human studies have demonstrated that as age and pubertal stage increase, physiological responses to stress increase as well. This has been demonstrated by higher levels of cortisol response to a socially stressful exercise in older adolescents compared with those at earlier pubertal stages,[2] and increased biological markers of beta adrenergic activity (blood pressure, cardiac output) in adolescents as compared with children when exposed to stress.[3]

Hormonal changes during puberty can interact with stress and substance use in complex ways. For example, the steroid 3 $\alpha$-OH-5[$\alpha$]$\beta$-pregan-20-one (THP) modulates stress via direct effects on the GABA$_A$ receptor. In both humans and rodents, levels of THP have been shown to increase after stress.[39] In both children and adults, THP potentiates the GABA$_A$ receptor, reducing anxiety and acting as a brake on stress levels. However, adolescents uniquely express high levels of the $\alpha4\beta\delta$ form of the GABA$_A$ receptor, which is *inhibited* by THP, meaning that in adolescents, THP actually increases and prolongs stress responses rather than reducing them.[40] Alcohol is a ready-made antidote for this added stress, as it activates $\alpha4\beta\delta$ GABA$_A$ receptors at relatively low concentrations.[41]

## UNIQUE SENSITIVITIES TO THE EFFECTS OF SUBSTANCES OF ABUSE

In general, animal studies have shown that adolescents are less sensitive to aversive effects of various addictive drugs as compared with adults.[17] For example, numerous animal studies have shown that adolescent rodents are less sensitive to the acute locomotor stimulatory effects of psychostimulants, compared with younger or older animals.[42] With regard to alcohol, Little and colleagues[43] found that adolescent rats were less likely to lose their righting reflex at the lowest dose of ethanol administration when compared with older and younger rats, and additionally, they regained their righting reflex significantly earlier than adult rats. Serum ethanol concentrations at the time of recovery of the righting reflex of adolescent rats were significantly higher than serum ethanol concentrations of adult rats at time of recovery of the righting reflex.[43] Similarly, Behar and colleagues[44] tested the effects of alcohol consumption on young adolescent boys, and the authors "were impressed by how little gross behavioral change occurred in the children after a dose of alcohol which had been intoxicating in an adult population." The implication of this is that adolescents may experience fewer subjective cues to limit intake, potentially resulting in the use of higher quantities, and consequently greater risk for dependence.

## NEUROBIOLOGICAL EFFECTS OF SUBSTANCE USE

Despite the decreased sensitivity demonstrated in animal studies of adolescents to many subjectively aversive effects of addictive substances, there are also a number of ways in which adolescents are more sensitive to substance-induced neuronal dysfunction. White and Swartzwelder[45] found both molecular and behavioral evidence of greater hippocampal memory impairment in adolescent rats compared with adult rats. They found that in hippocampal slices from adolescent rats, alcohol inhibited the induction of long-term potentiation and N-methyl-D-aspartate receptor–mediated synaptic potentials.[45] Adolescent rats injected with alcohol performed worse on a Morris water maze task compared with saline controls. Adult rats under the same test conditions showed recovery to normal performance after a drug-free period, whereas adolescent rats that had been injected with alcohol did not.[46] These findings are suggestive of persistent ethanol-related deficits specific to exposure during adolescence. There are a number of other long-term consequences of substance use during adolescence. De Bellis and colleagues[47] found that among adolescents and young adults with adolescent-onset alcohol use disorder, hippocampal volume was significantly smaller as compared with control subjects. This is perhaps because adolescents are more sensitive to the neurotoxic effects of alcohol.[48,49] To make matters worse, many of the brain areas most sensitive to alcohol-induced neurodegeneration, for example, the prefrontal cortex, are precisely the areas that normally exert inhibitory control over urges to abuse substances.[50,51]

## SUMMARY

There are many facets of the neurobiology of substance use that are distinct in adolescence as compared with adulthood. The adolescent brain is subject to intense subcortical reward processes, but is left with an immature prefrontal control system that is often unable to resist the pull of potentially exciting activities like substance use, even when fully aware of the dangers involved. Peer influences serve only to magnify these effects and foster more sensation-seeking, risky behavior. Unique neurobiology and social contexts often conspire to increase stress levels in adolescents, driving some to substance use as a way of coping with anxiety and other negative emotions. Adolescents are less sensitive to some of the acute negative consequences of substance use that often serve as a signal to limit intake, yet they are more sensitive to long-term effects, such as neurodegeneration and cognitive deficits that can, in turn, serve to promote further drug use. In many ways, substance use is a normative activity that adolescents are developmentally and biologically primed to undertake, but like other risky activities that serve similar adaptive functions at this critical life stage, indulging in substance use can have disastrous consequences for some individuals. Clinically, these unique aspects of neurobiology should be taken into consideration when designing prevention programs and clinical interventions for adolescent substance use disorders.

## REFERENCES

1. Shedler J, Block J. Adolescent drug use and psychological health. A longitudinal inquiry. Am Psychol 1990;45(5):612–30.
2. Sumter SR, Bokhorst CL, Miers AC, et al. Age and puberty differences in stress responses during a public speaking task: do adolescents grow more sensitive to social evaluation? Psychoneuroendocrinology 2010;35(10):1510–6.
3. Allen MT, Matthews KA. Hemodynamic responses to laboratory stressors in children and adolescents: the influences of age, race, and gender. Psychophysiology 1997;34(3):329–39.
4. Chambers RA, Taylor JR, Potenza MN. Developmental neurocircuitry of motivation in adolescence: a critical period of addiction vulnerability. Am J Psychiatry 2003;160(6):1041–52.
5. Grant BF, Dawson DA. Age of onset of drug use and its association with DSM-IV drug abuse and dependence: results from the National Longitudinal Alcohol Epidemiologic Survey. J Subst Abuse 1998;10(2):163–73.
6. Hyman SE, Malenka RC, Nestler EJ. Neural mechanisms of addiction: the role of reward-related learning and memory. Annu Rev Neurosci 2006;29:565–98.
7. Ikemoto S, Panksepp J. The role of nucleus accumbens dopamine in motivated behavior: a unifying interpretation with special reference to reward-seeking. Brain Res Brain Res Rev 1999;31(1):6–41.
8. Kelley AE. Ventral striatal control of appetitive motivation: role in ingestive behavior and reward-related learning. Neurosci Biobehav Rev 2004;27(8):765–76.
9. Robinson TE, Kolb B. Persistent structural modifications in nucleus accumbens and prefrontal cortex neurons produced by previous experience with amphetamine. J Neurosci 1997;17(21):8491–7.

10. Sowell ER, Peterson BS, Thompson PM, et al. Mapping cortical change across the human life span. Nat Neurosci 2003;6(3):309–15.
11. Dahl RE. Biological, developmental, and neurobehavioral factors relevant to adolescent driving risks. Am J Prev Med 2008;35(Suppl 3):S278–84.
12. Giedd JN, Blumenthal J, Jeffries NO, et al. Brain development during childhood and adolescence: a longitudinal MRI study. Nat Neurosci 1999;2(10):861–3.
13. Gogtay N, Giedd JN, Lusk L, et al. Dynamic mapping of human cortical development during childhood through early adulthood. Proc Natl Acad Sci U S A 2004; 101(21):8174–9.
14. McCutcheon JE, Conrad KL, Carr SB, et al. Dopamine neurons in the ventral tegmental area fire faster in adolescent rats than in adults. J Neurophysiol 2012;108(6):1620–30.
15. Rosenberg DR, Lewis DA. Changes in the dopaminergic innervation of monkey prefrontal cortex during late postnatal development: a tyrosine hydroxylase immunohistochemical study. Biol Psychiatry 1994;36(4):272–7.
16. Stanwood GD, McElligot S, Lu L, et al. Ontogeny of dopamine D3 receptors in the nucleus accumbens of the rat. Neurosci Lett 1997;223(1):13–6.
17. Bernheim A, Halfon O, Boutrel B. Controversies about the enhanced vulnerability of the adolescent brain to develop addiction. Front Pharmacol 2013;4:118.
18. Laviola G, Pascucci T, Pieretti S. Striatal dopamine sensitization to D-amphetamine in periadolescent but not in adult rats. Pharmacol Biochem Behav 2001; 68(1):115–24.
19. Galvan A, Hare TA, Parra CE, et al. Earlier development of the accumbens relative to orbitofrontal cortex might underlie risk-taking behavior in adolescents. J Neurosci 2006;26(25):6885–92.
20. Luna B. Developmental changes in cognitive control through adolescence. Adv Child Dev Behav 2009;37:233–78.
21. Belin D, Mar AC, Dalley JW, et al. High impulsivity predicts the switch to compulsive cocaine-taking. Science 2008;320(5881):1352–5.
22. Verdejo-Garcia A, Lawrence AJ, Clark L. Impulsivity as a vulnerability marker for substance-use disorders: review of findings from high-risk research, problem gamblers and genetic association studies. Neurosci Biobehav Rev 2008;32(4): 777–810.
23. Mahmood OM, Goldenberg D, Thayer R, et al. Adolescents' fMRI activation to a response inhibition task predicts future substance use. Addict Behav 2013;38(1): 1435–41.
24. Blakemore SJ, Choudhury S. Development of the adolescent brain: implications for executive function and social cognition. J Child Psychol Psychiatry 2006; 47(3–4):296–312.
25. Doremus-Fitzwater TL, Varlinskaya EI, Spear LP. Motivational systems in adolescence: possible implications for age differences in substance abuse and other risk-taking behaviors. Brain Cogn 2010;72(1):114–23.
26. Forbes EE, Ryan ND, Phillips ML, et al. Healthy adolescents' neural response to reward: associations with puberty, positive affect, and depressive symptoms. J Am Acad Child Adolesc Psychiatry 2010;49(2):162–72.e1-5.
27. Martin CA, Kelly TH, Rayens MK, et al. Sensation seeking and symptoms of disruptive disorder: association with nicotine, alcohol, and marijuana use in early and mid-adolescence. Psychol Rep 2004;94(3 Pt 1):1075–82.
28. Reyna VF, Farley F. Risk and rationality in adolescent decision making: implications for theory, practice, and public policy. Psychol Sci Public Interest 2006; 7(1):1–44.

29. Monk CS, McClure EB, Nelson EE, et al. Adolescent immaturity in attention-related brain engagement to emotional facial expressions. Neuroimage 2003; 20(1):420–8.

30. Yang TT, Menon V, Reid AJ, et al. Amygdalar activation associated with happy facial expressions in adolescents: a 3-T functional MRI study. J Am Acad Child Adolesc Psychiatry 2003;42(8):979–85.

31. Windle M, Spear LP, Fuligni AJ, et al. Transitions into underage and problem drinking: developmental processes and mechanisms between 10 and 15 years of age. Pediatrics 2008;121(Suppl 4):S273–89.

32. Dick DM, Pagan JL, Holliday C, et al. Gender differences in friends' influences on adolescent drinking: a genetic epidemiological study. Alcohol Clin Exp Res 2007; 31(12):2012–9.

33. Steinberg L. A social neuroscience perspective on adolescent risk-taking. Dev Rev 2008;28(1):78–106.

34. Gardner M, Steinberg L. Peer influence on risk taking, risk preference, and risky decision making in adolescence and adulthood: an experimental study. Dev Psychol 2005;41(4):625–35.

35. Chein J, Albert D, O'Brien L, et al. Peers increase adolescent risk taking by enhancing activity in the brain's reward circuitry. Dev Sci 2011;14(2):F1–10.

36. Wills TA. Stress and coping in early adolescence: relationships to substance use in urban school samples. Health Psychol 1986;5(6):503–29.

37. Kiess W, Meidert A, Dressendorfer RA, et al. Salivary cortisol levels throughout childhood and adolescence: relation with age, pubertal stage, and weight. Pediatr Res 1995;37(4 Pt 1):502–6.

38. Stroud LR, Foster E, Papandonatos GD, et al. Stress response and the adolescent transition: performance versus peer rejection stressors. Dev Psychopathol 2009;21(1):47–68.

39. Smith SS. The influence of stress at puberty on mood and learning: role of the $\alpha4\beta\delta$ GABAA receptor. Neuroscience 2013;249:192–213.

40. Shen H, Gong QH, Aoki C, et al. Reversal of neurosteroid effects at alpha4beta2delta GABAA receptors triggers anxiety at puberty. Nat Neurosci 2007;10(4):469–77.

41. Wallner M, Hanchar HJ, Olsen RW. Ethanol enhances alpha 4 beta 3 delta and alpha 6 beta 3 delta gamma-aminobutyric acid type A receptors at low concentrations known to affect humans. Proc Natl Acad Sci U S A 2003;100(25): 15218–23.

42. Spear LP. The adolescent brain and age-related behavioral manifestations. Neurosci Biobehav Rev 2000;24(4):417–63.

43. Little PJ, Kuhn CM, Wilson WA, et al. Differential effects of ethanol in adolescent and adult rats. Alcohol Clin Exp Res 1996;20(8):1346–51.

44. Behar D, Berg CJ, Rapoport JL, et al. Behavioral and physiological effects of ethanol in high-risk and control children: a pilot study. Alcohol Clin Exp Res 1983;7(4):404–10.

45. White AM, Swartzwelder HS. Hippocampal function during adolescence: a unique target of ethanol effects. Ann N Y Acad Sci 2004;1021:206–20.

46. Sircar R, Sircar D. Adolescent rats exposed to repeated ethanol treatment show lingering behavioral impairments. Alcohol Clin Exp Res 2005;29(8):1402–10.

47. De Bellis MD, Clark DB, Beers SR, et al. Hippocampal volume in adolescent-onset alcohol use disorders. Am J Psychiatry 2000;157(5):737–44.

48. Morris SA, Eaves DW, Smith AR, et al. Alcohol inhibition of neurogenesis: a mechanism of hippocampal neurodegeneration in an adolescent alcohol abuse model. Hippocampus 2010;20(5):596–607.

49. Crews FT, Braun CJ, Hoplight B, et al. Binge ethanol consumption causes differ-ential brain damage in young adolescent rats compared with adult rats. Alcohol Clin Exp Res 2000;24(11):1712–23.

50. Crews FT, Boettiger CA. Impulsivity, frontal lobes and risk for addiction. Pharmacol Biochem Behav 2009;93(3):237–47.

51. Medina KL, McQueeny T, Nagel BJ, et al. Prefrontal cortex volumes in adoles-cents with alcohol use disorders: unique gender effects. Alcohol Clin Exp Res 2008;32(3):386–94.

# Genetics of Substance Use Disorders

Cassie Yu, MD, Jon McClellan, MD*

## KEYWORDS

- Genomics • Genome-wide association • Alcohol • Nicotine • Addiction
- Alcohol dehydrogenase • Aldehyde dehydrogenase
- Nicotinic acetylcholine receptors

## KEY POINTS

- Substance abuse disorders are highly familial, with heritability estimates of 40% to 60%.
- Functional missense mutations in genes coding for alcohol-metabolizing enzymes (*ADH1B* and *ALDH2*) are associated with adverse responses to alcohol and are protective against alcohol dependence.
- A functional missense mutation in the nicotinic acetylcholine receptor *CHRNA5* decreases receptor sensitivity to nicotine and increases the risk for nicotine dependence.
- Substance abuse seems to be characterized by extreme genetic heterogeneity, most of which remains unexplained.

## INTRODUCTION

Substance abuse and dependence are highly heritable, and seem to have a strong genetic component. However, to date few definitive genetic variants moderating substance abuse risk have been identified. These conditions are characterized by substantial clinical heterogeneity and psychiatric comorbidity. Further, the expression of genetic vulnerability toward substance abuse depends in part on complex interactive social and cultural factors. Marked heterogeneity and the influence of environmental risk and protective factors complicates gene discovery.

In this article, we review contributions of genetics research on substance use disorders, starting with family, twin, and adoption studies. We then examine the genetics of alcohol, nicotine, and illicit drug use disorders individually. We also review issues underlying the basic genomic architecture of complex disease, and discuss strategies to guide future research characterizing genetic mechanisms underlying these conditions.

---

Disclosures: Dr J. McClellan has research grant funding from the NIH [Grant numbers: MH083989, MH096844]. The authors have no significant conflicts of interest to report.
Department of Psychiatry, University of Washington, Box 356560, Seattle, WA 98195, USA
* Corresponding author.
*E-mail address:* drjack@uw.edu

Child Adolesc Psychiatric Clin N Am 25 (2016) 377–385
http://dx.doi.org/10.1016/j.chc.2016.02.002
1056-4993/16/$ – see front matter
**childpsych.theclinics.com**

## FAMILY, TWIN, AND ADOPTION STUDIES

Substance abuse disorders are highly heritable.[1] Rates of substance abuse disorders are substantially increased in first-degree relatives of individuals with substance dependence (including opiates, cocaine, cannabis, and/or alcohol), as compared with controls.[2] In general, the use of alcohol, nicotine, and cannabis is strongly influenced by social and environmental factors during adolescence, with genetic factors playing an increasingly important role as substance use persists and progresses into young and middle adulthood.[3]

Twin and adoption studies suggest relatively stronger genetic versus environmental influences of alcohol use disorder. Rates of alcohol dependence were found to be significantly higher in a cotwin of an affected monozygotic twin pair, as compared with a cotwin of an affected dizygotic twin pair.[4] Children of alcoholics adopted by nonalcoholics and reared in a nondrinking environment have a higher risk of developing alcohol problems, as compared with children of nonalcoholics adopted by the same parents.[5]

Family and twin studies also support the role of genetic factors for smoking initiation and nicotine dependence.[6] Kendler and colleagues[7] demonstrated that male twin pairs have similar rates of tobacco use whether raised together or apart. In female twin pairs, the heritability estimates for tobacco use were higher in more recent birth cohorts, suggesting that, as cultural prohibitions for smoking relaxed, genetic factors played a greater role in women's smoking habits.

Although less well-studied, twin, family, and adoption studies also support the importance of both genetic and environmental factors for illicit substance use and abuse, including cannabis.[1] Specific patterns of substance abuse tend to correlate within families.[2]

However, because many people who misuse one drug misuse multiple drugs, distinguishing specific versus general risk factors of addiction is challenging.

## GENETIC ARCHITECTURE OF COMPLEX DISEASE

The prevailing model for much of psychiatric genetic research continues to be based on the common disease–common variant hypothesis. This model holds that common risk variants found in all human populations collectively confer a substantial portion of disease susceptibility for complex disease. Each variant risk allele confers a small effect, and by itself is not sufficient to cause disease. The total burden of risk variants, in combination with environmental risk factors, is hypothesized to explain the development of disease in most individuals.

Research over the past decade has challenged the common disease–common variant hypothesis. Complex disorders, including neuropsychiatric conditions, seem to be characterized by extreme genetic heterogeneity. Rare deleterious variants, including de novo mutations, or mutations that arose in recent generations, substantially contribute to disease risk. The common disease-rare variant model suggests that common illnesses are the collective sum of individually rare damaging mutations, such that most affected individuals or families may have a different genetic cause.[8]

Of course, rare and common alleles both contribute to disease risk and normal human variation. The genomic architecture of any illness or trait must stem from the same evolutionary forces that shape the human genome. In this regard, the nature of substance abuse presents an interesting dialectic. Although substance abuse and dependence are conceptualized clinically as categorical disorders, physiologic, psychological, and behavioral responses to psychoactive substances vary widely among humans. The ability to tolerate and metabolize substances is an adaptive trait, and yet addictive substances at sufficient dosages are toxic to all humans regardless of genotype.

Consider, for example, the influences of alcohol on human evolution. Hominids developed the capacity to metabolize alcohol several million years ago (*ADH4*)[9] as an adaption to diets that included fermented fruit. In developing human societies, alcoholic beverages in theory conferred an advantage in geographic regions with sources of water prone to endemic infectious diseases. Alcohol also has enormous impact on social structure by lessening inhibitions, increasing aggression, and encouraging reproductive behaviors. Therefore, depending on the individual, the setting, and the culture, the same substance may variably confer selective advantage, social disruption, and/or early demise. Inasmuch, both rare and common genetic variants may contribute to substance use and misuse.

## METHODS OF GENE DISCOVERY

To date, most substance abuse research has focused on the search for common risk variants using candidate gene, linkage and genome wide association approaches. Candidate gene studies focus on genes selected a priori based on hypothesized biological mechanisms underlying the disorder. The methods assess whether mutations within candidate genes, ideally those with known biological impact on gene function, are statistically associated with the phenotype under study.

Linkage studies classically identify markers genome-wide that segregate with illness in highly informative pedigrees. Genomic markers in close proximity tend to be inherited together. This concept is defined as linkage disequilibrium. By identifying genomic markers that segregate with a disorder, specific chromosomal regions harboring the causal mutation are linked to the condition.

Linkage strategies do not rely on prior knowledge of the underlying biology of the disorder, and have been exploited successfully to identify a number of different rare causal mutations in Mendelian disorders, and in complex disorders such as inherited breast cancer.[8] However, linkage methods for complex psychiatric disease often include large numbers of unrelated cases and controls, which adds significant clinical and genetic heterogeneity.

Genome-wide association studies (GWAS) are an extension of linkage methodology. GWAS studies characterize millions of common markers genome-wide, most often single nucleotide polymorphisms (SNPs), in very large cohorts of cases and controls. Variants associated with case status, after corrections for multiple testing, are assumed to either be causal variants or in linkage disequilibrium with causal variants. This approach will work if common causal mutations or haplotypes (inherited blocks of chromosomes) are shared across unrelated individuals. However, GWAS methods are significantly challenged if the illness is characterized by substantial genetic heterogeneity. In general, GWAS findings have been limited by lack of consistent replication, lack of established biological function for putative causal SNPs, exceedingly small effect sizes and the impact of population stratification on false-positive findings.[8]

## ALCOHOL USE DISORDERS
### Alcohol Metabolizing Gene Pathways

To date, the best-replicated genetic variants associated with alcohol use disorders involve alcohol-metabolizing enzymes.[10] Ethanol is metabolized via alcohol dehydrogenase (ADH) into acetaldehyde, which is then metabolized by aldehyde dehydrogenase (ALDH) into acetate, which is then excreted in urine. Higher acetaldehyde concentrations can cause adverse reactions including flushing and nausea.

The human genome has a total of 7 different ADHs and 3 different ALDHs.[11] ADH1 enzymes—*ADH1A, ADH1B, ADH1C*—encode enzymes involved with oxidative alcohol metabolism in the liver. *ADH1B*, located on chromosome 4, harbors a missense mutation (rs1229984) in exon 3 that defines 2 different functional alleles, ADH1B*1 and ADH1B*2. The ADH1B*2 has been shown by several studies to be protective against alcohol use disorders. The population frequency of the ADH1B*2 allele is higher in East Asians (70%–90% of the population), and lower among Europeans and Africans (approximately 5%). Carriers of ADH1B*2 have lower rates of alcohol dependence and consumption, regardless of ancestry.[12]

The ADH1B*2 allele metabolizes ethanol at a much higher rate. In theory, this variant will lead to increased concentrations of acetaldehyde levels after drinking alcohol, thus causing adverse effects that act as a deterrent. This mechanism has been demonstrated in animal studies.[13] However, in human studies, the ADH1B*2 variant was not associated with increased blood acetaldehyde concentrations.[14] Thus, although protective effects of ADH1B*2 allele are well-replicated, the mechanisms underlying its protective effects remain unclear.

Functional genetic variants in the acetaldehyde dehydrogenase gene family also have protective effects for alcohol abuse. The best-replicated SNP is a missense mutation in *ADLH2*, which substitutes lysine for glutamate at position 504. This allele, defined as the ALDH2*2, results in nearly inactive acetaldehyde metabolism activity. Carriers of this allele produce high levels of acetaldehyde after drinking alcohol, and experience unpleasant symptoms, including skin flushing. ALDH2*2 is common in East Asians, but rare in European and African populations.

### GABAergic System

The pharmacologic effects of alcohol on the brain are mediated in part by gamma aminobutyric acid (GABA), which is the primary inhibitory neurotransmitter in the central nervous system. GABA(A) receptors, which are involved with modulating anxiety and stress responses, have been widely studied in substance abuse research.[15] Different SNPs and haplotypes within the GABA(A) receptor subunits cluster on chromosome 4 have been associated with alcohol dependency in Native American,[16] European American,[17,18] and African American[19] cohorts. However, across studies, replication of specific variants has been inconsistent, and definitive causal variants within the region have not yet been identified.

### Linkage Studies

Linkage analyses have reported potential susceptibility loci for alcohol abuse, although the effects are modest and results vary across studies. The Collaborative Study on the Genetics of Alcoholism assessed multigenerational pedigrees with alcoholism in the United States, and detected signals suggestive of linkage at several chromosomal loci, including the ADH gene cluster on chromosome 4. Different chromosomal regions were implicated by a linkage study examining extended pedigrees from a Southwestern Native American tribe, including the GABRB1 gene locus on chromosome 4.[16]

### Genome-wide Association Studies

Several GWAS studies examining alcohol dependence have been published, each assessing hundreds to thousands of cases and controls.[20,21] Associations between SNPs in genes coding for alcohol-metabolizing enzymes and alcohol-related phenotypes have been noted consistently. Otherwise, although individual studies have reported associations with variants in proximity to genes of theoretic interest based on brain expression and function, replication is generally lacking. Furthermore, associated SNPs have been located mostly in noncoding regions, without established biological relevance. Some studies have incorporated pathway analyses to examine whether genes implicated by GWAS findings operate within key biological processes.[21] Genes that function in pathways important to brain development and neurotransmitter function have been highlighted. However, the specific genes and pathways implicated differ across different GWAS samples.

## NICOTINE USE DISORDERS
### Nicotinic Acetylcholine Receptors

To date, the best evidence for genetic risk factors related to nicotine dependence involves nicotinic acetylcholine receptors, which modulate the physiologic effects of nicotine. There are a total of 16 different nicotinic receptor subunit genes in humans that encode a set of nicotinic receptor subunit proteins.[22] Within the cluster of nicotinic acetylcholine receptor genes on chromosome 15q24: including the alpha 5, alpha 3, and beta4 subunits, *CHRNA5*, *CHRNA3*, and *CHRNB4* respectively; several SNPs have been associated with smoking behavior and nicotine dependence, as well as with smoking- related diseases of chronic obstructive pulmonary disease and lung cancer.[23,24]

The strongest known common genetic risk factor for nicotine dependence and smoking behavior is a missense mutation (rs16969968) in *CHRNA5* that changes the amino acid aspartate to asparagine at position 398. This mutation seems to decrease receptor sensitivity to nicotine. Carrying 1 asparagine allele increases the risk for nicotine dependence by 1.3-fold; homozygous carriers have a 2-fold risk as compared with those homozygous for the aspartate allele.[25] The association between this variant and nicotine dependence has been replicated in several independent studies. This SNP is also associated with a later age of smoking cessation, and an early age of onset of lung cancer.[26] In addition, a number of other rare and low frequency functional variants that impact *CHRNA5* have been shown to increase the risk of nicotine dependence in both European American and African American cohorts.[27]

### Cytochrome Enzyme CYP2A6

Nicotine is primarily metabolized to cotinine, mostly via the cytochrome P450 enzyme encoded by *CYP2A6*.[28] *CYP2A6* is highly polymorphic, with several different functional common alleles that vary in relative frequency across different ancestries. Rapid nicotine metabolism is associated with higher rates of cigarette use and nicotine dependence, and lower rates of smoking cessation. Several studies have reported reduced smoking behavior with decreased or absent CYP2A6 enzyme activity, including decreased number of cigarettes smoked, shorter smoking duration, and decreased withdrawal symptoms.[29]

### Linkage Studies

There have been more than 20 linkage studies addressing nicotine dependence. Collectively, these studies have reported a number of different putative risk loci. Replication across studies has been limited, with 4 genomic regions, on chromosomes 9q, 10q, 11p and 17p, implicated by independent samples. However, these loci do not corroborate findings from GWAS studies or from the nicotinic receptor subunit gene cluster findings on chromosome 15q24.

### Genome-wide Association Studies

Several GWAS studies have been conducted for nicotine dependence. A metaanalysis of GWAS studies, based on cohorts established by the Tobacco and Genetics Consortium (n = 74,053), confirmed prior findings regarding associations between variants in the nicotinic receptors gene cluster on chromosome 15q25 and different smoking behaviors.[30] In addition, noncoding SNPs in chromosomal regions 10q23 and 19q13, and an SNP in the first intron of *EGLN2* (egl-9 family hypoxia-inducible factor 2, involved in oxygen homeostasis) were associated with cigarettes smoked per day, and noncoding SNPs in proximity of *BDNF* (brain-derived neurotrophic factor) and *DBH* (dopamine beta hydroxylase) were associated with smoking initiation.

Loukola and colleagues[31] conducted GWAS analyses in Finnish cohorts examining for associations with a variety of different smoking behaviors, and for biomarkers of nicotine metabolism.[32] A number of different SNPs in the vicinity of *CLEC19A* (C-type lectin domain family 19, member A, a locus previously linked to attention deficit hyperactivity disorder) were associated with smoking quantity, while noncoding SNPs near the neuregulin receptor ERBB4 were associated with nicotine dependence. Neuregulin/ErB signaling pathways have been implicated in schizophrenia, as well as a suggested mechanism underlying the high comorbidity between schizophrenia and nicotine dependence.[33]

Although these studies suggest associations between smoking behaviors and different genes of theoretic interest to nicotine use, the functional significance for most of the candidate risk variants has not been established, effect sizes are small, and the findings differ across studies.

## ILLICIT SUBSTANCE USE DISORDERS

Research examining for genetic factors associated with addiction for substances other than alcohol and nicotine is limited. For cannabis use disorder, the gene encoding the central cannabinoid receptor (*CNR1*) has been most studied owing to its role in the cognitive and psychoactive effects of delta 9-tetrahydrocannabinol. Different noncoding SNPs in *CNR1* have been reported to be associated with cannabis dependence. Other SNPs in *CNR1* have been variably associated with cocaine dependence and intravenous drug use.[10]

Variation in the mu-opioid receptor (*OPRM1*) gene has been widely studied for associations with different types of substance abuse, given the presumed role of the endogenous opioid system in addiction based on its involvement with reward processing and dopamine signaling.[10] Different SNPs in *OPRM1*, including a functional missense mutation (rs1799971), have been variably associated with opioid, cocaine alcohol and nicotine use disorders. However, at this time none of the associated variants have been established clearly as risk factors for addictive disorders.

## SUMMARY

Despite extensive research, much of the genetic vulnerability to substance use disorders has yet to be explained. Although the focus has been on identifying biological underpinnings of addiction, the best replicated findings highlight mechanisms that self-limit the use of substances based on metabolic capacity or receptor sensitivity (eg, functional polymorphisms in *ADH1B* and *ALDH2* for alcohol, and in *CHRNA5* and *CYP2A6* for nicotine).

There are undoubtedly a vast number of different potential genetic mechanisms influencing risk for substance abuse and dependence, including direct pharmacogenetic effects (eg, differences in metabolism), variation in brain receptors/pathways that moderate the psychoactive and reward effects of specific substances, and vulnerabilities conferred by related psychopathology or personality characteristics (eg, risk taking behaviors, poor impulse control). Within each of these critical pathways and processes operates a multitude of genes and regulatory mechanisms that may contribute to substance abuse risk or protection.

With the advance of efficient sequencing technologies, whole exome and whole genome sequencing strategies are now feasible for large cohorts. These approaches allow for the identification of all classes of potential causal mutations, rare or common, genome-wide, including point mutations, small insertions and deletions and copy number variation. Sophisticated methodologies will combine informative cohorts (eg, highly affected pedigrees, extreme outliers in regards to metabolic profiles, or patterns of abuse) with state-of-the-art sequencing technologies to uncover causal mutations. In turn, each established causal mutation sheds light on related genes and critical pathways important to substance abuse and dependence.

## REFERENCES

1. Wang JC, Kapoor M, Goate AM. The genetics of substance dependence. Annu Rev Genomics Hum Genet 2012;13:241–61.
2. Merikangas KR, Stolar M, Stevens DE, et al. Familial transmission of substance use disorders. Arch Gen Psychiatry 1998;55:973–9.
3. Kendler KS, Schmitt E, Aggen SH, et al. Genetic and environmental influences on alcohol, caffeine, cannabis, and nicotine use from early adolescence to middle adulthood. Arch Gen Psychiatry 2008;65:674–82.
4. Kendler KS, Maes HH, Sundquist K, et al. Genetic and family and community environmental effects on drug abuse in adolescence: a Swedish National Twin and Sibling Study. Am J Psychiatry 2014;171(2):209–17.
5. Schuckit MA. An overview of genetic influences in alcoholism. J Subst Abuse Treat 2009;36:S5–14.
6. Li MD, Cheng R, Ma JZ, et al. A meta-analysis of estimated genetic and environmental effects on smoking behavior in male and female adult twins. Addiction 2003;98:23–31.
7. Kendler KS, Thornton LM, Pedersen NL. Tobacco consumption in Swedish twins reared apart and reared together. Arch Gen Psychiatry 2000;57:886–92.
8. McClellan J, King MC. Genetic heterogeneity in human disease. Cell 2010;141:210–7.
9. Carrigan MA, Uryasev O, Frye CB, et al. Hominids adapted to metabolize ethanol long before human directed fermentation. Proc Natl Acad Sci U S A 2015;112:458–63.
10. Bühler KM, Giné E, Echeverry-Alzate V, et al. Common single nucleotide variants underlying drug addiction: more than a decade of research. Addict Biol 2015;20:845–71.
11. Hurley TD, Edenberg HJ. Genes encoding enzymes involved in ethanol metabolism. Alcohol Res 2012;34:339–44.
12. Bierut LJ, Goate AM, Breslau N, et al. ADH1B is associated with alcohol dependence and alcohol consumption in populations of European and African ancestry. Mol Psychiatry 2012;17:445–50.

13. Rivera-Meza M, Quintanilla ME, Tampier L, et al. Mechanism of protection against alcoholism by an alcohol dehydrogenase polymorphism: development of an animal model. FASEB J 2010;24:266–74.

14. Peng GS, Yin SJ. Effect of the allelic variants of aldehyde dehydrogenase ALDH2*2 and alcohol dehydrogenase ADH1B*2 on blood acetaldehyde concentrations. Hum Genomics 2009;3:121–7.

15. Enoch MA. The role of GABA(A) receptors in the development of alcoholism. Pharmacol Biochem Behav 2008;90:95–104.

16. Long JC, Knowler WC, Hanson RL, et al. Evidence for genetic linkage to alcohol dependence on chromosomes 4 and 11 from an autosome-wide scan in an American Indian population. Am J Med Genet 1998;81:216–21.

17. Edenberg HJ, Dick DM, Xuei X, et al. Variations in GABRA2, encoding the alpha 2 subunit of the GABA(A) receptor, are associated with alcohol dependence and with brain oscillations. Am J Hum Genet 2004;74:705–14.

18. Covault J, Gelernter J, Hesselbrock V, et al. Allelic and haplotypic association of GABRA2 with alcohol dependence. Am J Med Genet B Neuropsychiatr Genet 2004;129B:104–9.

19. Ittiwut C, Yang BZ, Kranzler HR, et al. GABRG1 and GABRA2 variation associated with alcohol dependence in African Americans. Alcohol Clin Exp Res 2012;36:588–93.

20. Zuo L, Lu L, Tan Y, et al. Genome-wide association discoveries of alcohol dependence. Am J Addict 2014;23:526–39.

21. Hart AB, Kranzler HR. Alcohol dependence genetics: lessons learned from genome-wide association studies (GWAS) and post-GWAS analyses. Alcohol Clin Exp Res 2015;39:1312–27.

22. Dani JA, Bertrand D. Nicotinic acetylcholine receptors and nicotinic cholinergic mechanisms of the central nervous system. Annu Rev Pharmacol Toxicol 2007; 47:699–729.

23. Bierut LJ, Stitzel JA, Wang JC, et al. Variants in nicotinic receptors and risk for nicotine dependence. Am J Psychiatry 2008;165:1163–71.

24. Wassenaar CA, Dong Q, Wei Q, et al. Relationship between CYP2A6 and CHRNA5- CHRNA3-CHRNB4 variation and smoking behaviors and lung cancer risk. J Natl Cancer Inst 2011;103:1342–6.

25. Saccone NL, Culverhouse RC, Schwantes-An TH, et al. Multiple independent loci at chromosome 15q25.1 affect smoking quantity: a meta-analysis and comparison with lung cancer and COPD. PLoS Genet 2010;6. http://dx.doi.org/10.1371/journal.pgen.1001053.

26. Chen LS, Hung RJ, Baker T, et al. CHRNA5 risk variant predicts delayed smoking cessation and earlier lung cancer diagnosis–a meta-analysis. J Natl Cancer Inst 2015;107(5):djv100.

27. Olfson E, Saccone NL, Johnson EO, et al. Rare, low frequency and common coding variants in CHRNA5 and their contribution to nicotine dependence in European and African Americans. Mol Psychiatry 2015. http://dx.doi.org/10.1038/mp.2015.105.

28. Messina ES, Tyndale RF, Sellers EM. A major role for CYP2A6 in nicotine C-oxidation by human liver microsomes. J Pharmacol Exp Ther 1997;282:1608–14.

29. Minematsu N, Nakamura H, Furuuchi M, et al. Limitation of cigarette consumption by CYP2A6*4, *7 and *9 polymorphisms. Eur Respir J 2006;27:289–92.

30. Tobacco and Genetics Consortium. Genome-wide meta-analyses identify multiple loci associated with smoking behavior. Nat Genet 2010;42:441–7.

31. Loukola A, Wedenoja J, Keskitalo-Vuokko K, et al. Genome-wide association study on detailed profiles of smoking behavior and nicotine dependence in a twin sample. Mol Psychiatry 2014;19:615–24.
32. Loukola A, Buchwald J, Gupta R, et al. A genome-wide association study of a biomarker of nicotine metabolism. PLoS Genet 2015;11:e1005498.
33. Stefansson H, Sigurdsson E, Steinthorsdottir V, et al. Neuregulin 1 and susceptibility to schizophrenia. Am J Hum Genet 2002;71:877–92.

# Evidence-Based Prevention for Adolescent Substance Use

Erin Harrop, MSW[a], Richard F. Catalano, PhD[b],*

## KEYWORDS

- Prevention • Adolescent substance use • Young adult substance use • Risk factors
- Protective factors • Prevention science

## KEY POINTS

- In recent decades, prevention science has emerged as a unique field with growing empirical evidence of effectiveness.
- Prevention science is based on the identification of predictors, risk and protective factors, for problem behaviors that have been found in individual, peer, family, school, and community domains.
- There is a robust evidence base for prevention programs and policies that address these identified predictors.
- Effective prevention programs can be delivered in school, family, and community settings, and they include such things as school curricula for the promotion of social and emotional competence, parenting programs, mentoring programs, normative change campaigns, and policy development.
- The challenge now is to mobilize across disciplines and communities to advance the policies, programs, funding, and workforce preparation needed to use prevention science to promote behavioral health and prevent behavioral health problems among all young people, including those at greatest disadvantage or risk, from birth through age 24.

Adolescence is increasingly being recognized as a pivotal developmental period with defining characteristics and functions.[1] Further, during the transition from adolescence to young or emerging adulthood, there are more biological, psychological, and social changes occurring than in any other stage of life, except infancy.[2] During this time,

Conflict of Interest: E. Harrop has no conflicts of interest to declare. R.F. Catalano is on the board of Channing Bete Company, distributor of Guiding Good Choices and Supporting School Success, a component of the Raising Healthy Children program, 2 of the 22 programs referred to in this report.
[a] University of Washington School of Social Work, Seattle, WA 98026, USA; [b] Social Development Research Group, University of Washington School of Social Work, 9725 Third Avenue Northeast, Suite #401, Seattle, WA 98115, USA
* Corresponding author.
E-mail address: catalano@myuw.net

Child Adolesc Psychiatric Clin N Am 25 (2016) 387–410
http://dx.doi.org/10.1016/j.chc.2016.03.001
1056-4993/16/$ – see front matter © 2016 Elsevier Inc. All rights reserved.

childpsych.theclinics.com

adolescents are charged with many tasks that usher them into a period of adulthood, marked by greater independence. These developmental tasks include gaining skills to perform adult roles, separating from parents, achieving greater autonomy from adults, building social connections with peers, developing a positive body image, managing their emerging sexuality, and cultivating a more robust sense of identity.[2,3]

However, this period is not only marked by greater autonomy and growing responsibilities, but it is also marked by increasing experimental behaviors, through which adolescents explore the world. Neural changes in the brain during adolescence facilitate exploration and risk taking, while the cognitive functions of the brain are not yet fully developed, decreasing cognitive decision making, feelings of inhibition, and worry about the future, and increasing emotional-based decisions.[4] The benefits of this unique neural developmental pattern characteristic of adolescence include rapidly increasing knowledge about the world through a variety of new experiences and a heightened neural reward system. However, this period is also marked by greater vulnerability, as adolescents can be exposed to more potentially harmful situations as a result of their experimentation and exploration. A core challenge in adolescent and young adult health promotion is that "problem behaviors" related to experimentation are a normal part of adolescent development, yet they carry with them inherent threats to health.[5] These threats to health have severe consequences, including substance use problems, violence, vehicular accidents, risky sexual practices, self-harm, and even death. In fact, most adolescent and young adult deaths that occur globally are related to problem behaviors.[6] Laurence Steinberg, psychologist and expert on adolescent development, summarizes this unique developmental period in the following way:

> Brain science explains… why adolescence is a vulnerable period… There is a time lag between the activation of brain systems that excite our emotions and impulses and the maturation of brain systems that allow us to check these feelings and urgings—it's like driving a car with a sensitive gas pedal and bad brakes. When our capacity for self-regulation isn't strong enough to rein in our arousal, problems are more likely to result—problems such as depression, substance abuse, obesity, aggression, and other risky and reckless behavior.[7(p15)]

Due to the significant consequences of adolescent problem behaviors, researchers in the past 4 decades have increasingly focused on approaches to ameliorate these behaviors in hopes of improving adolescent health outcomes and mitigating mortality rates. Although many early prevention programs had disappointing success rates (and at times iatrogenic effects), programs in the past 3 decades have achieved more promising and effective outcomes.[8–12] This article specifically addresses the evidence base for prevention programs targeted at reducing substance use behaviors in adolescence and emerging adulthood. The article begins with a brief description of prevention science, followed by descriptions of key risk and protective factors specific to the adolescent and emerging adult periods. Following this, an overview of effective prevention programs and policies is described, including a brief presentation of prevention programs for adolescents and young adults with strong evidence of effectiveness. The article closes with an articulation of the challenges and opportunities currently emerging in the field.

## THE SCIENCE OF PREVENTING PROBLEMATIC BEHAVIORS

Prevention science had been created as a field by incorporating and organizing findings from research on life-course development, community epidemiology, and preventive intervention trials.[13] Prevention science is based on the premise that empirically verifiable precursors, often called risk and protective factors, affect the probability of later problems. Risk factors precede specific problematic health behaviors, and contribute to the likelihood of poor health outcomes. Similarly, protective factors precede certain health behaviors, and contribute to the likelihood of better health outcomes either directly or by reducing the effects of risk factors.[14,15]

Risk and protective factors exist across the life course, and occur in multiple socialization domains, including peer factors (eg, friends who use drugs), family factors (eg, family conflict), school factors (eg, academic performance), and community factors (eg, poverty, community laws and norms),[16] as well as individual factors (eg, early aggression and temperament). Thus, risk and protective factors span individual to structural factors, with multiple influences across socialization domains affecting the health outcomes of adolescents. The exposure to multiple risk factors appears to be cumulative. The more risk factors an adolescent has, the more likely a problematic health outcome is to occur.[14,17] However, risk factors also can be moderated or mediated by the presence of protective factors, which increase the likelihood of healthy development.[14,15] Additionally, risk and protective factors often influence more than one problem behavior.[16] Because risk and protective factors tend to cluster in the individual and risk/protective factors affect multiple problem behaviors, interventions that seek to change a single or a cluster of risk or protective factors may demonstrate effects on multiple outcomes because they are all predicted by the risk/protective factors addressed.[16] Thus, although this article focuses primarily on the prevention of substance use behaviors, many of the programs discussed have multiple beneficial outcomes, including reducing violence, enhancing mental health, and decreasing unwanted pregnancies.

Prevention programs are typically viewed as occurring on a spectrum from health promotion to indicated prevention (**Fig. 1**).[13] Substance use prevention programs can be aimed at a range of goals, from preventing initiation of substance use through preventing the development of substance use–related problems or substance use

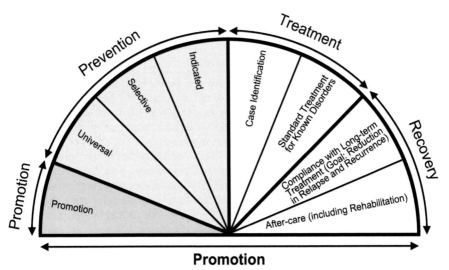

**Fig. 1.** Intervention spectrum. (*From* O'Connell ME, Boat T, Warner, KE. Preventing mental, emotional, and behavioral disorders among young people: progress and possibilities. Washington, DC: National Academies Press, 2009; with permission.)

dependence. Health promotion efforts involve the promotion of healthy behaviors, and do not explicitly target the reduction of problem behaviors. Prevention programs aim to reduce problem behaviors and are divided into 3 categories addressing different levels of risk within a population: universal, selective, and indicated prevention programs.[16] *Universal prevention programs* target reducing substance use in an entire population without regard to risk. Universal programs are frequently used because research has found that most cases of a complex disorder come from the large proportion of the population that is at low or moderate risk (genetic or environmental) for that disorder, and only a minority of cases occur in the small proportion of the population that is high risk. In a study of mortality from coronary disease, Geoffrey Rose coined the term prevention paradox to describe this phenomenon and demonstrated that a large number of people at a small risk may give rise to more cases of disease than the small number who are at a high risk.[18] Policy-level interventions, such as drinking-age laws and graduated licensing for drivers, are examples of universal prevention policies. *Selective programs* are targeted at populations that show increased levels of risk, such as programs delivered in neighborhoods with high levels of crime. Finally, *indicated programs* target individuals who have already begun to use, but have yet to show symptoms of abuse or dependence, such as adolescents who have initiated substance use but have not yet developed regular use associated with negative consequences.

## RISK FACTORS FOR SUBSTANCE USE

In the past 4 decades, much work has been done to identify risk and protective factors for adolescent substance use and other problems.[19] Risk factors have been shown to be consistent predictors across groups, including gender, ethnicity, community, and country.[20] Risk factors are grouped by socialization domain, and organized into community factors, school factors, family factors, and individual/peer factors. **Table 1** summarizes risk factors for adolescent substance use and other problems and provides information from a recent review of risk factors for young adult substance use.[21] We first provide an overview of risk factors associated with adolescent substance use and other problems, followed by a brief summary of risk factors specific to young adult substance use.

### Risk Factors for Substance Use in Adolescence

Characteristics of communities can increase the likelihood that adolescents within those communities will use substances. When a community has laws and norms that are favorable to substance use, such as low enforcement of drinking ages or frequent community events featuring alcohol, youths in these communities are more likely to use substances.[15] Another key factor is availability. Availability of substances varies from community to community, with some communities having greater availability (eg, more liquor or marijuana stores). Communities with higher availability have increased rates of youth substance use.[22] It has also been found that perception of availability is also an important factor. If youth merely perceive that drugs and alcohol are more available, this perception (however inaccurate) is also associated with higher rates of youth drug use.[23] Perhaps influencing adolescents' perception of substance availability or acceptability, media portrayals of substance use in communities (ranging from alcohol advertisements to movies featuring substance use) have also been linked to substance abuse and earlier initiation of substance use.[24]

Other community factors that are less directly linked to substance use can also impact youth substance use. For example, communities with higher rates of mobility have been linked with higher rates of drug problems.[25] Extreme economic deprivation also can be a risk factor for later substance abuse problems, particularly when children in those communities experience both poverty and early behavioral problems.[25] Additionally, adolescents living in neighborhoods lacking organization, with less surveillance of public places, and fewer strong social institutions, also show increased rates of substance use.[26]

In the school domain, academic failure, as early as mid-elementary school, has been linked with increased risk of substance use and substance-related problems in adolescence.[27] Low commitment to school or having low expectations for achievement or finding school is unrewarding, are all associated with increased substance use.[28]

In the family domain, parental attitudes toward drug use are similarly predictive of later adolescent use. Adolescents are more likely to engage in substance use behavior when their parents have favorable or approving attitudes toward drug and alcohol use.[29,30] Parental history of drug or alcohol abuse also predicts adolescent substance use, and increases the likelihood that a teen will progress from experimentation with substances to more significant substance-related problems.[31,32] Also, coming from a family with a substance-abusing parent has been linked to dependence for a wide range of substances, with twin studies in which children separated at birth from substance-using parents show increased risk of problems, suggesting that there may be an underlying heritable, possibly genetic, component to substance use.[33–36] Family management problems, including poor supervision and monitoring, lack of clear behavioral expectations, and inconsistent or harsh punishment are associated with increased risk of adolescent substance abuse problems.[29,37,38] Additionally, adolescents raised in families with high levels of conflict are also more likely to use substances and later develop substance use problems.[39]

In the individual and peer domain, several constitutional factors have emerged as consistent predictors of later substance use. Individuals characterized as sensation seekers or risk takers, having low harm avoidance and higher impulsivity, are more likely to engage in substance use behaviors.[15,40] Similarly, adolescents who display more frequent and higher levels of childhood aggressive behavior, and antisocial behavior in early adolescence, are also more likely to engage in substance use behaviors.[22,41–43] Not surprisingly, having friends who engage in antisocial behavior, and being friends with peers who use substances, also predicts later substance use.[44,45] Rebelliousness has also been linked with regular cigarette and alcohol use, in addition to current use of marijuana.[46] An adolescent's own attitude toward alcohol and other drugs is also predictive of later drug use, with adolescents who view substance use more favorably being more likely to initiate substance use.[47] As in the case of many risky behaviors, the earlier an adolescent initiates use of substances, the more likely he or she is to develop substance abuse problems later in life.[48]

As can be seen in **Table 1**, risk factors for adolescent substance abuse also predict other adolescent problems. This implies that interventions that address risk factors for substance abuse will likely affect multiple problems.[19] In sum, "This commonality also suggests that preventive interventions that address precursors of multiple problems are an efficient approach."[13(p1654)]

### Risk Factors for Substance Use in Emerging Adulthood

Emerging adulthood (usually defined as the period from age 18 to age 25) is an important time in life because it sets the stage for later adult development.[49–52] Many researchers[52–55] have identified this stage as another key developmental time period characterized by rapid transitions in social context. This developmental period is

**Table 1**
Risk factors for adolescent and young adult problem behaviors

| Risk Factors | Adolescent Substance Use | Delinquency | Teen Pregnancy | School Dropout | Violence | Depression and Anxiety | Young Adult Substance Use |
|---|---|---|---|---|---|---|---|
| **Community** | | | | | | | |
| Availability of drugs | ✓ | — | — | — | ✓ | — | ✓ |
| Availability of firearms | — | ✓ | — | — | ✓ | — | — |
| Community laws and norms favorable to drug use, firearms, and crime | ✓ | ✓ | — | — | ✓ | — | ✓ |
| Media portrayal of violence | ✓ | — | — | — | ✓ | — | — |
| Low neighborhood attachment and community disorganization | ✓ | ✓ | — | — | ✓ | — | — |
| Extreme economic deprivation | ✓ | ✓ | ✓ | ✓ | ✓ | — | — |
| Transitions and mobility | ✓ | ✓ | — | ✓ | — | ✓ | — |
| **School** | | | | | | | |
| Academic failure beginning in late elementary school | ✓ | ✓ | ✓ | ✓ | ✓ | ✓ | ✓ |
| **Family** | | | | | | | |
| Family management problems | ✓ | ✓ | ✓ | ✓ | ✓ | ✓ | ✓ |
| Family conflict | ✓ | ✓ | ✓ | ✓ | ✓ | ✓ | ✓ |
| Favorable parental attitudes and involvement in the problem behavior | ✓ | ✓ | — | — | ✓ | — | ✓ |
| Family history of the problem behavior | ✓ | ✓ | ✓ | ✓ | ✓ | ✓ | ✓ |

| Individual/Peer | | | | | | |
|---|---|---|---|---|---|---|
| Early and persistent antisocial behavior | ✓ | ✓ | ✓ | ✓ | ✓ | ✓ |
| Alienation and rebelliousness | ✓ | ✓ | ✓ | ✓ | — | — |
| Favorable attitudes toward the problem behavior | ✓ | ✓ | ✓ | ✓ | — | ✓ |
| Early initiation of the problem behavior | ✓ | ✓ | ✓ | ✓ | — | ✓ |
| Individual/Peer | | | | | | |
| Friends who engage in the problem behavior | ✓ | ✓ | ✓ | ✓ | ✓ | ✓ |
| Constitutional factors | ✓ | ✓ | — | ✓ | ✓ | ✓ |
| Internalizing | — | — | — | — | — | ✓ |
| Adolescent substance use | — | — | — | — | — | ✓ |
| Not living with parents or spouse | — | — | — | — | — | ✓ |
| Being unmarried | — | — | — | — | — | — |
| College attendance | — | — | — | — | — | ✓ |
| Being unemployed | — | — | — | — | — | ✓ |

Adapted from Catalano RF, Haggerty KP, Hawkins JD, et al. Prevention of substance use and substance use disorders: the role of risk and protective factors. In: Kaminer Y, Winters KC, editors. Clinical manual of adolescent substance abuse treatment. Washington, DC: American Psychiatric Publishing; 2011. p. 30–1; with permission.

characterized by new social contexts that involve greater freedom and less social control than experienced during adolescence. Along with changing societal roles, there is a simultaneous weakening of societal safety net supports.[56] Among the transitions facing young adults, many have significant developmental impacts: they may leave home, exit the compulsory educational system, begin college, enter the workforce, and form families.[56] Navigating these transitions requires skills and resources that can be compromised by substance use.

Concurrent with this new found independence is an increase in rates of substance use and abuse, sexual risk behaviors, and the beginning of a decline from the peak of criminal involvement. Longitudinal data from the Monitoring the Future survey indicates that rates of heavy alcohol, marijuana, and daily smoking peak in the mid-20s and decline slowly thereafter.[56,57] Rates of abuse and dependence on alcohol and illicit drugs follow a similar trend.[3] Additionally, rates of driving under the influence peak during young adult years.[57] Increasing transitions that offer more freedom and less control, and the concomitant increase in substance use and misuse suggests that young adults may need additional supports. Further, there is a substantial portion of the population whose substance use persists or even escalates beyond the mid-20s.[58–61] Substance misuse, if sustained, progresses to dependence and contributes to failure to successfully adopt adult roles and responsibilities, as well as the emergence of other mental health problems.[62–66] Thus, understanding the risk and protective factors specific to young adults is critical as we seek to reduce the impact of substance-related problems.

Many predictors of young adult substance abuse are those already described during childhood and adolescence that persist as predictors; however, many are unique to the young adult period (see **Table 1**). Stone and colleagues[21] document the predictors of young adult substance use. During young adulthood, in the community domain, the availability of drugs, community laws and norms favorable to substance use, and lower income and parental education increased the risk for young adult substance use. Extreme economic deprivation during childhood also predicted young adult use. In the family domain, family history of substance use, family management problems, family conflict, and favorable parental attitudes toward substance use from childhood and adolescence predicted young adult substance abuse. For example, White and colleagues' study of risk factors in emerging adulthood found that good parental monitoring of behavior that occurred in high school continued to decrease risk for alcohol and marijuana use into young adulthood. This research suggests that not only can preventive family-based efforts produce positive outcomes for adolescents who are still in the home, but also these preventive interventions' effects have been found to persist into young adulthood.[67] Efforts to involve parents to assist adolescents in the transition to more independent living have also shown effects.[68] Family conflict during young adulthood also predicted young adult substance use. School failure at any age (during childhood, adolescence, or in young adulthood) is linked with increased substance use in young adulthood. However, lack of commitment to school specifically emerged as a predictor of young adult substance use only during adolescence. In the individual domain, antisocial behavior and favorable attitudes toward substance use at any age predicted young adult substance abuse. Constitutional factors and early initiation of substance use were predictors of young adult substance use from the childhood period only. Having friends who use substances (during adolescence and young adulthood) was predictive of young adult substance abuse.

In addition to these risk factors, there are several specific risk factors that have emerged as uniquely important in emerging adulthood. Living situation often changes when a young person reaches emerging adulthood. Although some young adults continue to live at home with parents while beginning college or starting their employment journey, many young people live away from their parents for the first time, either on a college campus or in housing on their own or with peers. Living situation has been found to be closely connected to substance use, with young adults living away from home experiencing significantly more substance use than young adults who continue to live with their parents.[69] This finding remains significant regardless of college attendance.[69]

Interestingly, although grades during high school are related to decreased rates of substance use in adolescence, these same high school grades are related to increased risk for substance use in emerging adulthood.[28,67] This could be because those with higher grades in high school are more likely to attend college and that aspects of the college environment encourage heavy drinking, and increase accessibility of alcohol.[70,71] White and colleagues[67] also found that although college attendance increased alcohol use for young adults overall, young adults attending college who still lived at home with parents experienced a smaller increase in alcohol use behaviors compared with those who did not live with their parents. Also, being unmarried[72] and being unemployed during emerging adulthood are both risk factors for young adult substance abuse. Being unemployed was also associated with greater risk for developing substance use disorders.[73,74]

## PROTECTIVE FACTORS FOR SUBSTANCE USE IN ADOLESCENCE AND EMERGING ADULTHOOD

Opportunities for prevention exist not only in programs that seek to decrease risk factors, but also in seeking to increase protective factors. Protective factors can directly lower the likelihood of substance use problems or mediate or moderate risk. During adolescence, in the community and school domains, opportunities for prosocial involvement, such as after-school clubs, youth organizations, and community events, act protectively against substance use, with adolescents experiencing less risk for substance use.[46] Similarly, recognition for involvement in prosocial activities at school is also protective against substance use behaviors.[46] At the family level, a similar trend emerges, where opportunities for prosocial involvement in the family, such as game nights and opportunities to help with chores, are similarly associated with fewer substance use behaviors, as is family recognition of prosocial involvement.[46] Resnick and colleagues[75] found adolescents with a higher sense of attachment or connection to their families also displayed lower rates of multiple problem behaviors, including substance use, sexual initiation, violence, and suicidal behaviors; the same was true for adolescents with a higher perception of attachment to their schools. Finally, at the individual level, Beyers and colleagues[46] found that higher religiosity, social skills, and healthy beliefs and clear standards were all protective factors for adolescent substance use. Healthy beliefs and clear standards were also protective for young adults. Considerably less is known about protective factors in young adulthood, as less research has explored protection for young adult substance abuse.

## EVIDENCE-BASED PREVENTION PROGRAMS WITH IMPACT ON SUBSTANCE USE
### Overview of Prevention Program Development

According to Mrazek and Haggerty,[76] prevention programs are typically developed through a series of stages in prevention science. The first stage, epidemiology studies, involves understanding the prevalence of problem behaviors or disease, along with the associated predictors of those problem behaviors or diseases. Developing theory that can explain how these predictors work together to cause negative health outcomes and behaviors is the next step. Once risk and protective factors have been identified, and theoretical explanations for how they work together have been established, prevention programs can be developed by constructing a logic model. Logic models should indicate which risk and protective factors will be addressed by the program, and the activities through which the intervention is expected to reduce risk and enhance protection. Promising targets for preventive interventions are those factors that predict multiple problems and/or those predictors that tend to cluster in individuals. The logic model should specify the changes expected, including short-term changes related to the intervention activities themselves (eg, improved parenting skills), intermediate-term outcomes on risk and protection (eg, reduction in family management problems and increases in family bonding), and long-term impacts on the problems targeted (eg, decreased initiation or substance misuse).

The next step is to develop the activities suggested by the logic model that may change the targeted risk and protective factors, and then conduct a pilot or feasibility trial of the intervention. After making the changes to the intervention suggested by the pilot study, efficacy trials can be developed in which the prevention intervention is tested through a controlled trial with either a quasi-experimental or experimental design. If the efficacy trial demonstrates that the prevention program has had the expected short-term, intermediate-term, and long-term impacts, an effectiveness trial should be conducted. Effectiveness trials are conducted to see if efficacious programs can still produce expected outcomes in real-world settings delivered outside of the controlled setting of the efficacy trial. This is necessary because experimental settings often fail to mimic real-world conditions, and before widespread dissemination, it is important to evaluate whether or not the prevention program continues to have positive effects in real-world settings. Finally, once effectiveness is demonstrated, diffusion trials can be conducted to address issues that arise in the implementation and dissemination of prevention programs at scale (eg, do they reach large proportions of the target population, are they delivered with fidelity to the intervention protocols, are they sustained).

### Key Factors in Developing and Implementing Prevention Interventions

When designing and developing a prevention intervention, several key factors must be considered. First, target risk factors should be identified. Second, a theory of behavior change should guide the development of the intervention (eg, Social Cognitive Theory,[77] the Social Development Strategy,[78] the Health Belief Model[79]). Third, a prevention intervention should occur before the initiation or escalation of problem behaviors.[80] Timing is essential in prevention research, as many substance use behaviors begin in early adolescence and peak in emerging adulthood, thus preventive efforts should begin before the onset of the targeted substance use behavior (initiation, regular use, abuse, and dependency).[80]

### Effective and Efficacious Prevention Programs

There have been many reviews of efficacy trials of prevention programs.[19] A relatively large number of prevention programs have demonstrated in controlled trials short-term and long-term impacts on preventing substance use. Several lists of efficacious prevention programs have been developed by government and nongovernmental bodies (Blueprints for Healthy Youth Development[81] National Registry of Evidence-based Programs and Practices,[82] Office of Juvenile Justice and Delinquency Prevention,[83] What Works Clearinghouse,[84] Centers for Disease Control and Prevention Community Guides,[85] Coalition for Evidence-Based Policy[86]). One of the most rigorous of these lists, Blueprints for Healthy Youth Development,[81] has been developed by the Center for the Study and Prevention of Violence. We have chosen to use this list to illustrate the types of efficacious prevention programs that have been trialed and have effects on substance use. This Web-based tool keeps a record of prevention programs that have been empirically supported, and rates them according to several criteria, including impact; evaluation quality; intervention specificity regarding target population; risk and protective factors identified and intervention activities; and whether the program has training, technical assistance, and cost information. It has 3 categories of programs: Promising, Model, and Model Plus. To meet the standards of a *Promising* program, interventions must show positive findings in at least 1 high-quality randomized controlled trial or 2 high-quality quasi-experimental trials. Promising programs must also identify the specific behavioral outcomes and associated risk factors, and be ready for dissemination with all of the necessary manuals, trainings, and other assistance needed to implement the program in a community. *Model* programs meet all of these criteria, but in addition have been tested in at least 2 randomized controlled trials. Finally, *Model Plus* programs meet all the forgoing criteria and have also been supported in an independent replication by someone who was not one of the program developers.

Table 2 shows the Blueprint programs demonstrating effectiveness at the Promising, Model, and Model Plus levels delivered in middle childhood, adolescence, and emerging adulthood, respectively. Prevention programs are typically delivered in 1 of 3 settings: school, family, and community. A brief overview of programs in these domains follows, with more complete program identification available in **Table 2**.

School-based programs are delivered any time from preschool (eg, Positive Action[87]) up through postsecondary education (eg, alcohol BASICS [Brief Alcohol Screening and Intervention for College Students] education[88]). School-based programs take many forms, but effective school-based programs typically incorporate one or several of the following elements: teacher instructional and classroom management skills; curricula that teaches social, emotional, and cognitive skills; and tutoring.[19] School-based programs can focus both on risk factors, such as academic failure, and protective factors, such as increasing student bonding or connectedness to the school, or increasing the availability of prosocial opportunities at the school. Life Skills Training[89] and Positive Action[87] are examples of Model Plus and Model school-based prevention programs.

Family-based programs throughout childhood and adolescence have been shown to reduce substance use in adolescence. Universal parenting programs focus on parenting skills during childhood and adolescence, including aspects such as establishing clear standards for behavior, family management skills, strategies for dealing with anger, and creating prosocial opportunities for children. Guiding Good Choices,[90,91] Familias Unidas,[92] and Strengthening Families 10-14[93,94] are examples of family-based programs that have demonstrated strong empirical findings. Some parenting programs work with families having more difficulties. Functional Family Therapy (FFT) is an indicated prevention program that works with families that have a delinquent adolescent at risk for institutionalization. Like universal parenting programs, FFT works on family communication and supportiveness and behavior management, but in addition works on decreasing intense negativity and dysfunctional patterns of family behavior.[95]

Community programs typically use prevention coalitions to implement community-level interventions and pursue policy changes that support reductions in substance use. Community-level interventions include such things as normative change campaigns[96] (eg, billboards stating the percentages of adolescents who do not use alcohol or drugs) and community mentoring programs, such as Big Brothers Big

**Table 2**
**Blueprints substance use prevention programs for adolescents and young adults**

| Program | Description | Rating | Impact | Benefits Minus Cost Per Individual |
|---|---|---|---|---|
| *School programs* | | | | |
| Raising Healthy Children | Universal prevention for ages 5–18 (family and school setting). Targeting classroom teachers, parents, and students to promote opportunities, skills, and recognition. Parent training and teacher training provided, focusing on classroom management. | Promising | Academic performance, alcohol, antisocial aggressive behavior, illicit drug use, prosocial with peers. | N/A |
| EFFEKT | Universal prevention for ages 12–14 (family, school, and community setting). Targets parental attitudes about child alcohol use through information disseminated at meetings, through parent letters, and advertisement of healthy activities for children. | Promising | Alcohol, delinquency and criminal behavior. | N/A |
| Positive Family Support-Family Check-Up | Universal, selective, and indicated prevention for ages 12–14 (family, school setting). Six-week school curriculum addressing universal prevention, creation of a Family Resource Center teaching parenting behaviors and family management skills, and a family checkup with a trained therapist. | Promising | Alcohol, depression, sexual risk behaviors, tobacco. | ($251) |
| Positive Action | Universal prevention for ages 5–14 (school setting). Schoolwide program that includes climate change, curriculum lessons 2–4 times a week in grades K–8 focused on socioemotional development and reinforcement of positive actions. | Model | Academic performance, alcohol, anxiety, bullying, delinquency and criminal behavior, depression, emotional regulation, prosocial behavior, illicit drug use, sexual risk behaviors, tobacco, truancy, school attendance, violence. | $8583 |

| Program | Description | Classification | Outcomes | Cost |
|---|---|---|---|---|
| Achievement Mentoring— Middle School | Selective prevention for ages 12–14 (school setting); 2-y program in which teens meet in small groups and systematically work through behavior change through feedback, incentives, and a points-based program. | Promising | Academic performance, delinquency and criminal behavior, employment, illicit drug use, truancy, school attendance. | $4333 |
| Life Skills Training (LST) | Universal prevention for ages 12–18 (school setting). LST is a 3-y program delivered in middle school, focusing on decision making, goal setting, anger management, stress reduction, communication, peer pressure, and consequences of drug use. | Model Plus | Alcohol, delinquency and criminal behavior, illicit drug use, sexual risk behaviors, STIs, tobacco, violence. | $1199 |
| Project Northland | Universal prevention for ages 12–18 (school setting); 6-y intervention delivered in middle and high school, involving classroom curricula, peer leadership, youth-driven extracurricular activities, parent involvement programs, and community activism. | Promising | Alcohol. | $188 |
| Project Toward No Drug Abuse | Universal and selective prevention for ages 15–18 (school setting). Twelve 40-min sessions delivered in school over 3 wk focusing on communication, resource acquisition, and decision-making strategies. | Model | Alcohol, illicit drug use, tobacco, violent victimization. | $431 |
| Athletes Training and Learning to Avoid Steroids (ATLAS) | Universal prevention for young men ages 15–18 (school setting); 14-session program delivered to male athletes in high school about the dangers of steroids and other drug use, strength training, and sports nutrition. | Promising | Alcohol, illicit drug use, physical health and well-being. | N/A |
| SPORT Prevention Plus Wellness | Universal prevention for ages 15–18 (school setting). Health promotion program for high school adolescents to improve their physical fitness, nutrition, body image, and sleep habits, and avoid drug use, involving a health behavior screen, a one-on-one consultation, and a take-home fitness prescription. | Promising | Alcohol, illicit drug use, physical health and well-being, tobacco. | $1309 |

(continued on next page)

**Table 2**
*(continued)*

| Program | Description | Rating | Impact | Benefits Minus Cost Per Individual |
|---|---|---|---|---|
| Blues Program (Cognitive-Behavioral Group Depression Prevention) | Selective and indicated prevention program for ages 15–18 (school setting). Six, weekly 1-h groups delivered to high school students with depression, focusing on cognitive restructuring techniques and coping skills. | Model | Depression, illicit drug use. | ($126) |
| Brief Alcohol Screening and Intervention for College Students (BASICS) | Selected and indicated prevention for college students (school setting). A brief, motivational, cognitive-behavioral training delivered in schools as a selective and indicated prevention for alcohol-use problems. This program works with high-risk college students to enhance motivation to change, promote healthier choices, and teaches coping skills to moderate drinking behaviors. | Model | Alcohol use. | $1853 |
| InShape Prevention Plus Wellness | Universal prevention for college students (school setting). Cognitive-behavioral training delivered in school, aimed at improving physical, mental, and spiritual well-being through positive health habits. | Promising | Alcohol use, illicit drug use. | ($359) |
| *Family programs* | | | | |
| Guiding Good Choices | Universal prevention for ages 12–14 (family, school, community setting). Parenting program delivered over 5 sessions, focusing on family management strategies, adolescent refusal skills, coping with conflict, and prosocial family involvement. | Promising | Alcohol, delinquency and criminal behavior, depression, illicit drug use. | $981 |
| Strengthening Families 10–14 | Universal prevention for ages 12–14 (family, community, school setting). Seven-session program to enhance family protection and resiliency involving parent-child skill building, conflict resolution, communication, and activities to increase family cohesiveness and positive involvement of the child. | Promising | Alcohol, antisocial aggressive behavior, close relationships with parents, illicit drug use, internalizing, tobacco. | $2893 |

| Program | Description | Rating | Outcomes | Cost |
|---|---|---|---|---|
| Treatment Foster Care Oregon | Indicated prevention for ages 12–18 (family setting). Intensive in-home treatment for antisocial adolescents involving supervision, clear limits/consequences, positive reinforcement, an adult mentor, and daily/weekly family support. | Model | Delinquency and criminal behavior, illicit drug use, teen pregnancy, tobacco, violence. | $9126 |
| Functional Family Therapy (FFT) | Indicated prevention for ages 12–18 (family setting). FFT offers short-term, intensive therapeutic family services for 3 mo, focusing on supervision, discipline, and emotional support. | Model | Delinquency and criminal behavior, illicit drug use. | $26,973 |
| Familias Unidas Preventive Intervention | Selective prevention for Hispanic or Latino youth age 12–18 (family setting). Helps immigrant parents build a strong parent support network and learn culturally relevant parenting skills. | Promising | Externalizing, illicit drug use, sexual risk behaviors. | N/A |
| Multisystemic Therapy | Indicated prevention for ages 12–18 (family and community setting). Intensive family-based and community-based treatment that addresses serious antisocial behavior in juvenile offenders over 3–5 mo of treatment. | Model Plus | Close relationships with parents, delinquency and criminal behavior, illicit drug use, internalizing, mental health, prosocial behavior, violence. | $15,611 |
| Community programs | | | | |
| PROSPER (Promoting School-Community-University Partnerships to Enhance Resilience) | Universal prevention for ages 12–14 (school, community settings). Delivery system to foster implementation of evidence-based youth and family interventions, complete ongoing needs assessments, monitor implementation, and evaluate outcomes. | Promising | Alcohol, close relationships with parents, delinquency and criminal behavior, illicit drug use, tobacco. | N/A |
| Communities That Care | Universal prevention for infants through early adults (community setting). An encompassing community approach that selects and uses effective prevention programs that are individually tailored to the risk and protection factors unique to that community. | Promising | Alcohol use, delinquency and criminal behavior, tobacco use, and violence. | $1188 |

(continued on next page)

**Table 2**
*(continued)*

| Program | Description | Rating | Impact | Benefits Minus Cost Per Individual |
|---|---|---|---|---|
| Big Brothers Big Sisters of America | Selective prevention for ages 5–18 (community setting). Program matching adult mentors with an at-risk child to develop a caring and supportive relationship over 12 mo. | Promising | Alcohol, antisocial aggressive behavior, close relationships with parents, close relationships with peers, illicit drug use, prosocial behavior, truancy and school attendance. | N/A |
| Keep Safe | Selective prevention for ages 12–14 (community setting). Six-session group-based intervention for the foster-care youth and a 6-session, group-based intervention for the foster parents, focusing on goal setting, positive relationships, decision making, stability at home, and behavioral reinforcement techniques. | Promising | Illicit drug use, prosocial behavior, sexual risk behaviors, tobacco. | N/A |

N/A, not applicable; STI, sexually transmitted infections.

*Adapted from* University of Colorado Boulder Institute of Behavioral Science, Center for the Study and Prevention of Violence. Blueprints for Healthy Youth Development. Available at: http://www.blueprintsprograms.com/programs. Accessed July 25, 2015; with permission.

Sisters.[97,98] Communities That Care[99] is an example of a tested, effective community-level strategic approach to creating prevention infrastructure by building community coalition capacity to assess and prioritize risk, protection, and problems among their youth through school surveys; choosing effective prevention programs that match their priorities; and implementing chosen programs with fidelity. Communities That Care also provides tools for ongoing evaluation of the programs' effectiveness so that communities can track progress and make adjustments when needed, and explores funding mechanisms to sustain prevention efforts. In a randomized trial, researchers found that communities using the approach were able to reduce alcohol and tobacco use by approximately a third and delinquency by 25%.[100,101] Results have been largely replicated in a quasi-experimental statewide study in Pennsylvania.[102]

### Challenges in Prevention

Unfortunately, and too often, American society's response to major problems has been reactive. Such responses have evolved out of understandable efforts to deal with problems once they have emerged. The systems to deliver treatment interventions are quite developed for most of the common and costly substance use and allied psychological disorders once these problems have developed. Each year, more than 6 million young people receive treatment for mental, emotional, or behavioral problems. The financial costs of treatment services and lost productivity attributed to the related behavioral health problems of depression, conduct disorder, and substance abuse are estimated at $247 billion per year.[16] These costs are for a system that reaches only a small portion of those in need of treatment. Although treatment of existing problems is a critical service, evidence from more than 40 years of research suggests that we can prevent substance abuse and other problems from developing in the first place, and that disseminating proven prevention programs is likely to have substantial impact on rates of disorder and related harm. Given the number of tested, effective prevention programs, a population-wide reduction in substance use and negative consequences of substance use is possible. A recent discussion paper[103] published by the National Academy of Medicine suggested the following.

> Universal prevention has the potential to reach those who are not directly involved in the formal health and social service delivery sectors. Simultaneously ensuring that preventive interventions reach the highest-risk children and youth, who will benefit disproportionately from these efforts, will promote health equity. Preventing problems before they occur reduces human suffering and preempts costly punitive responses to these problems from education, law enforcement, child welfare, mental health, or juvenile justice systems. It is imperative that strategies to bring preventive interventions to scale pursue these dual objectives of overall population health and health equity for the most vulnerable and underserved populations (p. 10).

The challenge is how to get prevention programs widely implemented in communities. Despite the promise, a number of challenges arise in scaling up proven prevention programs. Given that services are organized and delivered by separate organizations (health care, public health, education, substance abuse, mental health, juvenile justice, and child welfare), community prevention coalitions are needed to bring together professionals, information, and funding to create teamwork and cooperation across different community sectors. Additionally, communities are different from one another, and it is unlikely that any one approach will provide the largest impact across communities.

To pick the best prevention programs for a given community, data need to be collected identifying the risk and protective factors of greatest importance to the youth living in each community. Because multiple risk factors for adolescent substance use and other problems have been identified in multiple socialization domains, there is need for efficient measurement. Researchers are now able to evaluate the presence of multiple risk factors with succinct questionnaires that produce valid and reliable results.[13] Such comprehensive surveys can be used to prioritize those risk factors that are most elevated or depressed and protective factors that are most depressed. Finally, evidence-based prevention programs will need sustainable funding, meaning cooperation across multiple agencies. Resnick and colleagues[104] suggest moving 10% of the total funds dedicated to children to efficacious prevention programs and policies.

## FUTURE DIRECTIONS FOR PREVENTION SCIENCE

Much progress has been completed in recent decades to improve the evidence base of prevention programs for substance use, including the identification and measurement of risk and protective factors, the development and testing of prevention programs, and recent work on testing prevention infrastructure. There is much work still to be done. Service systems addressing substance use focus mainly on intervention once substance use has become a problem; there are few resources dedicated to community-wide prevention programs, despite the growing support for these programs. To increase prevention funding, government officials, professionals, and the public should be educated about the evidence and cost effectiveness of prevention programs. Databases (such as the Blueprints database) should be expanded to include as many tested, effective prevention programs and policies as possible; consolidating research in easy-to-use tools can enhance the public's ability to choose efficacious programs when seeking to address substance use problems locally. Also, studies addressing the implementation and dissemination challenges of prevention programs would help to inform researchers and community organizers about the challenges of going to scale and creating sustainable change. Similarly, translational research on adaptation to unique needs of underserved or marginalized populations would significantly augment the research base and assist with promoting health equity.[102] Although research has demonstrated that risk factors are often common across national and racial boundaries, adaptations in program curriculum may assist with better fit and acceptability by different cultures; this could increase the cultural competence of prevention interventions and simultaneously expand intervention reach and impact. The development and growth of prevention coalitions may be an ideal place to further prevention science, as they offer local, place-specific knowledge that can enhance intervention effectiveness.[105] Finally, efforts to develop more prevention interventions specific to emerging adulthood should be pursued. Presently, Blueprints cites only 2 interventions that have demonstrated adequate empirical effectiveness on substance use for this population.[81] Given that substance use and its related problems peak during this time period,[56,57] additional prevention programs targeting young adult outcomes should be prioritized.

We end with a quote from a commentary from the National Academy of Medicine: "Prevention is the best investment we can make in behavioral health—and the time to make it is now."[103(p20)]

## REFERENCES

1. Holmbeck GN. A developmental perspective on adolescent health and illness: an introduction to the special issues. J Pediatr Psychol 2002;27(5):409–16.

2. Feldman SS, Elliott GR. At the threshold: the developing adolescent. Cambridge (MA): Harvard University Press; 1990.

3. Valencia LS, Cromer BA. Sexual activity and other high-risk behaviors in adolescents with chronic illness: a review. J Pediatr Adolesc Gynecol 2000;13(2): 53–64.

4. White AM. Understanding adolescent brain development and its implications for the clinician. Adolesc Med 2009;20(1):73–90.

5. Jessor R. Risk behavior in adolescence: a psychosocial framework for understanding and action. J Adolesc Health 1991;12(8):597–605.

6. Patton GC, Coffey C, Sawyer SM, et al. Global patterns of mortality in young people: a systematic analysis of population health data. Lancet 2009; 374(9693):881–92.

7. Steinberg LD. Age of opportunity: lessons from the new science of adolescence. Boston: Houghton Mifflin Harcourt; 2014.

8. Snow WH, Gilchrist LD, Schinke SP. A critique of progress in adolescent smoking prevention. Child Youth Serv Rev 1985;7(1):1–19.

9. Flay BR, Brannon BR, Johnson CA, et al. The television school and family smoking prevention and cessation project. I. Theoretical basis and program development. Prev Med 1988;17(5):585–607.

10. Ennett ST, Tobler NS, Ringwalt CL, et al. How effective is drug abuse resistance education? A meta-analysis of project DARE outcome evaluations. Am J Public Health 1994;84(9):1394–401.

11. Thomas BH, Mitchell A, Devlin MC, et al. Small group sex education at school: the McMaster Teen Program. In: Miller BC, Card JJ, Paikoff RL, et al, editors. Preventing adolescent pregnancy: model programs and evaluations. Sage focus editions, vol. 140. Thousand Oaks (CA): Sage; 1992. p. 28–52.

12. Ellickson PL, Bell RM. Drug prevention in junior high: a multi-site longitudinal test. Science 1990;247(4948):1299–305.

13. Catalano RF, Fagan AA, Gavin LE, et al. Worldwide application of prevention science in adolescent health. Lancet 2012;379(9826):1653–64.

14. Coie JD, Watt NF, West SG, et al. The science of prevention: a conceptual framework and some directions for a national research program. Am Psychol 1993; 48(10):1013–22.

15. Hawkins JD, Catalano RF, Miller JY. Risk and protective factors for alcohol and other drug problems in adolescence and early adulthood: implications for substance abuse prevention. Psychol Bull 1992;112(1):64–105.

16. O'Connell ME, Boat T, Warner KE, editors. Preventing mental, emotional, and behavioral disorders among young people: progress and possibilities. Washington, DC: National Academies Press; 2009.

17. Fergusson DM, Horwood LJ. Resilience to childhood adversity: results of a 21 year study. In: Luthar SS, editor. Resilience and vulnerability: adaptation in the context of childhood adversities. New York: Cambridge University Press; 2003. p. 130–55.

18. Rose G. Sick individuals and sick populations. Int J Epidemiol 2001;30(3): 427–32.

19. Catalano RF, Haggerty KP, Hawkins JD, et al. Prevention of substance use and substance use disorders: the role of risk and protective factors. In: Kaminer Y, Winters KC, editors. Clinical manual of adolescent substance abuse treatment. Washington, DC: American Psychiatric Publishing; 2011. p. 25–63.

20. Glaser RR, Horn MLV, Arthur MW, et al. Measurement properties of the Communities That Care® Youth Survey across demographic groups. J Quant Criminol 2005;21(1):73–102.

21. Stone AL, Becker LG, Huber AM, et al. Review of risk and protective factors of substance use and problem use in emerging adulthood. Addict Behav 2012; 37(7):747–75.

22. Duncan SC, Duncan TE, Strycker LA. A multilevel analysis of neighborhood context and youth alcohol and drug problems. Prev Sci 2002;3(2):125–33.

23. Maddahian E, Newcomb MD, Bentler PM. Risk factors for substance use: ethnic differences among adolescents. J Subst Abuse 1988;1(1):11–23.

24. Wills TA, Sargent JD, Gibbons FX, et al. Movie exposure to alcohol cues and adolescent alcohol problems: a longitudinal analysis in a national sample. Psychol Addict Behav 2009;23(1):23–35.

25. Sampson RJ, Lauritsen JL. Violent victimization and offending: individual, situational, and community level risk factors. In: Reiss Albert J Jr, Roth JA, editors. Understanding and preventing violence: vol. 3. Social influences. Washington, DC: National Academy Press; 1994. p. 1–114.

26. Elliott DS, Wilson WJ, Huizinga D, et al. The effects of neighborhood disadvantage on adolescent development. J Res Crime Delinq 1996;33(4):389–426.

27. Najaka SS, Gottfredson DC, Wilson DB. A meta-analytic inquiry into the relationship between selected risk factors and problem behavior. Prev Sci 2001;2(4): 257–71.

28. Kosterman R, Hawkins JD, Guo J, et al. The dynamics of alcohol and marijuana initiation: patterns and predictors of first use in adolescence. Am J Public Health 2000;90(3):360–6.

29. Peterson PL, Hawkins JD, Abbott RD, et al. Disentangling the effects of parental drinking, family management, and parental alcohol norms on current drinking by black and white adolescents. J Res Adolesc 1994;4(2):203–27.

30. Barnes GM, Welte JW. Patterns and predictors of alcohol use among 7-12th grade students in New York State. J Stud Alcohol 1986;47(1):53–62.

31. Haggerty KP, Skinner ML, MacKenzie EP, et al. A randomized trial of Parents Who Care: effects on key outcomes at 24-month follow-up. Prev Sci 2007; 8(4):249–60.

32. Pagan JL, Rose RJ, Viken RJ, et al. Genetic and environmental influences on stages of alcohol use across adolescence and into young adulthood. Behav Genet 2006;36(4):483–97.

33. Bierut LJ, Dinwiddie SH, Begleiter H, et al. Familial transmission of substance dependence: alcohol, marijuana, cocaine, and habitual smoking: a report from the Collaborative Study on the Genetics of Alcoholism. Arch Gen Psychiatry 1998;55(11):982–8.

34. Kendler KS, Prescott CA, Myers J, et al. The structure of genetic and environmental risk factors for common psychiatric and substance use disorders in men and women. Arch Gen Psychiatry 2003;60(9):929–37.

35. Agrawal A, Lynskey MT. The genetic epidemiology of cannabis use, abuse and dependence. Addiction 2006;101(6):801–12.

36. McGue M, Elkins I, Iacono WG. Genetic and environmental influences on adolescent substance use and abuse. Am J Med Genet 2000;96(5):671–7.

37. Brewer DD, Hawkins JD, Catalano RF, et al. Preventing serious, violent, and chronic juvenile offending: a review of evaluations of selected strategies in childhood, adolescence, and the community. In: Howell JC, Krisberg B, Hawkins JD,

et al, editors. A sourcebook: serious, violent, and chronic juvenile offenders. Thousand Oaks (CA): Sage; 1995. p. 61–141.

38. Patterson GR, Dishion TJ. Contributions of families and peers to delinquency. Criminology 1985;23(1):63–79.
39. Maggs JL, Patrick ME, Feinstein L. Childhood and adolescent predictors of alcohol use and problems in adolescence and adulthood in the National Child Development Study. Addiction 2008;103(Suppl 1):7–22.
40. King KM, Chassin L. Adolescent stressors, psychopathology, and young adult substance dependence: a prospective study. J Stud Alcohol Drugs 2008; 69(5):629–38.
41. Englund MM, Egeland B, Oliva EM, et al. Childhood and adolescent predictors of heavy drinking and alcohol use disorders in early adulthood: a longitudinal developmental analysis. Addiction 2008;103(Suppl 1):23–35.
42. Sher KJ, Walitzer KS, Wood PK, et al. Characteristics of children of alcoholics: putative risk factors, substance use and abuse, and psychopathology. J Abnorm Psychol 1991;100(4):427–48.
43. Zucker RA. Anticipating problem alcohol use developmentally from childhood into middle adulthood: what have we learned? Addiction 2008;103(Suppl 1): 100–8.
44. Elliott DS, Huizinga D, Ageton SS. Explaining delinquency and drug use. Beverly Hills (CA): Sage; 1985.
45. Oxford ML, Harachi TW, Catalano RF, et al. Preadolescent predictors of substance initiation: a test of both the direct and mediated effect of family social control factors on deviant peer associations and substance initiation. Am J Drug Alcohol Abuse 2001;27(4):599.
46. Beyers JM, Toumbourou JW, Catalano RF, et al. A cross-national comparison of risk and protective factors for adolescent substance use: the United States and Australia. J Adolesc Health 2004;35(1):3–16.
47. Arthur MW, Hawkins JD, Pollard JA, et al. Measuring risk and protective factors for substance use, delinquency, and other adolescent problem behaviors: The Communities That Care Youth Survey. Eval Rev 2002;26(6):575–601.
48. Robins LN, Przybeck TR. Age of onset of drug use as a factor in drug and other disorders. In: Jones CL, Battjes RJ, editors. Etiology of drug abuse: implications for prevention (NIDA Research Monograph No. 56). Rockville (MD): National Institute on Drug Abuse; 1985. p. 178–92.
49. Arnett JJ. Emerging adulthood. A theory of development from the late teens through the twenties. Am Psychol 2000;55(5):469–80.
50. George LK. Sociological perspectives on life transitions. Annu Rev Sociol 1993; 19:353–73.
51. Hogan DP, Astone NM. The transition to adulthood. Annu Rev Sociol 1986;12: 109–30.
52. Shanahan MJ. Pathways to adulthood in changing societies: variability and mechanisms in life course perspective. Annu Rev Sociol 2000;26:667–92.
53. Osgood DW. On your own without a net: the transition to adulthood for vulnerable populations. Chicago: University of Chicago Press; 2005.
54. Schulenberg JE, Maggs JL. A developmental perspective on alcohol use and heavy drinking during adolescence and the transition to young adulthood. J Stud Alcohol 2002;Suppl 14:54–70.
55. Schulenberg JE, Sameroff AJ, Cicchetti D. The transition to adulthood as a critical juncture in the course of psychopathology and mental health. Dev Psychopathol 2004;16(4):799–806.

56. Park MJ, Mulye TP, Adams SH, et al. The health status of young adults in the United States. J Adolesc Health 2006;39(3):305–17.

57. Substance Abuse and Mental Health Services Administration. Results from the 2012 National Survey on Drug Use and Health: summary of national findings, NSDUH series H-46, HHS publication No. (SMA) 13–4795. Rockville (MD): Substance Abuse and Mental Health Services Administration; 2013.

58. National Institute on Alcohol Abuse and Alcoholism. Five year strategic plan fy07-11. Bethesda (MD): National Institute on Alcohol Abuse and Alcoholism; 2006.

59. Prejean J, Song R, An Q, et al. Subpopulation estimates from the HIV incidence surveillance system–United States, 2006. MMWR Morb Mortal Wkly Rep 2008; 57(36):985–9.

60. Johnston LD, O'Malley PM, Bachman JG, et al. Monitoring the Future national survey results on drug use, 1975-2007. Volume II: college students and adults age 19–50 (NICH Publication No. 09-7403). Bethesda (MD): National Institute on Drug Abuse; 2009.

61. Jackson KM, Sher KJ, Schulenberg JE. Conjoint developmental trajectories of young adult alcohol and tobacco use. J Abnorm Psychol 2005;114(4):612–26.

62. Gmel G, Rehm J, Room R, et al. Dimensions of alcohol-related social and health consequences in survey research. J Subst Abuse 2000;12(1–2):113–38.

63. Hingson R, Winter M. Epidemiology and consequences of drinking and driving. Alcohol Res Health 2003;27(1):63–78.

64. Leonard KE, Roberts LJ. Alcohol in the early years of marriage. Alcohol Health Res World 1996;20(3):192–6.

65. Roman PM, Johnson JA. Alcohol's role in work-force entry and retirement. Alcohol Health Res World 1996;20(3):162–9.

66. Quigley LA, Marlatt GA. Drinking among young adults: prevalence, patterns, and consequences. Alcohol Health Res World 1996;20(3):185–91.

67. White HR, McMorris BJ, Catalano RF, et al. Increases in alcohol and marijuana use during the transition out of high school into emerging adulthood: the effects of leaving home, going to college, and high school protective factors. J Stud Alcohol 2006;67(6):810–22.

68. Ichiyama MA, Fairlie AM, Wood MD, et al. A randomized trial of a parent-based intervention on drinking behavior among incoming college freshmen. J Stud Alcohol Drugs 2009;16(16):67–76.

69. Mason WA, Kosterman R, Haggerty KP, et al. Gender moderation and social developmental mediation of the effect of a family-focused substance use preventive intervention on young adult alcohol abuse. Addict Behav 2009; 34(6–7):599–605.

70. Presley CA, Meilman PW, Leichliter JS. College factors that influence drinking. J Stud Alcohol 2002;Suppl 14:82–90.

71. White HR, Jackson K. Social and psychological influences on emerging adult drinking behavior. Alcohol Res Health 2004/2005;28(4):182–90.

72. Duncan GJ, Wilkerson B, England P. Cleaning up their act: the effects of marriage and cohabitation on licit and illicit drug use. Demography 2006;43(4): 691–710.

73. Oesterle S, Hill KG, Hawkins JD, et al. Positive functioning and alcohol-use disorders from adolescence to young adulthood. J Stud Alcohol Drugs 2008;69(1): 100–11.

74. Casswell S, Pledger M, Hooper R. Socioeconomic status and drinking patterns in young adults. Addiction 2003;98(5):601–10.

75. Resnick MD, Bearman PS, Blum RW, et al. Protecting adolescents from harm. Findings from the National Longitudinal Study on Adolescent Health. JAMA 1997;278(10):823–32.
76. Mrazek PJ, Haggerty RJ, Committee on Prevention of Mental Disorders, Institute of Medicine, editors. Reducing risks for mental disorders: frontiers for prevention intervention research. Washington, DC: National Academy Press; 1994.
77. Bandura A. Social foundations of thought and action: a social cognitive theory. Englewood Cliffs (NJ): Prentice-Hall; 1986.
78. Hawkins JD. Science, social work, prevention: finding the intersections. Soc Work Res 2006;30(3):137–52.
79. Becker MH. The health belief model and personal health behavior. Thorofare (NJ): C.B. Slack; 1974.
80. McGorry PD, Purcell R, Goldstone S, et al. Age of onset and timing of treatment for mental and substance use disorders: implications for preventive intervention strategies and models of care. Curr Opin Psychiatry 2011;24(4):301–6.
81. Center for the Study and Prevention of Violence. Blueprints for Healthy Youth Development. 2015. Available at: http://www.blueprintsprograms.com/. Accessed August 3, 2015.
82. SAHMSA. NREPP: SAHMSA's National Registry of Evidence-Based Programs and Practices. 2015. Available at: http://www.nrepp.samhsa.gov/. Accessed August 23, 2015.
83. Office of Juvenile Justice and Delinquency Prevention. Model programs guide. Available at: http://www.ojjdp.gov/mpg/. Accessed August 23, 2015.
84. Institute of Education Sciences. What works clearinghouse. Available at: http://ies.ed.gov/ncee/wwc/. Accessed August 23, 2015.
85. Centers for Disease Control and Prevention. The guide to community preventive services: The Community Guide: what works to promote health. 2015. Available at: http://www.thecommunityguide.org/. Accessed August 23, 2015.
86. Coalition for Evidence-Based Policy. Coalition for Evidence-Based Policy. 2015. Available at: http://coalition4evidence.org/. Accessed August 23, 2015.
87. Flay B, Allred C, Ordway N. Effects of the Positive Action program on achievement and discipline: two matched-control comparisons. Prev Sci 2001;2(2): 71–89.
88. Dimeff LA. Brief Alcohol Screening and Intervention for College Students (BASICS): a harm reduction approach. New York: Guilford Press; 1999.
89. Botvin G, Griffin K. Life Skills Training: empirical findings and future directions. J Prim Prev 2004;25(2):211–32.
90. Park J, Kosterman R, Hawkins JD, et al. Effects of the "Preparing for the Drug Free Years" curriculum on growth in alcohol use and risk for alcohol use in early adolescence. Prev Sci 2000;1(3):125–38.
91. Mason WA, Kosterman R, Hawkins JD, et al. Reducing adolescents' growth in substance use and delinquency: randomized trial effects of a preventive parent-training intervention. Prev Sci 2003;4(3):203–312.
92. Prado G, Pantin H, Briones E, et al. A randomized controlled trial of a parent-centered intervention in preventing substance use and HIV risk behaviors in Hispanic adolescents. J Consult Clin Psychol 2007;75(6):914–26.
93. Kumpfer KL, Whiteside HO, Greene JA, et al. Effectiveness outcomes of four age versions of the Strengthening Families Program in statewide field sites. Group Dyn 2010;14(3):211–29.

94. Spoth R, Redmond C, Shin C, et al. Substance-use outcomes at 18 months past baseline: the PROSPER Community-University Partnership Trial. Am J Prev Med 2007;32(5):395–402.
95. Barton C, Alexander J, Waldron H, et al. Generalizing treatment effects of Functional Family Therapy: three replications. Am J Fam Ther 1985;13(3):16–26.
96. Wechsler H, Nelson TE, Lee JE, et al. Perception and reality: a national evaluation of social norms marketing interventions to reduce college students' heavy alcohol use. J Stud Alcohol 2003;64(4):484–94.
97. Tierney JP, Grossman JB, Resch NL. Making a difference: an impact study of Big Brothers Big Sisters. Philadelphia: Public/Private Ventures; 1995.
98. Herrera C, Grossman JB, Kauh TJ, et al. Mentoring in schools: an impact study of Big Brothers Big Sisters school-based mentoring. Child Dev 2011;82(1): 346–61.
99. Hawkins JD, Catalano RF Jr. Communities That Care: action for drug abuse prevention. 1st edition. San Francisco (CA): Jossey-Bass; 1992.
100. Hawkins JD, Oesterle S, Brown EC, et al. Results of a type 2 translational research trial to prevent adolescent drug use and delinquency: a test of Communities That Care. Arch Pediatr Adolesc Med 2009;163(9):789–98.
101. Hawkins JD, Oesterle S, Brown EC, et al. Youth problem behaviors 8 years after implementing the Communities That Care prevention system. A community-randomized trial. JAMA Pediatr 2014;168(2):122–9.
102. Feinberg ME, Jones D, Greenberg MT, et al. Effects of the Communities That Care model in Pennsylvania on change in adolescent risk and problem behaviors. Prev Sci 2010;11(2):163–71.
103. Hawkins JD, Jenson JM, Catalano R, et al. Unleashing the power of prevention (Discussion Paper). Washington, DC: Institute of Medicine and National Research Council; 2015. Available at: http://nam.edu/wp-content/uploads/2015/06/DPPowerofPrevention.pdf.
104. Resnick MD, Catalano RF, Sawyer SM, et al. Seizing the opportunities of adolescent health. Lancet 2012;379(9826):1564–7.
105. Fagan AA, Hawkins JD, Catalano RF. Engaging communities to prevent underage drinking. Alcohol Res Health 2011;34(2):167–74.

# Assessment and Treatment of Adolescent Substance Use Disorders: Alcohol Use Disorders

Cecilia Patricia Margret, MD, PhD, MPH[a],*, Richard K. Ries, MD[b]

## KEYWORDS

- Adolescence • Binge use • Screening • Interventions • Pharmacotherapy
- Prevention • Biomarkers • Continuum of care

## KEY POINTS

- The article discusses the current prevalence of alcohol use disorder among youth and its biopsychosocial correlates that modify the prevalence and natural progression.
- Clinical aspects of care are discussed to provide care teams with a knowledge basis of validated tools and treatment choices relevant for treating alcohol use disorders among youth.
- With the recent changes in DSM nosology, we discuss the importance of diagnostic considerations for alcohol use disorders.
- Clinical aspects such as confidentiality, differential levels of care, and criteria for best fitting treatments are discussed.

## INTRODUCTION

Alcohol drinking during the adolescence is a serious public health concern due to the significant risk of life-changing tragic consequences.[1] Adolescence is a dynamic phase of development when biopsychosocial factors shape an individual's potential into adulthood.[2] This transitional phase of impulsivity and novelty seeking is also known for its indulgence in risk taking.[3] Exposure to alcohol and drugs in this critical window, akin to kindling a fire, can soon derail into a lifetime of hazardous consequences and substance use problems.[4–6] Evidence shows that adolescents are at risk for drinking heavily starting as early as eighth grade, resulting in a high number of accidents, homicides, high-risk sexual behaviors, and changes in the brain[7] that predispose them to further substance use and psychiatric disorders.[8–10] Early alcohol use in the adolescent

[a] Department of Psychiatry and Behavioral Sciences, University of Washington, Seattle Children's Hospital, 4575 Sand Point Way Northeast, Suite 105, Seattle, WA 98105, USA; [b] Department of Psychiatry and Behavioral Sciences, Harborview Medical Center, University of Washington, 401 Broadway, 1st floor, Seattle, WA 98104, USA
* Corresponding author.
E-mail addresses: cecilia.margret@seattlechildrens.org; cmargret@uw.edu

Child Adolesc Psychiatric Clin N Am 25 (2016) 411–430
http://dx.doi.org/10.1016/j.chc.2016.03.008
1056-4993/16/$ – see front matter © 2016 Elsevier Inc. All rights reserved.

years quadruples the chance for substance use disorder than later use by college years,[11] highlighting the risks associated with early use. Recognizing these dangers related to problematic alcohol use by adolescents, the US surgeon general announced in 2007 a "Call to Action" to address the problem and develop appropriate interventions.[1] Over the last decade, since the call to action, researchers have identified several dimensions from developmental frameworks, from gene assays to gene–environmental interactions, that inform our understanding of underage drinking and unique treatment needs.[12] In this review, we focus on recent clinical advances to help providers understand and address alcohol use disorder among adolescents and children confidently using available tools.

We review the following:

i. Epidemiology of alcohol use and misuse among children and adolescents, studied by nationwide surveys monitoring this trend for decades,
ii. Risks that trigger onset and modify the course of problematic drinking,
iii. Common clinical considerations contingent on point of care sites, and
iv. The evidence-based screening tools and interventional modalities that are available.

## EPIDEMIOLOGY
### Prevalence

Alcohol is the most common drug used among youth under 17 years.[13] Based on recent national survey, the Monitoring The Future (MTF) series, 2 of every 3 students drink alcohol to varying degrees by 12th grade and 1 in 3 students report drinking by 8th grade.[13] Epidemiologic studies consistently show that adolescents have a higher tendency to engage in heavy drinking or bingeing when compared with adults.[13,14] Binge drinking is defined as consuming approximately 5 or more drinks in 2 hours. Heavy drinking is 5 drinks a day for at least 5 days.[14] According to nationwide survey of youth between 12 and 17 years, 23% (8.7 million) drink alcohol, 14% binge, and 3% report heavy drinking.[14,15] Both binge and heavy drinking are problematic trends among adolescents due to increased risk for hazardous injuries, suicides, poisoning, homicides,[8] and neuronal damages[16] which can result in death or a lifetime of disability.

Heavy drinking worsens with age. The MTF survey shows that 5% of 8th graders, 11% of 10th graders, and 17% of 12th graders[13] report heavy drinking when stratified by class. A study that explored high school seniors' drinking trend from the MTF series showed that some 12th grade students reported consuming 10 to 15 alcohol drinks in rapid succession, which can dramatically increase their risk for impairment.[17] A critical study by Donovan[18] in 2009 showed that bingeing on 5 drinks by adolescents resulted in blood alcohol concentrations that were 2 to 3 times the adult levels when drinking the same amount of alcohol. This finding highlighted how alcohol was metabolized differentially by adolescents when compared with adults. It also suggested the reclassifying of binge drinking for adolescents to 3 drinks at any given time, because the blood alcohol concentration varied based on age.[18]

Behavioral and genetic studies show that age at first drink bears the greatest risk and prognosis for later alcoholism.[19,20] Hingson & White[12] described that drinking before 14 years of age results in a 2-fold hazard risk for alcohol use problems within 10 years, independent of one's familial history, illicit drug use, depression, and disruptive behaviors. Early onset of drinking is a valid predictor of lifetime alcohol use and drug use disorders as evidenced by longitudinal studies showing strong association with heavy consumption, severe dependence, increased comorbidities, and familial history of problematic use of alcohol.[11,21]

Patrick and Schulenburg[17] observed few gender differences for underage drinking in youth under 17 years of age in general. Racial trends demonstrate that non-Hispanic white youth are the highest users of alcohol by high school, followed by Hispanic and African- American youth.[17]

The good news is that alcohol consumption by adolescence has declined to an all-time low since the 1970s. These changes are thought to be connected to zero tolerance laws, enforcing the legal drinking age, and changes in social perceptions, although they are not limited to these factors. The bad news is that harmful patterns of underage drinking continue to be associated with biopsychosocial consequences in adolescents, foreshadowing heavy use in adulthood.[22–24]

## Risk Factors

The explanatory model for alcohol use disorder is a complex interplay of biopsychosocial factors as noted by extensive evidence from twin, adoption, and family studies.[25] Understanding the risks in the natural trajectory of alcohol use among adolescents is pertinent for its prevention and appropriate interventions.

### Biological substrates

**Neurobiological substrate** The developing brain of an adolescent is vulnerable to detrimental effects from alcohol as it is to other licit and illicit drugs.[3,26,27] This is discussed in detail elsewhere in this issue (See Sharma A and Morrow JD: Neurobiology of Adolescent Substance Use Disorders).

**Temperament risks** Temperamental traits such as disinhibition and negative affectivity are known to be associated with problematic alcohol use.[28] Disinhibition is a strong predictor of early onset of alcohol use as early as 14 years[29,30]; negative affectivity as a causal agent remains inconclusive.[28] However, social anxiety and avoidant coping styles associated with negative affective states are strong correlates for alcohol use in adolescence.[31]

**Genetic factors** Fifty to seventy percent of alcohol use disorders in adults have been found to be the result of an inherited trait,[32–35] with replication to some extent among adolescents.[36] Genetic studies have evaluated candidate genes and their phenotypic characteristics that predispose alcohol use among adolescence. Research on genetic polymorphisms of several genes are underway, including but not limited to dopamine receptor gene (DRD4), serotonin transporter gene (5-HTTPLR), Mu-opioid receptor gene (OPRM1), aldehyde dehydrogenase (ALDH 2), and gamma amino butyric acid receptor (GABRA2), which show strong linkage with alcohol use among adolescents.[37] Interestingly, these candidate genes are also linked to impulsivity and anxiety, which also place the youth with these traits more vulnerable to problematic use.[38,39] Understanding these genetic influences that influence drinking behaviors is an evolving field[40] that may have implications for developing interventions specific to genotypes.

**Gene–environmental interactions** Current evidence from etiologic studies show that drinking initiation is shaped by environmental influences like peer use, siblings, or parenting styles, whereas persistent drinking patterns in adolescence and young adulthood are dictated by underlying genetic signatures.[34,36,41] Longitudinal findings from twin and adoption studies indicate that young children, who are genetically vulnerable, selectively interact with environmental factors, such as drinking with peers, and thereby increase their access to alcohol and their risk of developing alcohol use disorders.[36,42] Specifically, young adults with polymorphic changes to their DRD4 allele (known for alcohol use susceptibility) when choosing to drink with deviant peers, increase their chances for problematic use of alcohol in adulthood.[39] These findings that show the interplay of gene and environment variably modulate the development of alcohol use disorder. Understanding gene–host interactions promises the development of unique interventions specific to genotypic signatures that can alter the course of alcohol use progression from youth to adulthood.

### Psychiatric disorders and drug use related comorbidities
The literature shows strong evidence for the association of psychiatric morbidity and alcohol use among adolescents, with the onset of psychiatric disorders usually preceding alcohol problems chronologically.[43,44] Studies have observed consistently that depression, trauma,[45] low self-esteem,[17] conduct problems, and anxiety are robust predictors of problematic alcohol use[44,46] among adolescents. Temporally, psychiatric morbidity predisposes the individual to the development of early alcohol use and progression to misuse.[43] With regard to conduct disorders, the severity and age of onset of conduct problems are strongly linked to early onset of alcohol use among boys and girls, with some differential sensitivity based on racial groups. African American adolescents report less alcohol use than the majority population but they appear to be more vulnerable to this linear relationship between conduct disorder and alcohol use. The causes of these different racial findings are not clear.[28]

The use of drugs and other illicit substances along with alcohol is strongly associated with concurrent use in adolescence. Twin studies show that drugs and alcohol are mediated by common genetic influence[47] with a heritable factor close to 48% among adolescents.[48]

### Environmental influences
Environment usually dictates the first use and exposure to alcohol.[36] The factors discussed herein modify risks embedded with early alcohol use and its long-term consequences are stable across generation and demographics.

**Alcohol expectancies**  Social learning theory shows that having positive expectations from alcohol use by parents and peers tends to increase alcohol's appeal and use. Alcohol expectancies influence impressionable minds of children and adolescents and predict both initiation and use of alcohol.[28,49,50] Recently, social media[51] is also an added influence to promoting both positive and negative perceptions and expectation for alcohol among teens. Understanding the combined and individual impact of family, peers, media and social media on problematic drinking-related attitudes and behaviors among teens will help to develop preventive interventions that can modulate risks.

**Influence of peer and family**  Peer connectivity and development of self-identity independent of family norms are developmental landmarks for adolescents that tend to play significant roles in influencing alcohol use. Deviant peer influences, modeling, and perceived overestimation of peer drinking are influential pathways for adolescent drinking behaviors.[28] Moving away from family beliefs and traditions to secure one's identity is normative; on the other hand, discordant familial relationships, inconsistent parenting, less restrictive and supervised settings, strained communication between parent and child, and parental alcohol use[28,52–54] are known to significantly predispose adolescents toward alcohol use disorders.

Familial history of alcohol disorders, especially parents with active alcohol use disorders, increase the chances from 4 to 10 times for their children to develop alcohol-related problems.[1] These risks are thought to be mediated by means of having easy access to alcohol, normalized drinking behaviors at home, gaining positive expectancies to drinking by parental modeling, and last, learned temperamental characteristics from parents.[1]

**Influence of school and work** Studies have shown that good academic standing, educational expectations, and school bonding are protective of alcohol use among youth.[17] However, students working in part-time jobs displacing normative participation in school are noted to overuse alcohol, which results in increased school failure,[55] a trend commonly seen among Caucasians and Asian American youth.

**Influence of religion and sports** Individual affiliation with religious institutions or social trusts and high religiosity and social responsibility play strong protective influence to alcohol use, as does playing team sports.[17,56,57]

### Developmental determinants

The developmental processes of adolescence, including pubertal and brain changes, peer and family influences, and social role transitions, underlie the evolution of risky behaviors like drug use. Studies describe identity development, desire for autonomy, and peer pressure as modifiable risk factors underlying initiation and problematic use of alcohol.[58] Treatment planning and prevention approaches that use developmental framework are recommended to be more meaningful and effective.[59]

## CLINICAL CONSIDERATIONS

In this section, we consider some clinical presentations related to alcohol use in children and adolescents, across different clinical settings.

### Primary Care

Alcohol and drug use among adolescents starts often as an exploratory experience that burgeons into significant behavioral or social problems, and usually follows a deceptively insidious course. Hence the common clinical presentations related to alcohol use are nonspecific issues and must be recognized as the "tip of the iceberg" that need further probe or referral as per intensity of problem. The primary care provider is an accessible point of care and approachable for youth, relative to other systems of care.[10,60,61] Hence, building capacity within the primary care provider's office for early screening and brief intervention is increasingly recognized as an effective interventional point of care.[10,60] Medically toxic states like alcohol tolerance, or alcohol-related medical comorbidities such as pancreatitis and liver dysfunction, are less common among children and adolescents, during primary care provider visits, because of more episodic than heavy regular use pattern in adults. Common symptoms related to alcohol use encountered in primary care are:

- Increased irritability, exacerbating mood, anxiety, and attention deficit hyperactivity disorder/attention deficit disorder;
- Poor academic performance, school avoidance, and absences;
- Changes in peer connectivity, anhedonia; and isolative tendencies;
- Family conflicts, running away from home, and abuse/trauma;
- Accidents and injuries, suicidal, or homicidal attempts;
- Disruptive, oppositionality, conduct and delinquent behaviors, and legal involvements;
- Unprotected sex, unintended pregnancy, and sexually transmitted disease(s);
- Chronic pain, gastrointestinal disturbances, and changes in eating and sleeping patterns;

- Slurred speech, memory impairments, and poor coordination; and
- Comorbid other substance use (prescriptive and nonprescription).

Stigma related to substance use disorders and psychiatric morbidity often precludes self-referral to addiction treatment specialist, which is why the recommendation for screening and brief intervention within primary care is emphasized.

### Critical Care Issues

#### Overdosing

Adolescent alcohol and drug use has led to an estimated cost burden of US$24 billion per year,[28] specific to death and emergency room visits. The Drug Abuse Warning Network report from 2010 shows 45% of annual emergency room visits by youth 20 years and younger is related to drug misuse, of which one-third is solely due to alcohol use.[9] Alcohol overdose or poisoning presents as stupor, coma, confusion or seizures, respiratory depression, and hypothermia warranting immediate attention. Research shows that underage drinkers tend to drink more than adults, overshooting blood alcohol concentrations beyond safety limits that result in overdoses.[18] Alcohol intoxication can be easily fatal because alcohol often potentiates the toxicity of other drugs, even in small doses.[62,63]

#### Impaired decision making

The Centers for Disease Control and Prevention have warned that youth are more vulnerable for death from alcohol related impaired driving at all blood alcohol concentrations than the older or general population. Alcohol use results in poor decision making, driving without seatbelts, and/or riding with other intoxicated drivers. Impaired driving is a serious risk that warrants immediate intervention. Parents should be counseled to give clear guidance on driving expectations including refraining from driving after drinking any amount of alcohol, to draw up a driving contract, take the adolescents' car keys when found to be drinking or violating the contract, and/or to consider having the adolescent referred for alcohol and drug assessment and treatment when drinking or drug use is suspected.[10] Alcohol-related impaired judgment also increases risks for sexual victimization, aggression, and unprotected sex resulting in unintended teen pregnancies and sexually transmitted diseases. Adolescents should be counseled on these health risks as well and how to prevent them and seek help when needed.

### Psychiatric Care

Alcohol use with comorbid psychiatric disorder is not an exception but the norm. Outpatient psychiatric care providers should be aware of worsening cognitive, behavioral, mood, and anxiety symptoms with the concurrent substance use. Careful elucidation of psychiatric symptom evolution with onset of substance use helps in the differential diagnosis. Screening and treatment planning must always prioritize safety planning for suicide, homicide, and high-risk behaviors, given the alcohol-related propensity for suicides[28] and injuries. Trauma, either as physical or sexual abuse, is highly correlated with alcohol use, both as a precedent to and as consequence of drinking.[64]

### Inpatient Care

Hospitalizations related to alcohol use are commonly associated with alcohol overdose, suicide, and alcohol-related injury. Inpatient survey from 1999 to 2008 shows that alcohol related overdoses are increasing for youth in age groups less than 17 and 18 to 24 years.[63] This highlights need for robust interventions for youth with problematic alcohol use and comorbid drug use problems that often trigger suicidal behaviors. Inpatient treatment serves as a safe place for treatment of alcohol withdrawal or intoxication syndromes and for observation of alcohol-induced mood and anxiety symptoms to help clarify diagnoses and help with further treatment planning.

## SCREENING AND ASSESSMENT
### Screening Tools

Early screening and detection of underage drinking is critical, given the life-threatening and pervasive risks on behavior and health. It is important to differentiate between experimental use which is alcohol or drug use by an adolescent 3 times or less compared to the next level, regular use which in adolescents quickly progresses to problematic use and dependence.[65] The recognition of underage drinking as a serious public health problem with health risks was first called to light in 2007[1] by a US Surgeon General who promoted study of several effective screening tools and interventions, a few which are discussed herein. Currently, despite mixed evidence on universal screening in primary care by from the US Preventive Services Task Force, the majority of the nationwide medical associations lean toward universal screening and brief interventions in primary care or any point of care medical system owing to the low cost and low risks. In this article, we discuss the prominent screening tools that validated for use in youth, to sensitively identify alcohol use in various clinical settings.

The National Institute of Abuse, Alcohol and Alcoholism in collaboration with the American Academy of Pediatrics[10] recommend an empirically derived 2 age-specific questions for screening alcohol use of patient and their peers to strongly predict alcohol misuse in youth under the age of 18. Based on number of drinks consumed, risk is stratified across ages 9 to 11, 12 to 15, and 16 to 18 for respective treatment interventions. For example, any drink for ages less than 11 years is considered high risk and brief motivational interviewing and referral to specialist are indicated. This screening modality has the advantage of being short and is quick to administer orally in a primary care setting with high success rates with motivational interviewing and referral-based stepped care.

Screening tools that specifically elicit alcohol misuse are as follows: the Adolescent Drinking Inventory, a 24 item that elicits bio-psychosocial profile and lack of control specific to alcohol; the Rutgers Alcohol Problem Index, which emphasizes functional domains affected by alcohol use; and the Adolescent Obsessive-Compulsive Disorder Scale, which explores alcohol use and compulsive drinking behaviors.

CRAAFT is a mnemonic scale that screens for alcohol and drugs. It is quick to administer or self-administered easily to elicit problems related to substance use and validated for use in adolescents. The Alcohol Use Disorders Identification Test (AUDIT), is a 10-item survey developed by the World health Organization, with a shorter version (AUDIT-C), for use in primary care. CRAAFT, AUDIT, and Problem Oriented Screening Instrument for Teenagers (POSIT), another screening survey, identify related problems and are highly validated for use among adolescents.[66,67] CAGEAID is a questionnaire that consists of 4 questions jointly used for alcohol and drugs, with 1 or more being positive warranting more probe. It is validated for use in primary care for adolescents over 16 years of age.

### Biomarkers
Biomarkers may one day serve as an adjunct to screening or self-report within appropriate confidentiality limits, but at this time they are unreliable as gold standards.

Breath alcohol tests, primarily used by law enforcement, are a noninvasive proxy for blood alcohol concentration, but is unreliable for clinical use or interpreting neurologic impairments.[68] Blood alcohol concentration is a reliable indicator when taken within 2 to 12 hours after use, showing good correlation with impairment and is used in emergency situations to assess for tolerance and morbidity levels. Blood alcohol concentrations in adolescent drinkers peak and double to 3 times the adult safety limits when adolescent drinkers consume heavily (5 drinks at 1 time), indicating a greater sensitivity to alcohol owing to underlying vulnerable physiology. A urine test, to date, is the most standardized, cost-effective, and noninvasive test to detect alcohol use within 7 to 12 hours of use. The initiation point-of-care test as a preliminary step is the qualitative immunoassay followed by quantitative assay for confirmation. Urine tests are used widely to screen, attenuate use, detect combinatorial drugs in toxindromes, monitor outcomes in treatment, and in conjunction with self-report to validate sensitivity. However, universal institution of this test, especially in school or medical visits, is limited owing to lack of sensitivity, confidentiality concerns, and threats to therapeutic relationship when the willingness to engage is replaced with coercion. Systemic biomarkers like liver function assays, mean corpuscular volume, and carbohydrate deficient transferrin are indirect alcohol markers, specific for chronic and heavy use among adults, with limited use in adolescent drinkers. For more precise estimates, detection of downstream metabolites like ethyl glucuronide and ethyl sulfate within 80 hours after consumptions, fatty acid ethyl esters up to 7 to 10 days in hair and skin cells, or phosphatidylethanol up to 4 days are sensitive, specifically to monitor abstinence and hold potential.[68,69]

Saliva, sweat, and hair samples are used to detect alcohol and hold promise with the caveat that they remain less standardized and more expensive to use. Neuroscience research[28,70] demonstrates electrophysiologic markers that can identify adolescent drug use and relate risk taking impulsivity as changes in electroencephalographic waveforms and event related potentials like P300 (event-related potential elicited in the process of decision making that has reduced amplitude). These electrophysiological events are correlates of phenotypical characteristics and hold potential to serve as biomarkers for externalizing and drinking problems.

Overall, these biomarkers are of limited use among adolescents because they lack sensitivities or standardization for use in a cost-effective manner, with clinical correlates and hence the search for an ideal biomarker continues. Trait markers such a disinhibition, impulsivity, novelty seeking, and electrophysiologic and radioimaging abnormalities that underlie these phenotypes have potential to serve as biomarkers to predict use patterns, but are still under study.[71]

### Assessment

Assessment helps to define the full scope of the problem with details of alcohol-related damage, functional impairment, strengths and weaknesses, and environmental context to inform a current state and coherent treatment plan in partnership with patient. Contingent on the goal of evaluation, a comprehensive assessment tool is chosen for research and or clinical quest. The Diagnostic Interview for Children and Adolescent–Revised, Diagnostic Interview Schedule for Children-IV, Adolescent Diagnostic Interview (Adolescent Drinking Inventory), and Customary Drinking and Drug Use Record are among the prominent scales related to the *Diagnostic and Statistical Manual of Mental Disorders* (DSM)-4 classification, to name a few. The scope of this article limits elaborate discussion of tools, which are discussed in detail by Winters[65] and Kaminer[72] for reference, because their relevance to the DSM-5 remains to be validated.

Clinically, a detailed psychiatric interview with patient is by far the most practical means to estimate accurately the burden of use and dysfunction. Self reports from children and adolescents would best be augmented with family and school reports report of behavior change. While adolescents have the ability to be as reliable as adults in reporting their use, they are likely to have limited insight into the cause and effect of their actions. This reinforces the need to have input from the adolescent's community which could include family, school, and collated information from other systems of care like diversion courts to build a broad construct for diagnosis and consideration of treatment. The American Society of Addiction Medicine suggests the use of a biopsychosocial template, which could be used as an assessment tool with its 6 dimensional aspects to assess: (1) acute intoxication, (2) biomedical, (3) emotional, (4) readiness to change, (5) relapse, and (6) recovery,[73] with the goal of repeat assessment and treatment planning to determine scope of service (outpatient vs residential services).

*Diagnostic nosology*
Because we have transitioned to the DSM-5 and base clinical diagnosis on this nosology, it is pertinent to understand the benefits and challenges. The current category for disorder integrates alcohol abuse and dependence disorders into a single disorder with a dimensional concept of severity contingent on symptoms accrued across 12 months. Craving has been added as a criterion and legal problem(s) is eliminated. Whether the new dimensional frame improves diagnosis and informs treatment decisions more among adolescents, remains to be studied. The combined nosology has already identified some critical considerations for adolescents. Winters and Kaminer postulate false positivity as a problem given the low threshold that the DSM-5 holds for diagnosing substance use disorders and the difficulty in elaborating terms such as hazardous use, withdrawal, and tolerance among adolescents. Alternatively this may be helpful in better early identification of adolescents at risk of a substance use disorder who are in need of early intervention treatment in contrast to the traditional adult model where prevention and early intervention are not options and the focus is on identifying those with a high burden of disease.[6]

**Confidentiality** Confidentiality is an important factor to be considered in the evaluation of adolescent alcohol use and problematic drinking behaviors. As per federal laws, adolescents are protected by their right to privacy of their disclosures related to substance use and treatments.[74] Clinical providers are encouraged to approach adolescents with thorough knowledge on confidentiality and limits to the same, before approaching adolescents on screening and introducing interventions to alcohol- and or drug-related use. Safety concerns are prime limits to confidentiality; however, adolescents are known to engage more successfully when they are well-supported by their parents and hence must be carefully explored.[75] As good clinical practice, obtaining consent to treatment and release of information with discussion of benefits versus risks of information sharing is considered important in the treatment of adolescents with substance use problems.

## SUMMARY OF CLINICAL MANAGEMENT
*Psychotherapy*

Methodological studies[76] indicate robust evidence for cognitive–behavioral therapy, family-based therapy, and brief motivational interventions with equivocal evidence for 1 method over the other. For the scope of this review, therapeutic approaches that are effective (large to medium effect size noted) in targeting adolescent substance use in general with consideration to alcohol use disorder[77] are discussed briefly, to enhance use of these tools as per indication in an integrative fashion.

### Brief motivational interviewing

Brief motivational interviewing has the best evidence track record with success among youth; it approaches effectiveness through Rogerian principles of empathy and nonjudgmental support. Used often in emergency services and in primary care practice to promote change and engage patient motivation with need for follow-up, which is critical for sustained effect. The effectiveness is known to be greatest in brief point of care situations, which are more likely in acute care with effective focus on harm reduction related to drunken driving, drinking and sexual high-risk behaviors, injuries, and so on. Its use is limited in severe substance use disorders population.[66,72,78]

### Twelve steps

Twelve step programs uses the Alcoholic Anonymous principles of helping those who wish to stop drinking as a community. The effectiveness is predictably related to cost effectiveness, social support for relapse prevention with recovery focus-based spiritual reflection, cohesive network with peers who are struggling, in a time that offsets environmental cues and provision of a 24/7 sponsor to personalize the 12 steps concepts. Empirical evidence indicates that 12 step programs for youth have been successful independently in achieving the goals of sustained abstinence and lowering relapse. Challenges to some extent may be a limited availability of age-matched groups, a nonprofessional community based-approach with extended time commitment, spiritual focus, and a limited understanding of the principles for effectiveness, which is under study.[72,74,79,80] Overall, when combined or used independently, 12 step programs have a strong advantage for sustaining abstinence.

### Cognitive–behavioral therapy

Cognitive–behavioral therapy uses operant and classical conditioning principles. Targets are triggers for use, misuse, and relapse, with promotion of skill-based learning through homework and modeling with use of social learning principles. Treatment effectiveness is based on self-efficacy, but has yet to show success among youth, but has some progress when combined with motivational interviewing. Used often in an integrated approach with other supplemental modalities to help achieve goal. Cognitive–behavioral therapy has been integrated with 12 steps and aftercare (relapse prevention strategies) and are noted to be more effective.[77]

### Family therapy

Family-based therapy is by far the best validated approach among youth using substances, its effectiveness stemming from an ecological standpoint and targeting the parent–child relationship, discipline, and parental substance use disorders. Multidimensional family therapy, a form of family therapy that has blended cognitive–behavioral therapy and multisystemic attributes, focuses on host and systems involved. It has high rank as an effective therapy for alcohol use disorder among youth with parenting practice as a mediator on influence, as noted in recent methodological review.[77,81,82] Brief strategic family therapy, a variant of family therapy that focuses on decreasing negative behaviors and with a prime focus on Hispanic community youth, has also been shown to be an effective approach, signifying the need to incorporate culturally appropriate family therapy strategies.[72,78] It is also known to be effective for most of the population with disadvantageous background and severity of misuse.

*Integrated care and other therapies*

A few other modalities that have also been found to be effective in outpatient care are integrated family and cognitive–behavioral therapy, behavioral treatment, and triple modality social learning, to name a few. Contingency management that uses the operant principle of positive reinforcement like rewards for abstinence (drug-free urine) has been effective when incorporated into behavioral programs.

In the inpatient population, residents have more severe use patterns, comorbid psychiatric problems with systemic problems within school, authority, law, and family disruptions that demands a unique blend of therapeutics for rehabilitation. The Training of Intervention Procedure manual talks about using the community as teacher and therapist, and a highly structured milieu as scaffolding for self-reliance, which is self-evolved and mutually modeled by peers/staff by social learning.[74] The targets are abstinence, removal from toxic milieu and repair if feasible, coping skills, and/or vocational rehabilitation for self-efficacy. Often, group and individual sessions are held, with deviant peer influences in group addressed by use of behavioral contract, contingency management, and recruitment of a diverse mix of youth.[72] Individually, self-image, sexuality, and guilt are key developmental themes that are known to benefit.

Youth with alcohol use disorder and substance use disorders in juvenile systems often benefit from diversion program that incorporate multisystemic therapy mandated by court with close monitoring and consideration of therapeutic community or reintegration into society.[74]

*Relapse prevention*

Finally, with more evidence in favor of neural basis of alcohol addiction and its chronic course, we know that relapse is common and calls for booster and aftercare planning, beyond the initial abstinence. This follow-up is critical for both outpatient and intensive residential treatments to sustain high yield and long-term remission.[72] A review[77] of effective therapies showed significant reduction of effect size at the 12-month follow-up, indicating a strong need for continuity of care, especially among adolescents when developmental vulnerabilities are dictating a natural progression of illness after initial insults. Basic strategies embedded for effective relapse preventions are cue recognition and avoidance, skills to promote assertive skills and cognitive restructuring from past experiences, in conjunction with medications that modulate neuronal excitability.[83]

*Pharmacotherapy*

---

The pharmacotherapy of alcohol use disorders is a less travelled path for adolescents, unlike the aggressive options available for adult population owing to the (i) differential patterns of use including binge drinking patterns that offset withdrawal or dependence states, (ii) emergence of disordered drinking in later adolescence or young adulthood, (iii) developing brain systems, and (iv) limited research on safety and efficacy of drug trials among adolescents.[84,85] However, medications are still considered pertinent because of alcohol-related plasticity on reward function, frontal lobe–related inhibition, and a limbic system that succumbs easily to cues and results in relapse.[86] Medication precludes toxic states like withdrawal and detoxification, reduces craving, prevents relapse, and manages comorbid psychiatric and medical problems, which tend to perpetuate chronic alcohol use.[86,87] The use of medications among adolescents is a judicious call, with caution to not replicate use on the basis of treating adolescents like "miniature adults." This section focuses on the principles of pharmacotherapy for addiction-related events, but not treatment of comorbid psychiatric disorders.

### Alcohol withdrawal and detoxification

Withdrawal is estimated at a very low prevalence[88] among adolescents, an event that occurs commonly among chronic users of alcohol. Withdrawal from a central nervous system depressant like alcohol causes both rebound hyperactivity of glutamate and gamma aminobutyric acid deficit states that can trigger a spectrum of symptoms, from physical discomfort to life-threatening seizures. Further, heavy binge drinking leading to greater hangover or withdrawal worsens neurocognitive abilities,[7,73,89] which results in poorer executive function, learning, and memory skills. Given the acute and chronic impact of alcohol use, acute withdrawal states warrant early treatment, just like in adults. Benzodiazepines, especially the long-acting types (diazepam), calm the withdrawal from alcohol, and nutritional and electrolytic rehabilitation is required for stabilization. Owing to abuse potential, lethality of withdrawal states and cross-tolerance with alcohol, toxic withdrawal is often managed in an inpatient setting.[87] Due to its limited occurrence in adolescents, extensive studies on safe use and limits of medications or interventions are limited. Other agents that are often considered, as alternatives, for uncomplicated withdrawal management are beta blockers like propranolol, clonidine, baclofen, and topiramate.

### Pharmacologic agents for medication-assisted addiction treatment

Understanding alcohol's influence on neural receptors and mechanisms of excitability or reinforcement of use has lent to the evolution of receptor-specific agents that are antagonistic in action and reduce relapse or craving. Incidentally, when alcohol was found to operate through endogenous opioids as its reinforcement pathway[90] from an animal study, naltrexone became (approved by the US Food and Drug Administration) an effective agent to significantly reduce relapse of alcohol use. Along the same lines, nalmefene (an opiate receptor) that has reduced impact on liver, unlike naltrexone, acamprosate (glutamate and $N$-methyl-D-aspartate receptor and dopamine pathway), baclofen (gamma aminobutyric acid), quetiapine (Seroquel; AstraZeneca, Westborough, MA; Dopamine), ondansetron (5-hydroxytryptamine−3, serotonin receptor), and topiramate (glutamate activist) are all receptor specific agents that are known to work in combination with naltrexone[86,91,92] or as standalone[86] agents to reduce alcohol craving among adults. Their use in relapse prevention and modulating chronic alcohol use is known to be effective in adolescents,[78] but there is a need for more controlled studies; their overall use in adolescents is limited.[87]

### Aversive therapy

An aversive agent interrupts the metabolism of a psychoactive substance causing unpleasant somatic symptoms that negatively reinforce the drinking or use of the psychoactive drug. Disulfiram, a classical aversive agent that is used in adults, inhibits metabolism of alcohol and accumulation of acetaldehyde resulting in physical discomfort such as nausea, flushing, and chest pain. This effect lasts for 2 weeks from its last intake by the patient, effectively averting from alcohol use. The use of disulfiram, despite its positive impact, among adolescents,[93] is limited in practice owing to the poor motivation to abstain and avoidance to experience discomfort. Further, the involvement of family and potential medical supervision challenges confidentiality, yet another deal breaker for treatment engagement among adolescents and like all treatment that fails without a collaborative approach this is another pertinent example.

### Treatment of comorbid conditions

Substance use among the adolescent population confers in itself a high risk for psychiatric comorbidities, such as conduct/disruptive problems, anxiety, and mood disorders compared with those who do not use drugs or alcohol.[94] Further, the study of lifetime occurrence of comorbidities among adolescents has shown that alcohol use usually follows the onset of psychiatric morbidity and in turn psychiatric morbidity sets the stage for earlier onset of alcohol use.[43] Further studies of natural progression have shown that cooccurring alcohol and psychiatric disorders among adolescence predicted long-term substance use disorder and increased incidences of borderline and antisocial personality disorders by young adulthood,[95] to name a few perpetuating influences on the morbid trajectory. These studies implicate the strong need to consider aggressive management of cooccurring disorders because they tend to have a bidirectional impact on the onset and chronic course of each disorder. Current evidence for treating comorbid conditions during active use of psychoactive substance is exploratory; however, given the comorbid burden of illness, it is important to include a detailed evaluation of predisposition, natural course of disorders, complicating factors of treatment, and plan toward an integrated care approach to treat the different entities.[78,96] Typically, due to the overlapping influence of alcohol on mood and anxiety symptoms, a brief remission is often recommended (abstinence from drugs and alcohol for 1 month) to delineate psychiatric symptoms for treatment. However, in practical translation of care, this is challenging to achieve unless done in a restrictive setting. The details of pharmacotherapy agents used are beyond the scope of this article and will be discussed in the October 2016 issue of this journal. However, it is pertinent to know that agents that are cross-tolerant with alcohol like benzodiazepines, and stimulants that are easily diverted or lend to abuse potential with history of alcohol use and hence are discouraged in concomitant treatment. In the past decade, studies have trialed the combination approach of psychopharmacological agents such as selective serotonin reuptake inhibitors (eg, fluoxetine), selective norepinephrine reuptake inhibitors (eg, atomoxetine), bupropion, or extended-release methylphenidate and lithium for cooccurring disorders of depression,[96] attention deficit hyperactivity disorder,[87,97,98] and mood disorders,[99] respectively, to treat psychiatric disorders and the ongoing active substance use. Results have shown that concurrent treatment is safe, but overall less impressive on substance use with no strong evidence for medication. Limiting the studies are usually the use of integrated approaches like cognitive–behavioral therapy or therapy that produces mixed results, with a need for robust evidence.[96] For example, an open trial of fluoxetine in adolescents with depression with cooccurring chronic depression and substance use disorders showed some promise,[100] whereas the impact of cognitive–behavioral therapy and fluoxetine as a combined approach among adolescents with major depressive disorder, substance use disorders, and chronic depression were less impressionable (effect size 0.78)[96] with mixed efficacy pointing to more benefits related to cognitive–behavioral therapy.

Current recommendations emphasize an integrated approach of therapy, rehabilitation, and medications to promote abstinence and abet cooccurring disorders in combination rather than a sequential approach during this critical period of develoment.[72,78]

## Levels of Care

Treatment of problematic alcohol use is a continuum of care, contingent on the following:

   i. Pattern of use;
  ii. Concurrent medical and psychiatric problems;
 iii. Coping skills;

iv. Interpersonal function; and
v. Support of environment.

Outpatient services vary from partial hospitalization, intensive outpatient therapy involving 9 to 20 hours per week for adults and 6 to 20 hours per week for adolescents, and plain outpatient support counseling contingent on the extent of the problematic use of alcohol and associated risks.[74] Adolescents with severe patterns of use, comorbidities, and triggers that threaten safety need the support of residential treatment (short term [<30 days] or long term [>30 days]). Detoxification and management of toxic state are often dealt in concurrently operated medical setting.

### Prevention

Given the mediation of environment in the initiation of adolescent onset of alcohol use, the role of prevention plays a significant role in impacting the overall trajectory of alcohol use. Universal and secondary prevention at school and primary care have been the most trialed areas to date. School-based programs like the Life Skills Program, Unplugged, and Good Behaviors Programs, which emphasize value of social skills and moral order are successful and carry much promise for wider implementation.[101] Nonschool universal interventions are yet to be robust in their impact.[102] The MTF Study showed that public policies such as public service advertising campaigns against drunk driving, increasing the minimum age for drinking, and awareness of designated drivers showed increased perceived risks of drinking effectively.[13,103,104] Media exposure is linked to moderate significance with alcohol use, with maximum impact on tobacco use.[105] Public health awareness and regulation of media content have shown implications in impacting the impressionable developing minds. In an overview, universal prevention focusing on environmental factors have held much promise whereas the host-related selective prevention approaches are variable and yet robust in impact. In conclusion, the problem of underage drinking is a serious and life-changing problem warranting early prevention and active treatment.

### REFERENCES

1. Office of the Surgeon General, National Institute on Alcohol Abuse, Alcoholism, Substance Abuse, Mental Health Services Administration. Publications and Reports of the Surgeon General. The Surgeon General's call to action to prevent and reduce underage drinking. Rockville (MD): Office of the Surgeon General (US); 2007. Available at: http://www.surgeongeneral.gov.

2. Pound P, Campbell R. Locating and applying sociological theories of risk-taking to develop public health interventions for adolescents. Health Sociol Rev 2015; 24(1):64–80.

3. Chambers RATJ, Potenza MN. Developmental neurocircuitry of motivation in adolescence: a critical period of addiction vulnerability. Am J Psychiatry 2003; 160(6):1041–52.

4. Selemon LD. A role for synaptic plasticity in the adolescent development of executive function. Transl Psychiatry 2013;3:e238.

5. Balogh KN, Mayes LC, Potenza MN. Risk-taking and decision-making in youth: relationships to addiction vulnerability. J Behav Addict 2013;2(1):1041–52.

6. Winters KC. Advances in the science of adolescent drug involvement: implications for assessment and diagnosis - experience from the United States. Curr Opin Psychiatry 2013;26(4):318–24.

7. Squeglia LM, Jacobus J, Tapert SF. The influence of substance use on adolescent brain development. Clin EEG Neurosci 2009;40(1):31–8.
8. Centers for Disease Control and Prevention. Alcohol and Public Health: Alcohol-Related Disease Impact (ARDI). Available at: https://nccd.cdc.gov/DPH_ARDI/default/default.aspx.
9. The DAWN report: Highlights of the 2012 Drug Abuse Warning Network (DAWN) Findings on Drug-Related Emergency Department Visits. Rockville, MD: Substance Abuse and Mental Health Services Administration, Center for Behavioral Health Statistics and Quality; 2012.
10. Alcohol Screening and Brief Intervention for Youth: A practitioner's Guide. 2015. Available at: www.niaaa.nih.gov/YouthGuide.
11. Grant BF, Dawson DA. Age of onset of drug use and its association with DSM-IV drug abuse and dependence: results from the National Longitudinal Alcohol Epidemiologic Survey. J Subst Abuse 1998;10(2):163–73.
12. Hingson R, White A. New research findings since the 2007 surgeon General's call to action to prevent and reduce underage drinking: a review. J Stud Alcohol Drugs 2014;75(1):158–69.
13. Johnston LD, O'Malley PM, Miech RA, et al. Monitoring the Future national survey results on drug use: 1975-2014: overview, key findings on adolescent drug use. Ann Arbor (MA): Institute for Social Research, The University of Michigan; 2015.
14. Substance Abuse and Mental Health Services Administration, Results from the 2013 National Survey on Drug Use and Health: Summary of National Findings, NSDUH Series H-48, HHS. Publication No. (SMA) 14–4863. Rockville (MD): Substance Abuse and Mental Health Services Administration; 2014.
15. Behavioral health trends in the United States: Results from the 2014 National Survey on Drug Use and Health (HHS Publication No. SMA 15-4927, NSDUH Series H-50). Rockville, MD: Center for Behavioral Health Statistics and Quality; 2015. Available at: http://www.samhsa.gov/data/.
16. Squeglia LM, Jacobus J, Tapert SF. The effect of alcohol use on human adolescent brain structures and systems. Handb Clin Neurol 2014;125:501–10.
17. Patrick ME, Schulenberg JE. Prevalence and predictors of adolescent alcohol use and binge drinking in the United States. Alcohol Res 2013;35(2):193–200.
18. Donovan JE. Estimated blood alcohol concentrations for child and adolescent drinking and their implications for screening instruments. Pediatrics 2009; 123(6):e975–81.
19. Hingson RW, Heeren T, Winter MR. Age at drinking onset and alcohol dependence: age at onset, duration, and severity. Arch Pediatr Adolesc Med 2006; 160(7):739–46.
20. Chen YC, Prescott CA, Walsh D, et al. Different phenotypic and genotypic presentations in alcohol dependence: age at onset matters. J Stud Alcohol Drugs 2011;72(5):752–62.
21. Dawson DA, Goldstein RB, Chou SP, et al. Age at first drink and the first incidence of adult-onset DSM-IV alcohol use disorders. Alcohol Clin Exp Res 2008;32(12):2149–60.
22. Merline AC, O'Malley PM, Schulenberg JE, et al. Substance use among adults 35 years of age: prevalence, adulthood predictors, and impact of adolescent substance use. Am J Public Health 2004;94(1):96–102.
23. Merline A, Jager J, Schulenberg JE. Adolescent risk factors for adult alcohol use and abuse: stability and change of predictive value across early and middle adulthood. Addiction 2008;103(Suppl 1):84–99.

24. Patrick ME, Schulenberg JE. How trajectories of reasons for alcohol use relate to trajectories of binge drinking: National panel data spanning late adolescence to early adulthood. Dev Psychol 2011;47(2):311–7.

25. Hopfer CJ, Crowley TJ, Hewitt JK. Review of twin and adoption studies of adolescent substance use. J Am Acad Child Adolesc Psychiatry 2003;42(6):710–9.

26. Bardo MT. High-risk behavior during adolescence: comments on part I. Ann N Y Acad Sci 2004;1021:59–60.

27. Dougherty DM, Lake SL, Mathias CW, et al. Behavioral impulsivity and risk-taking trajectories across early adolescence in youths with and without family histories of alcohol and other drug use disorders. Alcohol Clin Exp Res 2015; 39(8):1501–9.

28. Chartier KG, Hesselbrock MN, Hesselbrock VM. Development and vulnerability factors in adolescent alcohol use. Child Adolesc Psychiatr Clin N Am 2010; 19(3):493–504.

29. McGue M, Iacono WG, Legrand LN, et al. Origins and consequences of age at first drink. II. Familial risk and heritability. Alcohol Clin Exp Res 2001;25(8): 1166–73.

30. McGue M, Iacono WG, Legrand LN, et al. Origins and consequences of age at first drink. I. Associations with substance-use disorders, disinhibitory behavior and psychopathology, and P3 amplitude. Alcohol Clin Exp Res 2001;25(8): 1156–65.

31. Blumenthal H, Ham LS, Cloutier RM, et al. Social anxiety, disengagement coping, and alcohol-use behaviors among adolescents. Anxiety Stress Coping 2016;29(4):432–46.

32. Heath AC, Meyer J, Jardine R, et al. The inheritance of alcohol consumption patterns in a general population twin sample: II. Determinants of consumption frequency and quantity consumed. J Stud Alcohol 1991;52(5):425–33.

33. Agrawal A, Lynskey MT. Are there genetic influences on addiction: evidence from family, adoption and twin studies. Addiction 2008;103(7):1069–81.

34. Dick DM, Bierut LJ. The genetics of alcohol dependence. Curr Psychiatry Rep 2006;8(2):151–7.

35. Kalsi G, Prescott CA, Kendler KS, et al. Unraveling the molecular mechanisms of alcohol dependence. Trends Genet 2009;25(1):49–55.

36. Rhee SH, Hewitt JK, Young SE, et al. Genetic and environmental influences on substance initiation, use, and problem use in adolescents. Arch Gen Psychiatry 2003;60(12):1256–64.

37. Guerrini I, Quadri G, Thomson AD. Genetic and environmental interplay in risky drinking in adolescents: a literature review. Alcohol Alcohol 2014;49(2):138–42.

38. Olsson CA, Byrnes GB, Lotfi-Miri M, et al. Association between 5-HTTLPR genotypes and persisting patterns of anxiety and alcohol use: results from a 10-year longitudinal study of adolescent mental health. Mol Psychiatry 2005;10(9):868–76.

39. Mrug S, Windle M. DRD4 and susceptibility to peer influence on alcohol use from adolescence to adulthood. Drug Alcohol Depend 2014;145:168–73.

40. Cleveland HH, Schlomer GL, Vandenbergh DJ, et al. The conditioning of intervention effects on early adolescent alcohol use by maternal involvement and dopamine receptor D4 (DRD4) and serotonin transporter linked polymorphic region (5-HTTLPR) genetic variants. Dev Psychopathol 2015;27(1):51–67.

41. Rose RJ, Dick DM, Viken RJ, et al. Gene-environment interaction in patterns of adolescent drinking: regional residency moderates longitudinal influences on alcohol use. Alcohol Clin Exp Res 2001;25(5):637–43.

42. Dick DM, Bernard M, Aliev F, et al. The role of socioregional factors in moderating genetic influences on early adolescent behavior problems and alcohol use. Alcohol Clin Exp Res 2009;33(10):1739–48.
43. Rohde P, Lewinsohn PM, Seeley JR. Psychiatric comorbidity with problematic alcohol use in high school students. J Am Acad Child Adolesc Psychiatry 1996;35(1):101–9.
44. Sung M, Erkanli A, Angold A, et al. Effects of age at first substance use and psychiatric comorbidity on the development of substance use disorders. Drug Alcohol Depend 2004;75(3):287–99.
45. Rothman EF, Edwards EM, Heeren T, et al. Adverse childhood experiences predict earlier age of drinking onset: results from a representative US sample of current or former drinkers. Pediatrics 2008;122(2):e298–304.
46. Zimmermann P, Wittchen HU, Hofler M, et al. Primary anxiety disorders and the development of subsequent alcohol use disorders: a 4-year community study of adolescents and young adults. Psychol Med 2003;33(7):1211–22.
47. Young SE, Rhee SH, Stallings MC, et al. Genetic and environmental vulnerabilities underlying adolescent substance use and problem use: general or specific? Behav Genet 2006;36(4):603–15.
48. Han C, McGue MK, Iacono WG. Lifetime tobacco, alcohol and other substance use in adolescent Minnesota twins: univariate and multivariate behavioral genetic analyses. Addiction 1999;94(7):981–93.
49. Martino SC, Collins RL, Ellickson PL, et al. Socio-environmental influences on adolescents' alcohol outcome expectancies: a prospective analysis. Addiction 2006;101(7):971–83.
50. Miller PM, Smith GT, Goldman MS. Emergence of alcohol expectancies in childhood: a possible critical period. J Stud Alcohol 1990;51(4):343–9.
51. Moreno MA, Whitehill JM. Influence of social media on alcohol use in adolescents and young adults. Alcohol Res 2014;36(1):91–100.
52. Rossow I, Keating P, Felix L, et al. Does parental drinking influence children's drinking? A systematic review of prospective cohort studies. Addiction 2016;111(2):204–17.
53. Sher KJ, Grekin ER, Williams NA. The development of alcohol use disorders. Annu Rev Clin Psychol 2005;1:493–523.
54. Hernandez L, Rodriguez AM, Spirito A. Brief family-based intervention for substance abusing adolescents. Child Adolesc Psychiatr Clin N Am 2015;24(3):585–99.
55. Bachman JG, Staff J, O'Malley PM, et al. Adolescent work intensity, school performance, and substance use: links vary by race/ethnicity and socioeconomic status. Dev Psychol 2013;49(11):2125–34.
56. Wray-Lake L, Maggs JL, Johnston LD, et al. Associations between community attachments and adolescent substance use in nationally representative samples. J Adolesc Health 2012;51(4):325–31.
57. Terry-McElrath YM, O'Malley PM, Johnston LD. Exercise and substance use among American youth, 1991-2009. Am J Prev Med 2011;40(5):530–40.
58. Masten AS, Faden VB, Zucker RA, et al. A developmental perspective on underage alcohol use. Alcohol Res Health 2009;32(1):3–15.
59. Settles RE, Smith GT. Toward a developmentally centered approach to adolescent alcohol and substance use treatment. Curr Drug Abuse Rev 2015;8(2):134–51.
60. Sterling S, Kline-Simon AH, Wibbelsman C, et al. Screening for adolescent alcohol and drug use in pediatric health-care settings: predictors and implications for practice and policy. Addict Sci Clin Pract 2012;7:13.

61. Brown JD, Wissow LS. Discussion of sensitive health topics with youth during primary care visits: relationship to youth perceptions of care. J Adolesc Health 2009;44(1):48–54.

62. Devlin RJ, Henry JA. Clinical review: major consequences of illicit drug consumption. Crit Care 2008;12(1):202.

63. White AM, MacInnes E, Hingson RW, et al. Hospitalizations for suicide-related drug poisonings and co-occurring alcohol overdoses in adolescents (ages 12-17) and young adults (ages 18-24) in the United States, 1999-2008: results from the Nationwide Inpatient Sample. Suicide Life Threat Behav 2013;43(2):198–212.

64. Perepletchikova F, Krystal JH, Kaufman J. Practitioner review: adolescent alcohol use disorders: assessment and treatment issues. J Child Psychol Psychiatry 2008;49(11):1131–54.

65. Winters KC. Assessment of alcohol and other drug use behaviors among adolescents. In: Allen JP, Wilson VB, editors. Assessing Alcohol Problems, A guide for Clinicians and Researchers. 2nd edition. Bethesda, MD: US Department of Health and Human Services; 2003. p. 101–23.

66. Harris SK, Louis-Jacques J, Knight JR. Screening and brief intervention for alcohol and other abuse. Adolesc Med State Art Rev 2014;25(1):126–56.

67. Rumpf HJ, Wohlert T, Freyer-Adam J, et al. Screening questionnaires for problem drinking in adolescents: performance of AUDIT, AUDIT-C, CRAFFT and POSIT. Eur Addict Res 2013;19(3):121–7.

68. Levy S, Siqueira LM, Ammerman SD, et al. Testing for drugs of abuse in children and adolescents. Pediatrics 2014;133(6):e1798–807.

69. Substance Abuse and Mental Health Services Administration. The role of biomarkers in the treatment of alcohol use disorders, 2012 Revision. *Advisory*, Volume 11, Issue 2. Rockville, MD: Center for Substance Abuse Treatment, Substance Abuse and Mental Health Services Administration; 2012.

70. Carlson SR, McLarnon ME, Iacono WG. P300 amplitude, externalizing psychopathology, and earlier- versus later-onset substance-use disorder. J Abnorm Psychol 2007;116(3):565–77.

71. Hashimoto E, Riederer PF, Hesselbrock VM, et al. Consensus paper of the WFSBP task force on biological markers: biological markers for alcoholism. World J Biol Psychiatry 2013;14(8):549–64.

72. Bukstein OG, Kaminer Y. Adolescent substance use disorders: transition to substance abuse, prevention and treatment. In: Galanter M, Kleber HD, Brady KT, editors. The American Psychiatric Publishing textbook of substance abuse treatment. 5th edition. Washington, DC: American Psychiatric Association; 2015. p. 641–51.

73. Winward JL, Hanson KL, Bekman NM, et al. Adolescent heavy episodic drinking: neurocognitive functioning during early abstinence. J Int Neuropsychol Soc 2014;20(2):218–29.

74. Substance Abuse and Mental Health Services Administration (SAMHSA), CfBHSaQ. Treatment of adolescents with substance use disorders: treatment improvement protocol series (TIP 32). Rockville (MD): U.S. Department of Health and Human Services, SAMHSA; 2010.

75. Nackers KA, Kokotailo P, Levy SJ. Substance abuse, general principles. Pediatr Rev 2015;36(12):535–44.

76. Becker SJ, Curry JF. Outpatient interventions for adolescent substance abuse: a quality of evidence review. J Consult Clin Psychol 2008;76(4):531–43.

77. Tripodi SJ, Bender K, Litschge C, et al. Interventions for reducing adolescent alcohol abuse: a meta-analytic review. Arch Pediatr Adolesc Med 2010; 164(1):85–91.
78. Bukstein OG, Bernet W, Arnold V, et al. Practice parameter for the assessment and treatment of children and adolescents with substance use disorders. J Am Acad Child Adolesc Psychiatry 2005;44(6):609–21.
79. Kelly JF, Dow SJ, Yeterian JD, et al. Can 12-step group participation strengthen and extend the benefits of adolescent addiction treatment? A prospective analysis. Drug Alcohol Depend 2010;110(1–2):117–25.
80. Kelly JF, Dow SJ, Yeterian JD, et al. How safe are adolescents at alcoholics anonymous and narcotics anonymous meetings? a prospective investigation with outpatient youth. J Subst Abuse Treat 2011;40(4):419–25.
81. Liddle HA, Dakof GA, Turner RM, et al. Treating adolescent drug abuse: a randomized trial comparing multidimensional family therapy and cognitive behavior therapy. Addiction 2008;103(10):1660–70.
82. Henderson CE, Rowe CL, Dakof GA, et al. Parenting practices as mediators of treatment effects in an early-intervention trial of multidimensional family therapy. Am J Drug Alcohol Abuse 2009;35(4):220–6.
83. Coghill D, Bonnar S, Duke SL, et al. Child and Adolescent Psychiatry US. New York: Oxford University Press Inc.; 2009.
84. Stewart DG, Brown SA. Withdrawal and dependency symptoms among adolescent alcohol and drug abusers. Addiction 1995;90(5):627–35.
85. Simkin DR, Grenoble S. Pharmacotherapies for adolescent substance use disorders. Child Adolesc Psychiatr Clin N Am 2010;19(3):591–608.
86. O'Brien CP. Evidence-based treatments of addiction. In: Robbins TW, Everitt BJ, Nutt DJ, editors. The neurobiology of addiction. New York: Oxford University Press; 2010.
87. Clark DB. Pharmacotherapy for adolescent alcohol use disorder. CNS Drugs 2012;26(7):559–69.
88. Langenbucher J, Martin CS, Labouvie E, et al. Toward the DSM-V: the Withdrawal-Gate Model versus the DSM-IV in the diagnosis of alcohol abuse and dependence. J Consult Clin Psychol 2000;68(5):799–809.
89. Brown SA, Tapert SF, Granholm E, et al. Neurocognitive functioning of adolescents: effects of protracted alcohol use. Alcohol Clin Exp Res 2000;24(2):164–71.
90. Altshuler HL, Phillips PE, Feinhandler DA. Alteration of ethanol self-administration by naltrexone. Life Sci 1980;26(9):679–88.
91. Ait-Daoud N, Johnson BA, Javors M, et al. Combining ondansetron and naltrexone treats biological alcoholics: corroboration of self-reported drinking by serum carbohydrate deficient transferrin, a biomarker. Alcohol Clin Exp Res 2001;25(6):847–9.
92. Kranzler HR, Gage A. Acamprosate efficacy in alcohol-dependent patients: summary of results from three pivotal trials. Am J Addict 2008;17(1):70–6.
93. Niederhofer H, Staffen W. Comparison of disulfiram and placebo in treatment of alcohol dependence of adolescents. Drug Alcohol Rev 2003;22(3):295–7.
94. Kandel DB, Johnson JG, Bird HR, et al. Psychiatric comorbidity among adolescents with substance use disorders: findings from the MECA Study. J Am Acad Child Adolesc Psychiatry 1999;38(6):693–9.
95. Rohde P, Lewinsohn PM, Kahler CW, et al. Natural course of alcohol use disorders from adolescence to young adulthood. J Am Acad Child Adolesc Psychiatry 2001;40(1):83–90.

96. Riggs PD, Mikulich-Gilbertson SK, Davies RD, et al. A randomized controlled trial of fluoxetine and cognitive behavioral therapy in adolescents with major depression, behavior problems, and substance use disorders. Arch Pediatr Adolesc Med 2007;161(11):1026–34.

97. Riggs PD, Leon SL, Mikulich SK, et al. An open trial of bupropion for ADHD in adolescents with substance use disorders and conduct disorder. J Am Acad Child Adolesc Psychiatry 1998;37(12):1271–8.

98. Riggs PD, Winhusen T, Davies RD, et al. Randomized controlled trial of osmotic-release methylphenidate with cognitive-behavioral therapy in adolescents with attention-deficit/hyperactivity disorder and substance use disorders. J Am Acad Child Adolesc Psychiatry 2011;50(9):903–14.

99. Geller B, Cooper TB, Sun K, et al. Double-blind and placebo-controlled study of lithium for adolescent bipolar disorders with secondary substance dependency. J Am Acad Child Adolesc Psychiatry 1998;37(2):171–8.

100. Riggs PD, Mikulich SK, Coffman LM, et al. Fluoxetine in drug-dependent delinquents with major depression: an open trial. J Child Adolesc Psychopharmacol 1997;7(2):87–95.

101. Benningfield MM, Riggs P, Stephan SH. The role of schools in substance use prevention and intervention. Child Adolesc Psychiatr Clin N Am 2015;24(2):291–303.

102. Gates S, McCambridge J, Smith LA, et al. Interventions for prevention of drug use by young people delivered in non-school settings. Cochrane Database Syst Rev 2006;(1):CD005030.

103. O'Malley PM, Wagenaar AC. Effects of minimum drinking age laws on alcohol use, related behaviors and traffic crash involvement among American youth: 1976-1987. J Stud Alcohol 1991;52(5):478–91.

104. O'Malley PM, Johnston LD. Unsafe driving by high school seniors: national trends from 1976 to 2001 in tickets and accidents after use of alcohol, marijuana and other illegal drugs. J Stud Alcohol 2003;64(3):305–12.

105. Nunez-Smith M, Wolf E, Huang HM, et al. Media exposure and tobacco, illicit drugs, and alcohol use among children and adolescents: a systematic review. Subst Abus 2010;31(3):174–92.

# Cannabis Use Disorder in Adolescence

Annabelle K. Simpson, MD[a],*, Viktoriya Magid, PhD[b]

## KEYWORDS

- Cannabis • Marijuana • Abuse • Dependence • Adolescent • Teenager
- Cannabis use disorder

## KEY POINTS

- Cannabis use in the adolescent population poses a significant threat of addiction potential resulting in altered neurodevelopment.
- There are multiple mechanisms of treatment of cannabis use disorder including behavioral therapy management and emerging data on treatment via pharmacotherapy.
- Recognizing the diagnostic criteria for cannabis use disorder (according to DSM-5), cannabis withdrawal syndrome, and mitigating factors that influence adolescent engagement in cannabis use allows for comprehensive assessment and management in the adolescent population.

## INTRODUCTION

According to statistics collected by the Substance Abuse and Mental Health Services Administration (SAMHSA), Center for Behavioral Health Statistics and Quality, and National Survey on Drug Use and Health (NSDUH) 2014, cannabis remains the illicit drug substance that individuals most commonly abuse and/or develop dependence on within the age group 12 to 17 years old.[1,2] The illicit drug marijuana is derived from the cannabis sativa, indica, hybrid species, and/or ruderalis plants, which contain the psychoactive substance delta-9-tetrahydrocannabinol (THC). Throughout the body are cannabinoid receptors, CB1 and CB2, which are activated by endogenous cannabinoids. Cannabinoid receptors are located in the central nervous system (basal ganglia, hippocampus, cerebellum, and cortex) and systemically (immune cells and spleen). The mechanism of action of marijuana is the result of cannabis ligand binding to CB1 and CB2 receptors, resulting in psychoactive intoxication and other systemic effects in the peripheral tissue.

[a] Child and Adolescent Psychiatry, Seattle Children's Hospital, 4800 Sand Point Way Northeast, M/S: OA 5.154, Seattle, WA 98105, USA; [b] Department of Psychiatry and Behavioral Sciences, Medical University of South Carolina, 67 President Street, Charleston, SC 29425, USA
* Corresponding author.
E-mail address: Annabelle.Simpson@seattlechildrens.org

Child Adolesc Psychiatric Clin N Am 25 (2016) 431–443
http://dx.doi.org/10.1016/j.chc.2016.03.003                childpsych.theclinics.com
1056-4993/16/$ – see front matter © 2016 Elsevier Inc. All rights reserved.

## CLINICAL PRESENTATION AND DIAGNOSIS

According to the Diagnostic and Statistical Manual of Mental Disorders, fifth edition (DSM-5) cannabis intoxication, withdrawal, and use disorder are categorized by meeting specific diagnostic criteria.[3,4]

Cannabis intoxication occurs with recent use of cannabis and a diverse array of behavioral changes including impaired motor coordination, euphoria, anxiety, sensation of slowed time, and paranoia.[3] According to the DSM-5, to meet diagnostic criteria the patient is required to experience at least two of the following within a 2-hour period of using cannabis: conjunctival injection, increased appetite, dry mouth, and tachycardia; also, these signs and symptoms cannot be better explained by another general medical condition, substance intoxication, and/or mental health illness.

Cannabis withdrawal occurs as a result of multiple variables and is further discussed later.[3] The following signs and symptoms must be present to meet the diagnostic criteria for cannabis withdrawal according to the DSM-5. First, cessation of frequent and prolonged cannabis usage that is daily over the period of several months. Second, the exhibition/endorsement of three or more of the following signs and symptoms over the course of approximately 1 week:

1. Irritability, anger, or depression
2. Nervousness or anxiety
3. Sleep difficulty (ie, insomnia, disturbing dreams)
4. Decreased appetite or weight loss
5. Restlessness
6. Depressed mood
7. At least one physical symptom causing discomfort (ie, abdominal pain, shakiness/tremors, sweating, fever, chills, headache)

Third, the aforementioned psychological and/or physical symptoms must cause significant impairment to social, occupation, and/or other significant areas of life functioning. The signs and symptoms cannot be the result of withdrawal and/or intoxication from any other substance, general medical condition, and/or mental health illness.

According to DSM-5, cannabis use disorder is the significant impairment/distress in multiple areas of functionality and also development of tolerance and withdrawal to the drug over a 12-month period.[3]

- The development of a problematic behavior as consequence of the persistent use and/or increasing amounts of cannabis use
- Continued desire for the drug and failed attempts to decrease or control the use of the drug
- An excessive amount of the individual's time is spent involved in activities to obtain the drug
- Persistent use of cannabis negatively impacting the individual's ability to attend to roles at work, school, or home
- Persistent use of cannabis despite repeated social/interpersonal issues that are made worse by the continued use of cannabis
- Persistent use of cannabis in physically hazardous conditions
- Persistent use of cannabis despite the identification of a physical and/or psychological issue that was most likely secondary to cannabis use and/or exacerbated cannabis use
- Tolerance

- ○ The need of significantly increased quantity of cannabis to attain intoxication and/or desired effect
- ○ The occurrence of decreased intoxication effect with continued use of the same quantity of cannabis
- Withdrawal
  - ○ The experience of cannabis withdrawal signs and symptoms (diagnostic criteria previously discussed)
  - ○ The individual uses cannabis to pacify or circumvent the development of withdrawal symptoms

The diagnosis of cannabis use disorder requires specification of mild (two to three of the aforementioned), moderate (four to five of the aforementioned), and severe (greater than six of the aforementioned) symptomatology.[3]

## ADVERSE EFFECTS ASSOCIATED WITH USAGE OF CANNABIS

Short-term usage of cannabis has been associated with impairment of short-term memory, motor coordination, altered decision-making capacity, paranoia, and psychosis.[5] Long-term/heavy usage of cannabis has been associated with the development of addiction to the substance, psychosis, and significant decline in cognitive development. It has been postulated that the use of cannabis may result in uncovering psychosis in a user who might have genetic susceptibility toward the development of psychosis.

Furthermore, neuropsychological testing has demonstrated that long-term use of cannabis results in significant decline in executive functioning, memory, learning, and/or cognitive processing speed.[6] Additionally, impairments in verbal learning and memory have been demonstrated during acute intoxication and greater impairments demonstrated in chronic users; specifically, diminished immediate and delayed recall of words.[7]

The adolescent stage of neurocognitive development is thought to be the most vulnerable to pathology with the onset of cannabis use. During this stage in development, the brain undergoes neuronal maturation and also significant restructuring (in terms of synaptic pruning, myelination processing, and dendritic plasticity).[8] The commencement of usage during adolescence has been significantly associated with the eventual development of cannabis addiction. Additionally, heavy/regular use of cannabis during adolescence has been significantly correlated with decreasing the intelligence quotient (IQ).[9] In a cohort study conducted by Meier and colleagues[6] the greater the frequency and long-term duration of use, the greater the decline in IQ points; in comparison, individuals who had not engaged in cannabis usage showed a slight increase in IQ point. Of note, adult onset was not associated with decreased IQ points, even with persistent cannabis usage. Moreover, the cognitive impairments identified persisted even after greater than 1 year of abstinence.[8]

## CANNABIS WITHDRAWAL SYNDROME

Cannabis is the most commonly used illicit drug in the United States, with 35.1% of twelfth graders having used marijuana in the last year and 5.8% of twelfth graders reporting daily use.[10] There are many contributing factors to this including a lack of public awareness of addiction potential and withdrawal syndrome. Studies have shown that approximately 35% to 75% adolescents who sought treatment of cannabis use disorder underwent withdrawal syndrome during attempts to reduce or abstain from use.[11] The withdrawal syndrome included changes in mood (anxiety and depression), irritability, sensation of restlessness, appetite changes, sleep disturbance, and cannabis substance craving. Of note, because of the extended half-life of delta-9-THC (27–57 hours) and the metabolites of delta-9-THC (up to 5 days), particular symptoms of withdrawal may persist for several weeks and/or possibly months after reduction or discontinuation of cannabis use,[6] in particular cannabis craving and sleep disturbance. Additionally, individuals may experience functional impairments and exacerbation of underlying mood disorder (ie, anxiety and/or depression) during withdrawal from cannabis.[11]

In a study carried out by Greene and Kelly[11] of adolescent cannabis user population, 90 individuals were assessed and followed over the course of 1 year to further elucidate the withdrawal syndrome specific to cannabis. Follow-up assessments were carried out in-person and over the telephone; specifically, individuals were assessed for DSM-IV criteria of cannabis dependence and demographics data collected. During the course of this study, 40% of the adolescent participants experienced withdrawal symptoms. Those who experienced withdrawal symptoms along with greater problem recognition reported significantly decreased percentage days of abstinence, compared with individuals who did not experience withdrawal symptoms. Additionally, individuals who reported withdrawal symptoms also disclosed significantly greater preoccupation on cannabis, tolerance, deferring activities previously enjoyed, and were more likely to resume the use of cannabis despite the psychological and physiologic issues that were a direct result of their cannabis use. It was postulated that greater problem recognition, resulted in increased motivation to use adaptive behavior to curtail substance usage over the course of the 1-year follow-up.[11]

Furthermore, Greene and Kelly[11] demonstrated within their sample of participants that experienced withdrawal symptoms the most common outcomes of cannabis cessation included resuming usage (66.67%), sleep disturbance (30.56%), headache (13.89%), and irritability (13.89%). Other withdrawal symptoms that were less common included nausea, vomiting, gastrointestinal upset, fatigue, excess yawning, aggressive behavior, decreased appetite, anxiety, increased dreaming during sleep, decreased concentration, moodiness, impulsive behavior, loss of consciousness, restlessness, chest pains, and physical weakness. Finally, the experience of withdrawal syndrome is one factor significantly indicative of cannabis dependence and possible impediment to treatment of cannabis use disorder. Additionally, this study supports the importance of incorporating public awareness regarding withdrawal syndrome to enhance problem recognition skills and possibly decrease the development of persistent substance use and development of cannabis dependence.

## EPIDEMIOLOGY

Epidemiologic data were acquired from the NSDUH financially sponsored by SAMHSA, a department of the US Department Health and Human Services. Data collected revealed that cannabis users represented the highest percentage of illicit substance users in individuals age greater than 12 years old. Cannabis was the most common illicit drug used within the adolescent sample. Data collected revealed that over the course of 12 months there were 2.6 million people age 12 years or older who used cannabis for the first time second only to alcohol; average age of initiation was 18.5 years old. Within the adolescent age group (sample size of 667,000 participants) 2.7% of individuals met diagnostic criteria of cannabis use disorder over the course of the year.[1]

Cannabis use represented most first time users of any illicit substance from the NSDUH 2014 data sample. According to this data sample the total number of first time users of marijuana age 12 or older was 2.6 million within the past year, 1.2 million (approximately 46%) of these individuals were age 12 to 17, and 1.1 million (approximately 42%) of these individuals were 18 to 25 years old (transitional age group). Given this striking data of new users, subsequent analysis assessed the perception of risk, namely perceived availability of cannabis, determining whether the new users are soliciting cannabis versus being approached by dealers, perceived parental disapproval of cannabis use, perceived peer disapproval of cannabis use, and also exposure to substance prevention messages.[12–14]

Using these data collected in 2014, within the age group 12 to 17 years, 22.9% of adolescents perceived risk of harm from monthly cannabis use and 37.4% of adolescents perceived risk of harm from weekly cannabis use. In terms of perceived availability of cannabis approximately 47.8% disclosed that this drug would be obtainable with ease. Consideration of such data should be used when creating prevention programs/messages targeting this age group. Additionally, 87.5% of adolescents reported perceived parental disapproval in the use of cannabis or hashish. Of note, this factor is to be considered when initiating clinical management of families of known parental users/ambivalence toward cannabis use (consider in states legalizing cannabis use). In addition, 79.2% of adolescents reported that peers disapproved of the initiation of cannabis and/or hashish. Approximately 12.1% or one in eight adolescents were approached by a cannabis dealer. Note this value is not inclusive of initiates being approached by peers/dealers freely supplying the substance. Such individual perception and experiences are to be factored into public health initiatives when addressing neighborhood and/or cultural enclave normative substance behaviors.[12]

Moreover, in considering the efficacy of preventative messages to the adolescent population data obtained from the NSDUH 2014 addressed prevention messages (ie, via posters, pamphlets, radio, television). Approximately 72.9% of the adolescent group reported viewing various forms of prevention messages. Moreover, 7.1% of individuals from this age group were current cannabis users despite viewing prevention messages. Interestingly, 7.8% were current cannabis users who had not viewed prevention messages. It was noted, however, that over the course of data collected from 2002 to 2014, adolescents who were exposed to prevention messages showed a significantly decreased likelihood of engaging in substance use (inclusive of other illicit substances). Interestingly, prevention messages specifically viewed in school exhibited decreased cannabis users (6.6%) compared with those who had not viewed prevention messages in school who were cannabis users (9.9%).[12]

Furthermore, behavioral health trends within the adolescent population group (age 12–17) were elicited from this data sample. Of note adolescents who experienced an episode of major depressive disorder in the past year exhibited increased use of illicit substance within the year; specifically, 33% who had experienced an episode of depression and 15.2% who had not experienced an episode of depression.[1]

## EPIDEMIOLOGY: TRANSITIONAL AGE POPULATION

The comorbidity of mental health illness and substance use disorders is of significant value. Such individuals exhibit decline in quality of individual/family life and individual productivity in terms of school and work, and also increased use of health care services and criminal activities.[1] In discussion of negative effect of cannabis use in the adolescent population, a comprehensive discussion must include the effect on the transition age group's (18–25 years) daily functionality and health care systems use. According to the NSDUH data, between 2005 and 2011, the number of transitional age individuals who visited the emergency department for treatment of illicit substance use and/or misuse had increased. Additionally, according to data from NSDUH during the years 2011 to 2012, transitional age individuals who used cannabis on a daily basis accounted for 3.2 million individuals, second only to alcohol (4.8 million individuals) and greater than any other illicit substance.[15,16] Moreover, the 2011 Drug Abuse Warning Network (public health surveillance agency collecting data on mortality and morbidity related to substance use) collected data nationwide from metropolitan areas. Drug Abuse Warning Network 2011 data reported 845,000 transitional age individuals who were admitted to the emergency department secondary to drug-related issue. Within this data sample on an average day 422 visits were related to cannabis use, second only to alcohol (399 visits).[15]

Additionally, nationwide data regarding substance use were collected from the Treatment Episode Data Set and reported to SAMHSA. Over the course of 12 months during 2011, there were 403,756 individuals within the transitional age group admitted to a publicly funded substance use disorder treatment program. On an average day 308 of these individuals reported cannabis as their primary drug of choice second only to heroin and opiates (364 individuals). Interestingly, the principal referral source was the criminal justice system (459 admissions); self-referral/referral from other individuals (332 admissions), community organizations (135 admissions), alcohol/drug abuse care providers (99 admissions), other health care providers (51 admissions), schools (seven admissions), and employer/employee assistance programs (three admissions).[15]

## CLINICAL MANAGEMENT: PHARMACOTHERAPY AND BEHAVIORAL MANAGEMENT

Within the adolescent population, clinical management of cannabis use disorder involves the use of predominantly behavioral management approaches to achieve reduction in usage. In terms of the pharmacotherapy treatment of cannabis use disorder, the field continues to grow; however, there have been promising studies that have shown reduction in usage and treatment of withdrawal syndrome.

## EPIDEMIOLOGY OF CLINICAL MANAGEMENT

According to the NSDUH 2014 data, 21.5 million individuals age 12 or older had met criteria for a substance use disorder and 2.3 million received treatment targeting the substance use disorder, whereas 4.1 million individuals received treatment of issues related to their use of substances. Locations for treatment included self-help groups, outpatient rehabilitation, outpatient mental health center, inpatient rehabilitation, hospital inpatient, private physician's office, emergency department, and in prison/jail. Within the previously mentioned sample of individuals, it was reported that 1 million individuals received treatment of cannabis use during the 12-month period.

The NSDUH 2014 data revealed that 1.3 million adolescent individuals met criteria for substance use disorder treatment (drug and alcohol). Out of this sample 894,000 adolescents required treatment of an illicit substance use disorder. Also, 8.5% of the adolescents were able to receive treatment from a specialty facility within the 12-month period. Within this study, specialty treatment was defined as inpatient hospitalization, drug/alcohol rehabilitation (inpatient or outpatient), and/or mental health center. Moreover, this data sample identified 1.2 million adolescents who required substance use treatment, but had not received the treatment needed from a specialty facility within the past 12 months. From this sample, 32,000 or 2.7% expressed a perceived need for treatment, but did not receive specialty treatment services.

Additionally, it was revealed that 820,000 adolescents met criteria for treatment; however, 791,000 of these individuals did not perceive a need for treatment.

Within the population who were age 12 or older (inclusive of adults) and identified a need for treatment but had not received treatment, the following were reasons for treatment avoidance: (1) not ready to stop using (41.2%), (2) no health coverage and could not afford cost (30.8%), (3) concern of negative effect on job (if treatment were sought; 11.5%), (4) concern about negative opinions of community/neighbors (if treatment were sought; 11.1%), (5) lacked awareness of treatment sites (10.4%), and (6) unable to access program with the specific type of treatment needed (7.5%). The aforementioned barriers to treatment of substance use disorder and specifically cannabis use disorder are necessary to consider when addressing/creating clinical management protocol for substance users. Additionally, NSDUH 2014 data demonstrated that among population age 12 or older who perceived need for treatment but did not receive treatment, the following reasons were documented: lack of health coverage and beyond affordability for individual (35.3%), not ready to cease substance use (24.2%), health coverage excluded substance use disorder treatment (11%), lack of awareness of treatment sites (10.5%), lack of access to substance use treatment type needed (10.3%), and lack of transportation/inconvenient (10%).

Furthermore, according to the NSDUH 2014 data, approximately 3.4 million adolescents were provided with mental health services. Specialty mental health services were provided in various settings, which included specialty mental health setting (outpatient/inpatient), education setting, general medical setting, child welfare setting, juvenile justice setting, and/or specialty/nonspecialty settings (5.9%). The source of mental health services is a major consideration when creating and implementing prevention and treatment protocols.[17]

## BEHAVIORAL MANAGEMENT OF CANNABIS USE DISORDER

Taking into consideration the previously mentioned data it is striking the lack of perceived need for treatment, lack of motivation to cease substance use, and extrapolated from this data likely lack of knowledge about available specialty services. Multiple studies have investigated many behavioral therapy techniques in treating cannabis use disorder, in particular the cannabis youth treatment (CYT) study[18] and the study by Kamon and colleagues[19] investigating contingency management (CM) in the adolescent population to treat cannabis use disorder.

The CYT study investigated the following therapeutic modalities: motivational enhancement with cognitive behavioral therapy (MET-CBT), family support network psychotherapy approach, adolescent community reinforcement approach (ACRA), and multidimensional family therapy. Over the course of 12 months, these therapeutic interventions were evaluated working with a sample size of 600 adolescents (12–18 year old) and their families across four sites in several states (Connecticut, Pennsylvania, Florida, and Illinois). All four modalities of therapeutic intervention showed significant efficacy at 12-month follow-up in terms of significant increase in days of abstinence. The MET-CBT and ACRA showed the most significant change in terms of days of abstinence and cost-effectiveness. Interestingly, two programs of MET-CBT were compared: two sessions of individual MET and three group CBT sessions (6–7 weeks), and two sessions of individual MET and seven group CBT sessions (12–14 weeks). The 6- to 7-week MET-CBT program showed the most significant increase in days of abstinence as opposed to the 12- to 14-week program.[18]

The purpose of MET is to increase the individual's insight into the consequences and benefits of continued substance usage; the aim is to enhance the individual's motivation toward decreasing substance use secondary to appreciating that the benefits of doing so are greater than the consequence of continued usage. Throughout the CYT study MET addressed the ambivalence noted in adolescent cannabis users and worked to enhance their motivation toward reduction of use/abstaining from use. The purpose of the additional CBT group sessions is to aid the individual in gaining coping skills to target key problem areas: refusing drug offers, creating a social network that supports recovery, establishing alternative activities of interest unrelated to cannabis usage, developing a preemptive plan to manage high-risk situations, relapse, and also overall problem-solving skills enhancing maintenance of recovery.[18]

In addition, CM programs in combination with MET-CBT have shown significant improvement in abstinence/reduction of substance usage. CM is an intervention that uses various modules to address adolescents rarely seeking and/or following through to completing treatment of substance use disorder secondary to multiple reasons, such as parent disapproval and apprehension to involve parents in treatment, lack of perceived harm to self, and general ambivalence about substance cessation. Kamon and colleagues[19] used a CM program as an intervention to investigate influence on adolescents (12–18 years) using cannabis and/or alcohol and also exhibiting problem behaviors (ie, conduct disorder). This study implemented four interventions over the course of a 14-week period and followed up on sample size of 19 adolescent patients 30 days after the end of treatment. The four interventions included

1. Engaging adolescents into treatment and reinforcing abstinence with use of monetary-based incentive vouchers
2. Parents received training to assist in engaging their adolescent in initiating abstinence and maintaining abstinence and also address problem behaviors (ie, related to conduct disorder)
3. Skills training that reinforced and supported the adolescents' abstinence were enhanced with CM incentives directed toward parents to use the skills parents had learned via training sessions
4. Adolescent participants were engaged in individual therapy sessions via a MET-CBT intervention program

Urine toxicology revealed this form of therapy to be efficacious, abstinence rate increasing from 37% to 74% and persistence of abstinence 30 days posttreatment in 53% of adolescent participants.[19] This study identified a significant reduction in cannabis usage and increased abstinence days at 30-day follow-up from date of final assessment.

The CYT study also noted that adolescent participants responded with significantly increased abstinence using ACRA. This treatment yielded 34% of individuals in recovery; however, this treatment was not statistically significant when compared with MET-CBT/5 (two individual MET sessions followed by three CBT group therapy sessions) and multidimensional family therapy. Notably, ACRA and MET-CBT/5 was statistically significant in terms of lowered cost per day abstinent and cost per person in recovery. ACRA therapeutic intervention was carried out over the course of 12 to 14 weeks; the treatment involved 10 individual sessions with the adolescent participant and four parent/caregiver sessions (two of these involving the entire family). In addition to the individual, parent/caregiver, and family sessions, the family was supported with limited case management to address various family needs (ie, reminders, transportation, child care, make other community referrals if needed).

ACRA uses three main procedures during the individual sessions with the adolescent. First, functional analyses are carried out to identify antecedents and consequences to substance use and address prosocial behaviors. Second, the individual and therapist work together to identify simple, attainable, and well-defined goals of therapy. Third, the individual is encouraged to use a rating scale in monitoring quality of life, identify new goals, re-enforce prosocial behaviors, and carry out skills training for prevention of relapse and general problem solving. In addition, the four caregiver/parent sessions provide an overview of the ACRA program, educate caregiver/parent with skills to support adolescent abstinence, and then two sessions are devoted to the entire family. During the family sessions, the therapist facilitates and teaches a practice of positive communication between individuals within the family and also builds on problem-solving skills. These parent/caregiver sessions are thought to provide a scaffolding to enhance the support system received by the adolescent individual, thereby encourage use of skills and encourage abstinence.[18]

The aforementioned is a discussion of psychotherapy approaches that have been shown to be efficacious in treatment of cannabis use disorder. Targeting ambivalence toward abstinence, perception of harm, and eliciting obtainable goals are key to significantly impact substance use reduction and/or eventual abstinence.

## PHARMACOTHERAPY OF CANNABIS USE DISORDER

In addition to the psychotherapeutic approaches to treating cannabis use disorder, pharmacotherapy has shown tremendous promise in terms of addressing withdrawal syndrome and decreasing cannabis usage.

Gray and colleagues[20] carried out a clinical study investigating N-acetylcysteine (NAC) to aid cannabis use reduction. It was postulated that in an individual with cannabis use disorder, drug-seeking behavior is the result of glutamate dysregulation within the nucleus accumbens. Additionally, glutamate serves as a regulatory agent in the dopaminergic activity within the ventral tegmental area. The treatment with NAC serves to activate the cysteine/glutamate antiporter, which decreases the drug-seeking behavior; such had been exemplified in prior animal models in cocaine-dependent rats. Gray and colleagues[20] postulated that NAC would correct the downregulation of the cysteine/glutamate antiporter brought on by persistent cannabis use and thereby restore correct homeostasis to the dopaminergic system.

Gray and colleagues[20–22] carried out a randomized double-blind study including 116 participants who were between 15 and 21 years in age and on average had engaged in cannabis use for 4.2 years. The intervention of NAC, 1200 mg twice daily, in comparison with placebo twice daily was carried out over the course of 8 weeks and then participants were assessed at 12-week follow-up. Of note, the study used CM techniques and brief ($\leq$10 minutes) physician-delivered counseling encouraging cessation to maintain participant retention. The outcome of the study revealed that NAC in combination with CM as opposed to CM and placebo demonstrated significantly increased rates of participants submitting negative urine drug screens during treatment. Of note, adverse effects included vivid dreams and possibly severe heartburn (although this side effect occurred in only one participant).

In a subsequent study by Gray and colleagues[21] the previously mentioned outcomes were replicated in a group of transitional age individuals. The clinical study involved 24 participants age 18 to 21 years who sought treatment of cannabis use. The study took place over the course of 4 weeks to assess for tolerability and efficacy. Individuals were treated with NAC, 1200 mg twice daily, over the course of 4 weeks. There was noted significant reduction in cannabis use and craving as rated by the marijuana craving questionnaire self-report. Adverse effects reported included abdominal discomfort, myalgia, insomnia, headache, nasal congestion, nausea, decrease in weight, restlessness, and dizziness; these side effects were noted to be mild-moderate and did not result in participants discontinuing the medication. The NAC clinical studies have been prodigious in providing the area of cannabis pharmacotherapy treatment with potential for growth in treatment of adolescents with cannabis use disorder.[20–22]

Additional studies that have investigated the pharmacotherapy approaches to cannabis use disorder have occurred mainly in the adult population. Mason and colleagues[23] carried out a study of 50 participants, age 18 to 65 years (average, 33.9 years), who were individuals meeting criteria for DSM-IV cannabis dependence, who had used cannabis at least 1 week before treatment, and sought out outpatient research treatment. Gabapentin was used as the pharmacotherapy intervention for a period of 12 weeks; additionally, individuals participated in MET and CBT throughout the trial in addition to various self-referred group and/or individual counseling. Gabapentin and placebo were compared via a randomized double-blind treatment study. Gabapentin was titrated up to 1200 mg total daily dose over the course of 4 days and continued for a period of 12 weeks. The study participants were assessed for cannabis use (via self-report and urinary drug analysis), efficacy of medication on cannabis withdrawal symptoms, and also monitored for adverse effects. Over the course of the 12 weeks the participants exhibited a significant decrease in cannabis usage and at the 13-week follow-up the reduction of cannabis usage had sustained. Moreover, compared with placebo, the gabapentin group exhibited significant reduction in acute and persistent symptoms of cannabis withdrawal syndrome; specifically, significant reduction was noted in mood disturbance, craving, and sleep disturbance. Over the course of treatment gabapentin remained relatively well-tolerated; one participant complained of headache and dropped out of the study. Although the previously mentioned study evaluated the use of gabapentin in an adult population, primarily male, and greater duration of persistent cannabis use (compared with adolescent population), the results of this study may indicate potential for investigation in the adolescent and/or transitional age population.

Finally, further investigation needs to be carried out to investigate the risks and benefits of pharmacotherapy to treat cannabis use disorder, such as using short-term oral THC compounds (eg, dronabinol) to manage cannabis withdrawal syndrome. Additional agents that increase endocannabinoid neurotransmitter levels (eg, amandamide and 2-arachidonoylglycerol) may be used to minimize the cannabis withdrawal syndrome experienced by users. Once again, the efficacy, generalizability, and safety within the adolescent population remains to be determined.[24,25]

## SYNTHETIC CANNABINOIDS (HERBAL MARIJUANA ALTERNATIVES)

The discussion of cannabis is not complete without commentary on synthetic cannabinoids, which are herbal marijuana alternatives (eg, K2 or spice). Patients may disclose to health care providers and believe they have used marijuana when in fact the substance used is a synthetic cannabinoid. Additionally, on clinical presentation these substances are usually not identified in typical urine toxicology screenings despite the patient's clinical presentation suggesting intoxication.[8] These compounds are contained in many different vessels of produce, such as potpourri or incense, and can be purchased via Internet, local convenience stores, or gas stations. Essentially, the product to be sold contains various herbs (eg, red clover, vanilla) infused with various synthetic cannabinoid compounds. Individuals may use the substance with the expectancy of an intoxication that is similar to that of cannabis but more potent. Moreover, many of the synthetic cannabinoid compounds have been banned in 2011 and placed in the category of schedule I drugs resulting in a significant decrease in usage by approximately half since 2010.[10] Compared with 2011 in which 11.4% of adolescents reported usage this prevalence had decreased significantly in 2014% to 5.8% reported use by twelfth graders.[10] It should be noted, however, that synthetic cannabinoids remain accessible for purchase by adolescents.

There are seven major groups of synthetic cannabinoids: naphthoylindoles, naphthylmethylindoles, naphthoylpyrroles, naphthylmethilindenes, phenylacetylindoles, cyclohexylphenols, and classical cannabinoids.[26] Herbal marijuana alternatives are usually purchased as a substance that contains a combination of various herbs, multiple synthetic cannabinoids, and other additives. Synthetic cannabinoids bind to CB1 and CB2 with greater affinity compared with delta-9-THC in marijuana. Psychoactivation may take the form of anxiety, paranoia, poor eye contact, agitation, both grandiose and paranoid delusions, and also psychosis. Physiologic effects of intoxication include conjunctival injection, tachycardia, diaphoresis, and dry mouth. Although synthetic cannabinoids may not be detected by a typical hospital-administered urine drug screen (ie, rapid urine drug screen in the emergency department), there are other methods by which to detect these substances. Gas chromatography–mass spectrometry and liquid chromatography–tandem mass spectrometry are laboratory tests using blood serum samples to detect the parent synthetic cannabinoid compound and urine sample to detect the metabolites of synthetic cannabinoids. It has been suggested that these substances may be detectable up to 48 to 72 hours after usage; however, further investigation needs to be carried-out to confirm duration of action and half-life.[8]

## MEDICINAL BENEFITS

The medicinal benefits of marijuana within the human immunodeficiency virus/AIDS and cancer populations include management of neuropathic pain and nausea/emesis and also in multiple sclerosis populations in treating muscle spasticity.[22] It is important to understand that cannabis and cannabinoid ligands within the literature indicate the presence and absence of delta-9-THC, respectively. Marijuana or cannabis contains 460 active chemicals and greater than 60 cannabinoids.[22] It is important to understand that cannabis/medicinal marijuana vary in dose, potency, and chemical consistency. Furthermore, synthetic cannabinoids, namely dronabinol (marinol), is a cannabinoid that functions as a synthetic form of delta-9-THC. Other examples of cannabinoids that have been synthesized include nabilone (cesamer), similar to THC; nabiximols (sativex), which is derived from the cannabis plant and possesses an equal ratio of THC to cannabidiol concentrations within the drug formulation; and cannabidiol, a nonpsychoactive cannabinoid.[22] Current and future research continues to investigate the use of synthetic cannabinoids in the treatment of various pathologies including epilepsy, autism spectrum disorder, and cannabis use disorder to name a few. It is imperative to recognize the significant difference between cannabis used for intoxication or medicinal purposes versus the synthetic cannabinoids that have undergone rigorous scientific research investigation elucidating risks and benefits of using the substance as a pharmaceutical agent for various pathologies.

## DISCUSSION

Cannabis remains the most common illicit substance used within the adolescent population. Studies have shown that initiation of cannabis and development of cannabis use disorder result in persistent cannabis use disorder into adulthood. The persistence of cannabis use disorder negatively impacts cognitive development and has shown decreased IQ as a result of cannabis use disorder during adolescence. Furthermore, legalization of cannabis in various states may impact the perception of that population on risk of usage. These factors must be considered when creating prevention messages for adolescent populations. In terms of treatment of cannabis use disorder, MET-CBT and ACRA have shown significant reduction in cannabis usage. Additionally, new psychopharmacology studies in combination with behavioral therapy approaches (MET-CBT in combination with NAC pharmacotherapy) have shown tremendously promising results in reduction of cannabis usage within the adolescent population. Future studies need to further identify the appropriate use if any of cannabinoid agonist or cannabinoid antagonist within the adolescent population for treatment of cannabis use disorder. Neurobiologic development is ongoing into the transitional age years, and the pathology of the neurocircuitry that develops as a result of persistent cannabis use may take on a different character in an adolescent than an adult older than 35 years old who does not possess the extent of neural plasticity and neurocognitive development as in adolescence.

## REFERENCES

1. Center for Behavioral Health Statistics and Quality. Behavioral health trends in the United States: Results from the 2014 National Survey on Drug Use and Health (HHS Publication No. SMA 15–4927, NSDUH series H-50). 2015. Available at: http://www.samhsa.gov/data/. Accessed November 20, 2015.
2. Center for Behavioral Health Statistics and Quality. The Center for Behavioral Health Statistics and Quality report: profile of adolescent discharges from substance abuse treatment. Rockville (MD): Substance Abuse and Mental Health Services Administration; 2015.
3. American Psychiatric Association. Diagnostic and statistical manual of mental disorders: DSM-5. Cannabis-related disorders. Washington, DC: American Psychiatric Association; 2013. p. 509–19.
4. Budney AJ, Roffman R, Stephens RS, et al. Marijuana dependence and its treatment. Addict Sci Clin Pract 2007;4(1):4–16.
5. Substance Abuse and Mental Health Services Administration. Behavioral health barometer: United States, 2014. HHS Publication No. SMA-15-4895. Rockville (MD): Substance Abuse and Mental Health Services Administration; 2015.
6. Meier MH, Caspi A, Ambler A, et al. Persistent cannabis users show neuropsychological decline from childhood to midlife. Proc Natl Acad Sci U S A 2012; 109(40):E2657–64.
7. Solowij N, Battisti R. The chronic effects of cannabis on memory in humans: a review. Curr Drug Abuse Rev 2008;1(1):81–98.
8. Molina KM, Alegría M, Chen CN. Neighborhood context and substance use disorders: a comparative analysis of racial and ethnic groups in the United States. Drug Alcohol Depend 2012;125(Suppl 1):S35–43.
9. Volkow ND, Baler RD, Compton WM, et al. Adverse health effects of marijuana use. N Engl J Med 2014;370(23):2219–27.
10. Johnston LD, O'Malley PM, Miech RA, et al. Monitoring the future National Survey Results on Drug Use: 1975-2014: overview, key findings on adolescent drug use. Ann Arbor (MI): Institute for Social Research, The University of Michigan; 2015.
11. Greene MC, Kelly JF. The prevalence of cannabis withdrawal and its influence on adolescents' treatment response and outcomes: a 12-month prospective investigation. J Addict Med 2014;8(5):359–67.
12. Kroutil LA, Lipari R, Pemberton R. Risk and protective factors and initiation of substance use: results from the 2014 National Survey on Drug Use and Health.

National Survey on Drug Use and Health Data Review. 2015. Available at: http://www.samhsa.gov/data/. Accessed November 20, 2015.

13. Magid V, Settles R. Clinical guidelines for the detection, prevention and early intervention of adolescent substance use. Adolesc Psychiatry 2013;3(2):200–7.

14. Marshall K, Gowing L, Ali R, et al. Pharmacotherapies for cannabis dependence. Cochrane Database Syst Rev 2014;(12):CD008940.

15. Center for Behavioral Health Statistics and Quality. The Center for Behavioral Health Statistics and Quality report: a day in the life of young adults: substance use facts. Rockville (MD): Substance Abuse and Mental Health Services Administration; 2014.

16. Center for Behavioral Health Statistics and Quality. The treatment episode data set report: marijuana admissions to substance abuse treatment aged 18 to 30: early vs. adult initiation. Rockville (MD): Substance Abuse and Mental Health Services Administration; 2015.

17. Copello P, Elizabeth A, Han B, et al. Receipt of services for behavioral health problems: results from the 2014 National Survey on Drug Use and Health. National Survey on Drug Use and Health Data Review. 2015. Available at: http://www.samhsa.gov/data/. Accessed November 20, 2015.

18. Dennis M, Godley SH, Diamond G, et al. The Cannabis Youth Treatment (CYT) Study: main findings from two randomized trials. J Subst Abuse Treat 2004;27(3):197–213.

19. Kamon J, Budney A, Stanger C. A contingency management intervention for adolescent marijuana abuse and conduct problems. J Am Acad Child Adolesc Psychiatry 2005;44(6):513–21.

20. Gray KM, Carpenter MJ, Baker ML, et al. A double-blind randomized controlled trial of N-acetylcysteine in cannabis-dependent adolescents. Am J Psychiatry 2012;169(8):805–12.

21. Gray KM, Watson NL, Carpenter MJ, et al. N-acetylcysteine (NAC) in young marijuana users: an open-label pilot study. Am J Addict 2010;19(2):187–9.

22. Gray KM. New developments in understanding and treating adolescent marijuana dependence. Adolesc Psychiatry (Hilversum) 2013;3(4):297–306.

23. Mason BJ, Crean R, Goodell V, et al. A proof-of-concept randomized controlled study of gabapentin: effects on cannabis use, withdrawal and executive function deficits in cannabis-dependent adults. Neuropsychopharmacology 2012;37(7):1689–98.

24. Weinstein AM, Gorelick DA. Pharmacological treatment of cannabis dependence. Curr Pharm Des 2011;17(14):1351–8.

25. Vandrey R, Stitzer ML, Mintzer MZ, et al. The dose effects of short-term dronabinol (oral THC) maintenance in daily cannabis users. Drug Alcohol Depend 2013;128(1–2):64–70.

26. Rosenbaum CD, Carreiro SP, Babu KM. Here today, gone tomorrow... and back again? A review of herbal marijuana alternatives (K2, Spice), synthetic cathinones (bath salts), kratom, Salvia divinorum, methoxetamine, and piperazines. J Med Toxicol 2012;8(1):15–32.

# Tobacco Use Disorders

Deepa R. Camenga, MD, MHS[a],*, Jonathan D. Klein, MD, MPH[b]

## KEYWORDS

- Smoking • Tobacco products • Tobacco use disorder • Adolescent • Young adult
- Smoking cessation

## KEY POINTS

- Tobacco use is prevalent among adolescents, and alternative tobacco product (ie, electronic cigarettes and hookah) use rates are increasing.
- Adolescents with psychiatric and/or substance use disorders are at particularly high risk of experiencing tobacco dependence and having difficulty with quitting.
- Several practice guidelines recommend that clinicians ask adolescents about tobacco use and provide a strong messages regarding the importance of abstinence from all tobacco products.
- Clinical management of tobacco use consists of behavioral and pharmacologic interventions, which can be used in combination.

## INTRODUCTION/BACKGROUND

Tobacco use is a pervasive public health problem and the leading cause of preventable morbidity and mortality in the United States.[1] The treatment of adolescent cigarette smoking and tobacco use disorders, in particular, continues to be a substantial public health priority. Adolescence is a critical period for neurodevelopment, and nicotine exposure during adolescence causes addiction, sustained tobacco use into adulthood, and may have lasting adverse consequences for brain development.[1–3] Almost all (88%) adult smokers start before the age of 18, and adolescents have difficulty quitting successfully.[1] Although rates of cigarette use have decreased in the past decade, according the Center for Disease Control's 2014 National Youth Tobacco Survey, 9.2% of high school students and 2.5% of middle school students reported current (past month) cigarette use (**Fig. 1**).[4] Additionally, as rates of cigarette smoking are decreasing, rates of alternative tobacco product (including electronic cigarettes [e-cigarettes] and hookah) and dual (using cigarettes with another product) or polytobacco use (using any 3 or more products) remain prevalent.[5,6] Many adolescents are also exposed to second

Disclosures: The authors have nothing to disclose.
Funding: Funded by NIH (K12DA033012).
[a] Department of Emergency Medicine, Yale School of Medicine, 464 Congress Avenue, Suite 260, New Haven, CT 06519, USA; [b] American Academy of Pediatrics, Julius B. Richmond Center, Elk Grove Village, IL 60007, USA
* Corresponding author.
E-mail address: deepa.camenga@yale.edu

| Abbreviations | |
|---|---|
| AAP | American Academy of Pediatrics |
| DSM | Diagnostic and Statistical Manual of Mental Disorders |
| NRT | Nicotine replacement therapy |
| SLT | Smokeless tobacco |

hand tobacco smoke.[7] Adolescents with psychiatric and/or substance use disorders are at particularly high risk for becoming tobacco dependent and are even less likely to quit than other youth.

The 2012 US Surgeon General's Report "Preventing Tobacco Use among Youth and Young Adults" describes tobacco use as a "multi-determined behavior," with many biological, psychosocial, and environmental factors influencing its progression.[1] (**Box 1**). Successful prevention programs have aimed to ameliorate the impact of these factors by promoting self-efficacy and refusal skills and decreasing access to tobacco products; however, tobacco use continues to substantially impact the health and well-being of youth.[8,9] If smoking continues at the current rate among youth in this country, 5.6 million of today's Americans younger than 18 (1 out of 13 youth) will die early from a smoking-related illness.[10] This article reviews the epidemiology of tobacco use (including cigarette, alternative tobacco product, and dual/poly-tobacco use patterns) among adolescents and review the highlights of the clinical presentation, diagnosis, and management of tobacco use disorders in youth.

## EPIDEMIOLOGY
### Cigarette Use

Every day, approximately 3200 youths younger than 18 years old initiate cigarette smoking, and 700 youths begin daily smoking.[1] There has been a decrease in cigarette

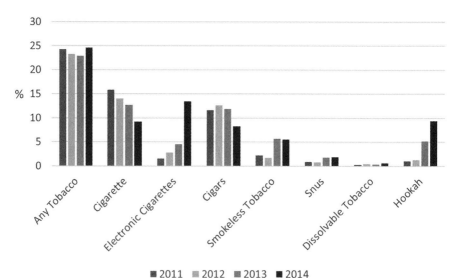

**Fig. 1.** Estimated percentage of high school students who used tobacco in the preceding 30 days, by tobacco product—National Youth Tobacco Survey, United States, 2011 to 2014. (*Adapted from* Arrazola RA, Singh T, Corey CG, et al. Tobacco use among middle and high school students - United States, 2011–2014. MMWR Morb Mortal Wkly Rep 2015;64(14):383.)

---

**Box 1**
**Risk factors for tobacco use**

- Lower socioeconomic status
- Lower levels of academic achievement
- High levels of access to tobacco products
- Lack of skills (self-efficacy, refusal skills) necessary to avoid tobacco
- Perceptions that tobacco use is normative and not harmful
- Use of tobacco by significant others and approval of tobacco use among those persons
- Lack of parental support

*From* US Department of Health and Human Services. Preventing tobacco use among youth and young adults: a report of the surgeon general. Atlanta (GA): US Department of Health and Human Services; Centers for Disease Control and Prevention; National Center for Chronic Disease Prevention and Health Promotion; Office on Smoking and Health; 2012. p. 427.

---

smoking rates over the last 40 years. The decrease in cigarette smoking is likely owing to many factors, including restrictions on advertising, taxation of cigarettes, and smoke-free laws.[10] In 2014, 9.8% of high school students and 2.5% of middle school students reported past month cigarette use. In 2013, 18.9% of 18- to 24-year-olds reported current cigarette use.[4] Historically, cigarettes have been the most common tobacco product that is used exclusively among youth (rather than in combination with another tobacco products).[6] Cigarette smoking rates differ by race/ethnicity as well as geographic regions. In 2013, the prevalence of past month cigarette smoking was higher among white students than black or Hispanic students.[11] Cigarette smoking rates are also higher among youth residing in non-metropolitan areas.[12]

### Electronic Cigarettes

E-cigarettes are currently the most commonly used tobacco product by US adolescents.[4] There are several different types of e-cigarettes, including disposable, cartridge, and tank-style e-cigarettes, and adolescents may refer to them by a variety of names including vape pens, e-pens, e-hookah, and vape sticks (**Table 1**). E-cigarette liquid ("e-juice") contain contains nicotine, propylene glycol, vegetable glycerin, flavorants, and various additives.[13] Puffing the e-cigarette ("vaping") activates a heating element in the atomizer, and the liquid in the cartridge is vaporized into a mist that is inhaled. When youth initiate e-cigarette use, they often start with a flavored e-cigarette.[14] Cartridges with nicotine typically contain 0 to 36 mg of nicotine per milliliter of solution.[15] Therefore, a 5-mL vial of an 18 mg/mL solution contains 90 mg of nicotine. If accidentally or deliberately ingested, this would dose of nicotine could result in intoxication or death.[16]

In 2014, 13.4% of high school students and 3.9% of middle school students reported current e-cigarette use.[4] From 2011 to 2014 the prevalence of ever e-cigarette use tripled among both middle school and high school students, indicating increased experimentation.[4] E-cigarettes especially appeal to cigarette smokers; however, a growing proportion of e-cigarette users are nonsmokers.[17] Leventhal and colleagues[18] demonstrated among a school-based cohort of 14-year-old high school students in Los Angeles, California that, among students who had never used a combustible tobacco product (including cigarettes), ever use of e-cigarettes at baseline (as compared with never use of e-cigarettes) was positively associated with combustible cigarette and hookah use 6 months later. These emerging findings

**Table 1**
**Electronic cigarettes**

| | |
|---|---|
| <br>Brands: Njoy, One Joy, Aer Disposable, Flavorvapes | Disposable e-cigarette<br>Cigarette-shaped device consisting of a battery and a cartridge containing an atomizer to heat a solution (with or without nicotine). Not rechargeable or refillable and is intended to be discarded after product stops producing aerosol. Also called an E-hookah. |
| <br>Brands: Blu, Greensmoke, Eonsmoke | Rechargeable e-cigarette<br>Cigarette-shaped device consisting of a battery that connects to an atomizer used to heat a solution typically containing nicotine. Often contains an element that regulates puff duration and/or how many puffs may be taken consecutively. |
| <br>Brands: Vapor King Storm, Totally Wicked Tornado | Pen-style, medium-sized rechargeable e-cigarette<br>Larger than a cigarette, often with a higher capacity battery, may contain a pre-filled cartridge or a refillable cartridge (often called a clearomizer). These devices often come with a manual switch allowing to regulate length and frequency of puffs. |
| <br>Brands: Volcano Lavatube | Tank-style, large-sized rechargeable e-cigarette<br>Much larger than a cigarette with a higher capacity battery and typically contains a large, refillable cartridge. Often contains manual switches and a battery casing for customizing battery capacity. Can be easily modified. |

*From* Grana R, Benowitz N, Glantz SA. Background paper on E-cigarettes (electronic nicotine delivery systems). Center for Tobacco Control Research and Education, University of California, San Francisco, a WHO Collaborating Center on Tobacco Control. Prepared for World Health Organization Tobacco Free Initiative. December 2013; with permission. Available at: http://pvw.escholarship.org/uc/item/13p2b72n. Accessed March 21, 2016.

contribute to the public health community's concern that e-cigarettes may serve as a gateway product to combustible tobacco use, as well as a product with unknown safety and long-term health effects.[19,20] The increasing prevalence of e-cigarette use may be attributed to heavy marketing and advertising in youth-dominated media outlets such as social networking and Internet sites, their low price, and the misperception that e-cigarettes are a safer alternative to traditional cigarettes.[21,22]

## Cigars, Cigarillos, and Little Cigars

The US Department of the Treasury defines cigars as "any roll of tobacco wrapped in leaf tobacco or in any substance containing tobacco."[23] The US Department of Treasury has classified cigars into 2 types:

1. Little cigars (weighing <3 lb per thousand);
2. Large cigars and cigarillos (weighing more than 3 lb per thousand).

Little cigars are comparable to cigarettes with regard to shape and size, they often have a filter, and adolescents may describe them as cigarettes during a clinical interview.[24]

According to the 2014 National Youth Tobacco Survey, 8.2% of high school students and 1.9% of middle school students reported current cigar use. The prevalence of current cigar use among high school males (10.8%) was approximately double that of high school females (5.5%).[4] The Centers for Disease Control and Prevention recently reported that between 2011 and 2014, cigar use decreased, which reflects the general trend of decreasing popularity of traditional combustible tobacco products among youth.

Cigar use often co-occurs with cigarette use.[25,26] The combination of cigars and cigarettes is the most common combination of dual product use among older adolescents and young adults. Similar to e-cigarettes, youth often report that cigars are appealing owing to flavors.[14]

## Smokeless Tobacco

Despite recent declines in cigarette use among youths, declines in smokeless tobacco (SLT) have stalled in recent years.[2] In the United States, popular forms of SLT have included chewing tobacco or moist snuff. Chewing tobacco is made of long strands of tobacco, whereas snuff tobacco is a fine-grained and comes in a moist blend that usually is used orally.[2]

Snus and dissolvables are novel SLT products that have become increasingly available over the last 10 years. Snus are made of non-fermented, heat-cured, finely grained tobacco and are spit-free and consumed via pouches, which are placed between the cheek and gum.[27] Snus have been used in Sweden since the early 19th century, but were introduced to the United States in 2006.[28] Snus are now marketed by major US tobacco companies with cigarette brand names (eg, Marlboro Snus, Camel Snus).[28] Dissolvables are another novel SLT that comes in pellets, strips, or sticks. They are designed to be held and dissolved in the mouth for between 3 (strips) and 30 (sticks) minutes.[29] Similar to snus, dissolvables were recently introduced in US markets and bear cigarette brand names (eg, Camel Orbs, Camel Strips).[30]

In 2014, 5.5% of high school students and 1.6% of middle school students reported current SLT use, and a majority used chew/dip. Snus and dissolvables are less popular, with 1.9% and 0.6% of high school students reporting current use, respectively. White males have the highest prevalence of SLT use as measured by multiple national surveys, including the National Survey on Drug Use and Health, Monitoring the Future, and the National Youth Tobacco Survey.[4,11,12] Similar to other tobacco products, advancing age, male cigarette smoking, and perceived friend approval, as well as male gender predict SLT use.[31,32]

### Hookah

Hookah, also known as narghile, hubble-bubble, shisha, and waterpipe, delivers a form of combustible tobacco. Commonly flavored, inhaling through the waterpipe pulls the burning tobacco's smoke through the waterpipe's water reservoir and then through a tube to which the mouthpiece is attached. Many adolescents believe that hookah smoking is relatively safe.[33] Compared with the smoke from a single cigarette, the smoke from one hookah session contains up to 40 times the tar, 2 times the nicotine, 10 times the carbon monoxide and 30 to 50 times the carcinogenic polycyclic aromatic hydrocarbons.[33–35]

In 2014, 5.4% of high school students and 1.3% of middle school students reported current hookah use,[4] with rates increasing between 2011 and 2014. Hookah use increases with age and has increased in popularity among young adults. A survey of a national sample of young adults found that 25% of the sample had ever used hookah and 4% reported use in the past 30 days.[26] Predictors of hookah smoking in college and high school students include peer pressure/social acceptability, the perception that hookah is not harmful or addictive, the presence of a family member who uses hookah, and curiosity.[26]

### Dual Use and Polytobacco Use

Rates of dual and polytobacco use are increasing. In 2012, 6.7% of middle and high school students reported use of only one tobacco product, while 3.6% reported use of 2 tobacco products and 4.3% reported use of 3 or more tobacco products.[6] In 2014, 13% of youth report using 2 or more tobacco products in the past month.[6] Compared with those who exclusively use cigarettes, those who use cigarettes and any other form of tobacco are more likely to be male, have greater receptivity to tobacco advertising, and are more likely to use flavored tobacco products.[6] Dual use of e-cigarettes and cigarettes in particular is also associated with the use of alcohol and other drugs, rebelliousness, sensation seeking, and behavioral dysregulation.[36] Polytobacco use is additionally associated black, non-Hispanic ethnicity, living with someone who uses tobacco, and perceived prevalence of peers using tobacco.[6]

### Comorbidity with Mental Health or Developmental Disorders

Adolescents with mental health or developmental disorders may be particularly vulnerable to tobacco use. This comorbidity may be explained by a common vulnerability to both psychiatric disorders and smoking (familial/genetic or environmental), the need for self-medication, and/or common neurobiological alterations.[1] Although the link between mental health disorders and tobacco use has been described extensively in adults, there are few data describing the association among youth. Among adolescents receiving inpatient psychiatric treatment, the prevalence of cigarette of smoking has been reported to be as high as 60%.[37] A 2002 review by Upadhyaya and colleagues[38] found that adolescent cigarette smoking is highly associated with disorders involving disruptive behavior (such as oppositional defiant disorder, conduct disorder, and attention deficit hyperactivity disorder), major depressive disorders, and drug and alcohol use. More recently, a longitudinal study of 814 adolescent lifetime cigarette smokers assessed the presence of psychiatric disorders with the diagnostic interview schedule for children version IV.[39,40] Adolescents and their parents completed 5 waves of data over 2 years. Overall, 33.9% reported any psychiatric disorder (**Table 2**). Additionally, 60.5% of adolescents meeting *Diagnostic and Statistical*

**Table 2**
Rate of adolescent lifetime psychiatric disorders and nicotine dependence

|  | By Wave 5 | |
|---|---|---|
|  | Baseline% | Total% |
| Nicotine dependence[b] | | |
| Ever 1+ criterion | 27.9 | 53.7 |
| Ever 3+ criteria | 10.4 | 26.1 |
| Total $n \leq$ | (714) | (814) |
| Anxiety[a] | | |
| Social phobia | 3.7 | 6.3 |
| Panic | — | — |
| Attacks, no disorder | 2.2 | 3.8 |
| Disorder | 2.6 | 3.4 |
| Generalized anxiety | 2.3 | 4.1 |
| Any anxiety | 8.6 | 14.1 |
| Mood[b] | | |
| Major depression | 14.5 | 17.9 |
| Dysthymia | 1.0 | 1.7 |
| Any mood | 15.0 | 18.8 |
| Disruptive[a] | | |
| Attention-deficit hyperactivity | 2.1 | 2.9 |
| Oppositional defiant | 11.4 | 14.2 |
| Conduct | 14.2 | 21.2 |
| Any disruptive | 21.4 | 29.5 |
| Any psychiatric disorder | 33.9 | 43.2 |
| Total $n$ | (814) | (814) |

[a] Baseline: wave 3 reports.
[b] Baseline: wave 1 reports.
*Adapted from* Griesler PC, Hu MC, Schaffran C, et al. Comorbid psychiatric disorders and nicotine dependence in adolescence. Addiction 2011;106(5):1014; with permission.

*Manual of Mental Disorders*, fourth edition (DSM-IV), criteria for nicotine dependence reported a history of a psychiatric disorders, whereas only 30.3% of adolescents with 0 symptoms of nicotine dependence reported any psychiatric disorder.

Data regarding the temporality of psychiatric disorders and tobacco use remains equivocal.[1] The aforementioned longitudinal cohort of adolescent smokers found that psychiatric disorders (including mood disorders) preceded the onset of tobacco use (1.3–2.4 years lower) and first nicotine dependence criterion (2.5–3.7 years lower).[40] However, a 2009 systematic review of longitudinal studies examining association between depression and smoking in adolescents concluded that the relationship between depression and smoking is bidirectional.[41]

There are only a few studies that examine the co-occurence of psychiatric disorders with dual use or alternative tobacco product use. A longitudinal cohort study of 486 high school students who reported past month cigarette smoking found that cigar, cigarillo, and little cigar users showed higher levels of depression, anxiety, and antisocial behavior than nonusers, even after adjustment for frequency of cigarette smoking.[42]

### Comorbidity with Substance Use Disorders

Use of illicit drugs or alcohol greatly increase the likelihood of tobacco use and dependence among adolescents. Studies have found that up to 80% of youth with substance use disorders report past month tobacco use, many report daily smoking, and many become highly dependent, long-term tobacco users.[38,43] For example, a recent study of 34 substance use treatment programs found that 48% of the 1062 adolescents included met criteria for tobacco dependence, 58% reported weekly tobacco use, and the sample reported a mean of 5 cigarettes smoked per day.[44] Several studies have demonstrated that levels of tobacco use persist despite decreases in alcohol or drug use during substance use treatment,[43,45] indicating the targeted interventions for smoking cessation are needed for youth receiving substance use treatment.

## CLINICAL PRESENTATION

The general examination may reveal signs that increase the probability of tobacco use. For example, the presence of smoke-odored clothing, a bottle for chew/dip spit, or cigarette packs may clue the clinician to ask more detailed questions about tobacco use. Adolescents rarely present with clinical signs that are present in adults, such as stained teeth or fingernails, wrinkles, or a hoarse voice. Adolescents in nicotine withdrawal may present with irritability, anxiety, and agitation, and may ask "how long will I be here (because I need to smoke a cigarette)?"

Tobacco contains the psychoactive drug nicotine, which is central nervous system stimulant. The immediate effects of nicotine administration are tachycardia, hypertension, increased respiration, enhanced memory storage, improved concentration, and appetite suppression. Nicotine produces withdrawal symptoms about 1 hour after the last dose. Withdrawal symptoms are not life threatening, are usually self-limited, and include irritability, annoyance, anxiety, and cravings for nicotine.

## DIAGNOSIS

The primary method of diagnosing tobacco use is through the confidential psychiatric or medical interview. The type of tobacco product used, and the frequency and intensity of use is gauged through adolescent self-report. The 2015 American Academy of Pediatrics' (AAP) *Clinical Practice Policy to Protect Children from Tobacco, Nicotine and Tobacco Smoke* endorses several questions from the American College of Chest Physicians Tobacco Treatment Toolkit to screen for and characterize adolescent tobacco use (**Box 2**).[20] Of note, the clinician should specifically ask about noncigarette

---

**Box 2**
**Questions to screen for the severity of tobacco use in adolescents**

- Do any of your friends use tobacco? Do you friends use e-cigarettes, e-hookah, or vape? *(This question may help open the conversation, especially for younger adolescents.)*

- Have you ever tried a tobacco product? Which tobacco products have you used? Have you tried an e-cigarette, e-hookah, or vape?

- How many times have you tried (name of tobacco product)?

- How often do you use (name of tobacco product)?

*Adapted from* Farber HJ, Walley SC, Groner JA, et al; Section on Tobacco Control. Clinical practice policy to protect children from tobacco, nicotine, and tobacco smoke. Pediatrics 2015;136(5):1008–17.

tobacco products, such as hookah and e-cigarettes, because adolescents may not immediately identify them as tobacco products.[20]

Tobacco Use Disorder is a diagnosis in the fifth edition of the DSM (DSM-5) assigned to individuals who are dependent on the drug nicotine. The DSM-5 replaces the DSM-IV-TR categories of nicotine abuse and dependence with an overarching category called tobacco use disorder. The criteria for DSM-5 tobacco use disorder are the same as those for other substance use disorders. However, adolescents who smoke rarely experience significant social/occupational dysfunction owing to tobacco use, because many of their friends and family members may smoke, thus normalizing the behavior.

Clinicians may choose to assess the severity of cigarette smoking dependence through use of the Hooked on Nicotine Checklist or the modified Fagerstrom Test for Nicotine Dependence (both available through the Alcohol and Drug Abuse Institute-University of Washington Library http://lib.adai.washington.edu/). Adolescents may score positively on these assessments (indicating symptoms of tobacco dependence) soon after they start smoking intermittently, and do not need to be daily or long-term smokers to report signs of addiction.[29,46] Data from the 2012 National Youth Tobacco Survey demonstrated that adolescent tobacco users reported symptoms of dependence even with low levels of tobacco use.[30]

Breath carbon monoxide can be used to assess the presence of smoking in the last 24 hours; however, in practice, it is rarely used outside of intensive smoking cessation treatment programs (such as contingency management–based programs). Cotinine, a metabolite of nicotine, can be found in urine, saliva, and blood for up to 7 days after tobacco use, but is rarely used in clinical practice to guide treatment.

According to the 2006 American Psychiatric Association's *Practice Guideline for Treatment of Patients with Substance Use Disorders*,[47] additional points should be incorporated into the assessment of tobacco use in patients with psychiatric disorders to determine the appropriate time for treatment initiation (**Box 3**).

In the case of severe psychiatric comorbidity, the clinician must weigh the risks of benefits of initiating or delaying treatment for tobacco dependence.[20,47] Regardless of the timing, all adolescents with comorbid psychiatric disorders should be offered the opportunity to participate in smoking cessation treatment at some point during their psychiatric treatment course.

## BRIEF SUMMARY OF CLINICAL MANAGEMENT

Many professional organizations endorse the importance of cigarette and tobacco cessation counseling. The 2006 American Psychiatric Association Substance Use

---

**Box 3**
**Considerations for patients with co-occuring psychiatric disorders**

- Psychiatric reasons for concern about whether this is the best time for cessation; that is, new therapies, patient currently in crisis, other pressing psychiatric problem.
- The likelihood that cessation would worsen the non–nicotine-related psychiatric disorder.
- Signs or symptoms of other undiagnosed psychiatric or substance use disorders that might interfere with efforts to quit tobacco use.
- The patient's current ability to use coping skills for cessation.

*From* Kleber HD, Weiss RD, Anton RF, et al. Treatment of patients with substance use disorders, second edition. American Psychiatric Association. Am J Psychiatry 2006;163(8 Suppl):73.

Treatment Guidelines encourage mental health clinicians to assess smoking status with all patients and to assist smokers in quitting.[47] Additionally, both the 2008 Public Health Service's Guideline[48] and the 2015 AAP policy statement on tobacco[20] recommend that all clinicians ask adolescent and young adult patients about tobacco use and provide a strong message regarding the importance of total abstinence from tobacco use. These guidelines acknowledge that smoking cessation may be more difficult for smokers with psychiatric disorders, and treatment may need to be more intensive.

The clinical management of tobacco use consists of behavioral and pharmacologic interventions, which can be used in combination.[48] In general, behaviorally based programs for smoking cessation in adolescents may be most beneficial for adolescents with mild degrees of dependence. The addition of pharmacotherapy can be considered for moderate to severely tobacco-dependent adolescents who want to stop smoking.[20]

### Behavioral Interventions for Tobacco Use Disorders

Although a comprehensive review of the behavioral interventions for tobacco use disorders is beyond the scope of this review, several systematic reviews have outlined the evidence base surrounding these interventions for adolescents. Stanton and Grimshaw's 2013 Cochrane Review "*Tobacco cessation interventions for young people*" found that most studies used complex interventions that incorporated strategies from multiple health behavior theories.[49] Common modalities included motivational enhancement, cognitive–behavioral therapy, and stage-based interventions using the transtheoretical model. The metaanalysis demonstrated that transtheoretical model resulted in a pooled risk ratio of 1.56 at 1 year (95% CI, 1.21–2.01) for cessation, motivational enhancement resulted in an risk ratio of 1.60 (95% CI, 1.28–2.01), and trials of cognitive–behavioral therapy did not result in statistically significant changes in abstinence.

The US Public Health Service 2008 Guideline and the AAP 2015 Clinical Practice Policy recommends brief counseling for treating adolescent smokers.[20,48] The guidelines recommend the 5A model of care (Ask, Advise, Assess, Assist, Arrange follow-up). In this model, the clinician is encouraged to Ask all adolescents about tobacco use and about secondhand smoke exposure. Next, the clinician should Advise cessation through use of a strong message describing the personal health risks for the patient and the benefits of quitting. Advice should also address protection of oneself and others from secondhand smoke exposure. Through use of the questions/measures described, the clinician should then Assess level of nicotine addiction, as well as readiness to make a quit attempt and/or initiate treatment. Then the clinician should assist the patient in formulating an appropriate tobacco cessation plan, which could include use of behavioral treatments and pharmacotherapy. Last, clinicians should Arrange for follow-up within 2 weeks wherein they discuss the patient's progress with the quit attempt.

### Pharmacotherapy

Nicotine replacement therapy (NRT; including patch, gum, inhaler and nasal spray), bupropion, and varenicline are approved for the treatment of smoking cessation in adults (see **Table 3**).[50] However, there are limited studies that evaluate the efficacy of various pharmacotherapies for adolescent smoking cessation; therefore, the Food and Drug Administration's labeling indicates these medications for adults older than 18 years.

**Table 3**
**Smoking cessation pharmacotherapy**

| Medication | Dosing | Initial Treatment Duration | Adverse Effects | Contraindications | Available | Studied in Adolescents? |
|---|---|---|---|---|---|---|
| *Nicotine replacement therapy* | | | | | | |
| Nicotine patch | If >10 cigarettes/d → 21-mg patch daily; if ≤10 cigarettes/d → 14-mg patch. | 8 wk | Local skin reactions, insomnia and/or vivid dreams | Pregnancy,* severe skin conditions | OTC | Yes |
| Nicotine gum | 4-mg piece if smoking ≥25 cigarettes/d, otherwise 2-mg piece. Use every 1–2 h PRN. | 12 wk | Mouth soreness, hiccups, dyspepsia, jaw ache | Pregnancy, unstable angina or arrhythmias | OTC | Yes |
| Nicotine lozenge | 4-mg lozenge if smoking first cigarette within 30 min of waking, otherwise 2-mg lozenge. Use every 1–2 h PRN. | 12 wk | Nausea, hiccups, heartburn, headache, cough | Pregnancy, unstable angina or arrhythmias | OTC | No |
| Nicotine inhaler | 1 puff PRN, up to 6–16 cartridges/d. | 24 wk | Mouth and throat irritation, cough, rhinitis | Pregnancy, severe reactive airway disease, unstable angina or arrhythmias | Rx | No |
| Nicotine nasal spray | 1 spray each nostril, every 1–2 h PRN. | 12–24 wk | Nasal irritation, nasal congestion, change in sense of smell and taste | Pregnancy, severe reactive airway disease, severe nasal disease, unstable angina or arrhythmias | Rx | Yes |
| *Nonnicotine replacement therapies* | | | | | | |
| Varenicline | 0.5 mg daily × 3 d, then 0.5 mg twice a day × 4 d, then 1 mg twice a day. | 12 wk | Nausea, insomnia, vivid dreams; rare cases of agitation, changes in behavior, and suicidal ideation | Pregnancy, use cautiously in patients with psychiatric illness | Rx | No |
| Bupropion sustained release | 150 mg daily × 3 d, then increase to 150 mg twice a day. | 7–12 wk | Insomnia, dry mouth; lowers seizure threshold | Pregnancy, seizure disorder, eating disorder. Use of an MAO inhibitor in the past 14 d | Rx | Yes |

*Abbreviations:* MAO, monoamine oxide; OTC, over the counter; PRN, as needed; Rx, prescription.

\* The 2008 Tobacco Treatment Guidelines suggest that pregnant smokers should be encouraged to quit without medication and should be offered intensive behavioral counseling support at the first prenatal visit and throughout the course of the pregnancy.[53] Nicotine replacement products are FDA pregnancy class D agents. Varenicline and bupropion are FDA pregnancy class C agents.

*Adapted from* Baldassarri SR, Toll BA, Leone FT. A comprehensive approach to tobacco dependence interventions. J Allergy Clin Immunol Pract 2015;3(4):484; with permission.

In 2013, the Cochrane Group for Systemic Reviews reviewed studies evaluating the efficacy of interventions to promote smoking cessation in youth.[51] The review identified 1 study evaluating the efficacy of NRT in adolescents who met the inclusion criteria of being a randomized controlled trial/controlled trial. This double-blind, double-dummy, randomized trial of 120 adolescent daily smokers compared nicotine patch (21 mg), nicotine gum (2 and 4 mg), and a placebo patch and gum. All study participants also received cognitive–behavioral group therapy. Intent-to-treat analyses of all randomized participants showed biochemically confirmed prolonged abstinence rates of 18% for the active patch group, 6.5% for the active gum group, and 2.5% for the placebo group, with a statistically significant difference between the patch and placebo group.[52] A metaanalysis of 8 studies evaluating the efficacy of NRT for smoking cessation in adolescents found that abstinence rates ranged from 6.5% for the nicotine gum to 28% for the nicotine patch at 10 weeks; however, these abstinence rates were not significant when compared with placebo.[53] Compliance with NRT varied, ranging from 29% to 85%; however, adverse event rates were low.

The 2013 Cochrane Review also identified 2 studies evaluating bupropion for adolescent smoking cessation and did not find a benefit of this pharmacotherapy.[51] Although varenicline is approved for use in adults greater than 18 years (and should be used with caution in adults with co-occuring psychiatric disorders) there are no current published studies of its use in adolescents.[54] Given this evidence, the AAP recently recommended that clinicians should consider using NRT for adolescents with moderate to severe substance use disorder.[20] Additionally, given the lack of data regarding the safety and efficacy of e-cigarettes, the AAP also recommends that providers advise adolescents that these products should not be used for tobacco cessation.[20]

## CONSIDERATIONS WITH CO-OCCURING PSYCHIATRIC DISEASE OR SUBSTANCE USE DISORDERS

There are few published studies evaluating smoking cessation interventions in adolescents with co-occuring psychiatric or substance use disorders. A metaanalysis of smoking cessation trials in adults with depression, found that the addition of psychosocial mood management to standard smoking cessation treatment improved long term abstinence rates in adults with both current and past depression.[55] However, there are no systematic evaluations of smoking cessation treatments in adolescents with depression. A randomized trial of 191 adolescents hospitalized in an inpatient psychiatric unit found similar rates of abstinence when comparing motivational interviewing and brief advice for treating nicotine dependence.[56] At 12 months, quit rates were 14% and 9% for the motivational intervention and brief advice conditions, respectively.

A systematic review of 17 studies evaluating smoking cessation treatments among adults in substance use treatment or recovery found that NRT, behavioral support, and combination approaches seemed to increase smoking abstinence in those treated for substance use disorders.[57] However, similar to psychiatric disorders there are few studies that evaluate effective interventions for adolescents with substance use disorders. For example, a controlled efficacy study of 54 adolescents in substance abuse treatment compared a 6-session tobacco cessation intervention with a wait-list control group. Adolescents receiving the tobacco cessation intervention had significantly greater point prevalence abstinence at 3-month follow-up than did those in the control group, in addition to fewer days of substance use.[58] Overall, studies in adults and adolescents have shown that tobacco cessation during substance use treatment is associated with increased abstinence from other substances, decreased substance use overall, and lowered risk for relapse of alcohol and drugs.[59,60]

## SUMMARY

Despite great advances in tobacco control, tobacco use and secondhand smoke exposure continues to substantially impact youth. Rates of cigarette use are decreasing; however, use of e-cigarettes, hookah, and other alternative tobacco products are increasing. Youth with psychiatric or substance use disorders are particularly vulnerable to develop tobacco use disorders. All clinicians should screen adolescents for all forms of tobacco use, and provide behavioral and, when indicated, pharmacologic support for quitting. There is a small body of literature evaluating smoking cessation interventions in youth with psychiatric or substance use disorders, and future research should aim to refine smoking cessation techniques for this important population. Given the large body of evidence supporting the deleterious health effects of tobacco use during adolescence, clinicians should give a strong message on the importance of tobacco abstinence.

## REFERENCES

1. US Department of Health and Human Services. Preventing tobacco use among youth and young adults: a report of the surgeon general. Atlanta (GA): US Department of Health and Human Services; Centers for Disease Control and Prevention; National Center for Chronic Disease Prevention and Health Promotion; Office on Smoking and Health; 2012.
2. Smith RF, McDonald CG, Bergstrom HC, et al. Adolescent nicotine induces persisting changes in development of neural connectivity. Neurosci Biobehav Rev 2015;55:432–43.
3. Fuhrmann D, Knoll LJ, Blakemore SJ. Adolescence as a sensitive period of brain development. Trends Cogn Sci 2015;19(10):558–66.
4. Arrazola RA, Singh T, Corey CG, et al. Tobacco use among middle and high school students - United States, 2011-2014. MMWR Morb Mortal Wkly Rep 2015;64(14):381–5.
5. Arrazola RA, Dube SR, Kaufmann RB, et al. Tobacco use among middle and high school students United States, 2000-2009. MMWR Morb Mortal Wkly Rep 2010; 59(33):1063–8.
6. Lee YO, Hebert CJ, Nonnemaker JM, et al. Youth tobacco product use in the United States. Pediatrics 2015;135(3):409–15.
7. Homa DM, Neff LJ, King BA, et al. Vital signs: disparities in nonsmokers' exposure to secondhand smoke–United States, 1999-2012. MMWR Morb Mortal Wkly Rep 2015;64(4):103–8.
8. Thomas RE, McLellan J, Perera R. School-based programmes for preventing smoking. Cochrane Database Syst Rev 2013;(4):CD001293.
9. Grucza RA, Plunk AD, Hipp PR, et al. Long-term effects of laws governing youth access to tobacco. Am J Public Health 2013;103(8):1493–9.
10. US Department of Health and Human Services. The health consequences of smoking- 50 years of progress: a report of the surgeon general. Atlanta (GA): US Department of Health and Human Services; Centers for Disease Control and Prevention; National Center for Chronic Disease Prevention and Health Promotion; Office on Smoking and Health; 2014.
11. Kann L, Kinchen S, Shanklin SL, et al. Youth risk behavior surveillance–United States, 2013. MMWR Surveill Summ 2014;63(Suppl 4):1–168.

12. Johnston LD, O'Malley PM, Bachman JG, et al. Subgroup trends among adolescents in the use of various licit and illicit drugs, 1975-2013 (monitoring the future occasional paper 81). Ann Arbor (MI): Institute of Social Research; The University of Michigan; 2014.

13. Grana R, Glantz SA. Background paper on E-cigarettes (electronic nicotine delivery systems). Available at: http://escholarship.org/uc/item/13p2b72n2013. Accessed October 20, 2015.

14. Ambrose BK, Day HR, Rostron B, et al. Flavored tobacco product use among us youth aged 12-17 years, 2013-2014. JAMA 2015;314(17):1871–3.

15. Cameron JM, Howell DN, White JR, et al. Variable and potentially fatal amounts of nicotine in e-cigarette nicotine solutions. Tob Control 2014;23(1):77–8.

16. Hajek P, Etter J-F, Benowitz N, et al. Electronic cigarettes: review of use, content, safety, effects on smokers, and potential for harm and benefit. Addiction 2014; 109(11):1801–10.

17. Bunnell RE, Agaku IT, Arrazola RA, et al. Intentions to smoke cigarettes among never-smoking US middle and high school electronic cigarette users: national Youth Tobacco Survey, 2011-2013. Nicotine Tob Res 2015;17(2):228–35.

18. Leventhal AM, Strong DR, Kirkpatrick MG, et al. Association of electronic cigarette use with initiation of combustible tobacco product smoking in early adolescence. JAMA 2015;314(7):700–7.

19. Grana RA. Electronic cigarettes: a new nicotine gateway? J Adolesc Health 2013; 52:135–6.

20. Farber HJ, Walley SC, Groner JA, et al, Section on Tobacco Control. Clinical practice policy to protect children from tobacco, nicotine, and tobacco smoke. Pediatrics 2015;136(5):1008–17.

21. Ambrose BK, Rostron BL, Johnson SE, et al. Perceptions of the relative harm of cigarettes and e-cigarettes among U.S. youth. Am J Prev Med 2014;47(2 Suppl 1):S53–60.

22. Kong G, Morean ME, Cavallo DA, et al. Reasons for electronic cigarette experimentation and discontinuation among adolescents and young adults. Nicotine Tob Res 2015;17(7):847–54.

23. U.S. Department of Treasury, Alcohol and Tobacco Tax Trade Bureau. Available at: http://www.ttb.gov/tobacco/tobacco-products.shtml. Accessed March 23, 2016.

24. Delnevo CD, Hrywna M. "A whole 'nother smoke" or a cigarette in disguise: how RJ Reynolds reframed the image of little cigars. Am J Public Health 2007;97(8): 1368–75.

25. Cohn A, Cobb CO, Niaura RS, et al. The other combustible products: prevalence and correlates of little cigar/cigarillo use among cigarette smokers. Nicotine Tob Res 2015;17(12):1473–81.

26. Villanti AC, Cobb CO, Cohn AM, et al. Correlates of hookah use and predictors of hookah trial in U.S. young adults. Am J Prev Med 2015;48(6):742–6.

27. Galanti MR, Rosendahl I, Wickholm S. The development of tobacco use in adolescence among "snus starters" and "cigarette starters": an analysis of the Swedish "BROMS" cohort. Nicotine Tob Res 2008;10(2):315–23.

28. Mejia AB, Ling PM. Tobacco industry consumer research on smokeless tobacco users and product development. Am J Public Health 2010;100(1):78–87.

29. DiFranza JR, Coleman M, St Cyr D. A comparison of the advertising and Accessibility of cigars, cigarettes, chewing tobacco, and Loose tobacco. Prev Med 1999;29(5):321–6.

30. Apelberg BJ, Corey CG, Hoffman AC, et al. Symptoms of tobacco dependence among middle and high school tobacco users: results from the 2012 national youth tobacco survey. Am J Prev Med 2014;47(2, Supplement 1):S4–14.

31. Tomar SL, Hatsukami DK. Perceived risk of harm from cigarettes or smokeless tobacco among U.S. high school seniors. Nicotine Tob Res 2007;9(11):1191–6.

32. Agaku IT, Ayo-Yusuf OA, Vardavas CI, et al. Use of conventional and novel smokeless tobacco products among US adolescents. Pediatrics 2013;132(3): e578–86.

33. Eissenberg T, Shihadeh A. Waterpipe tobacco and cigarette smoking: direct comparison of toxicant exposure. Am J Prev Med 2009;37(6):518–23.

34. Sepetdjian E, Shihadeh A, Saliba NA. Measurement of 16 polycyclic aromatic hydrocarbons in narghile waterpipe tobacco smoke. Food Chem Toxicol 2008; 46(5):1582–90.

35. Shihadeh A, Saleh R. Polycyclic aromatic hydrocarbons, carbon monoxide, "tar", and nicotine in the mainstream smoke aerosol of the narghile water pipe. Food Chem Toxicol 2005;43(5):655–61.

36. Wills TA, Knight R, Williams RJ, et al. Risk factors for exclusive e-cigarette use and dual e-cigarette use and tobacco use in adolescents. Pediatrics 2015; 135(1):e43–51.

37. Ramsey SE, Brown RA, Strong DR, et al. Cigarette smoking among adolescent psychiatric inpatients: prevalence and correlates. Ann Clin Psychiatry 2002; 14(3):149–53.

38. Upadhyaya HP, Deas D, Brady KT, et al. Cigarette smoking and psychiatric comorbidity in children and adolescents. J Am Acad Child Adolesc Psychiatry 2002;41(11):1294–305.

39. Shaffer D, Fisher P, Lucas CP, et al. NIMH Diagnostic Interview Schedule for Children Version IV (NIMH DISC-IV): description, differences from previous versions, and reliability of some common diagnoses. J Am Acad Child Adolesc Psychiatry 2000;39(1):28–38.

40. Griesler PC, Hu MC, Schaffran C, et al. Comorbid psychiatric disorders and nicotine dependence in adolescence. Addiction 2011;106(5):1010–20.

41. Chaiton MO, Cohen JE, O'Loughlin J, et al. A systematic review of longitudinal studies on the association between depression and smoking in adolescents. BMC Public Health 2009;9:356.

42. Schuster RM, Hertel AW, Mermelstein R. Cigar, cigarillo, and little cigar use among current cigarette-smoking adolescents. Nicotine Tob Res 2013;15(5):925–31.

43. Cole J, Stevenson E, Walker R, et al. Tobacco use and psychiatric comorbidity among adolescents in substance abuse treatment. J Subst Abuse Treat 2012; 43(1):20–9.

44. Coleman-Cowger VH, Catlin ML. Changes in tobacco use patterns among adolescents in substance abuse treatment. J Subst Abuse Treat 2013;45(2):227–34.

45. Shelef K, Diamond GS, Diamond GM, et al. Changes in tobacco Use among adolescent smokers in substance abuse treatment. Psychol Addict Behav 2009;23(2):355–61.

46. Scragg R, Wellman RJ, Laugesen M, et al. Diminished autonomy over tobacco can appear with the first cigarettes. Addict Behav 2008;33(5):689–98.

47. Kleber HD, Weiss RD, Anton RF, et al. Treatment of patients with substance use disorders, second edition. American Psychiatric Association. Am J Psychiatry 2006;163(8 Suppl):5–82.

48. Fiore MC, Jaen CR, Baker TB, et al. Treating tobacco use and dependence: 2008 update. Clinical practice guideline. Rockville (MD): US Department of Health and Human Services; Public Health Services; 2008.
49. Stanton W, Baade P, Moffatt J. Predictors of smoking cessation processes among secondary school students. Subst Use Misuse 2006;41(13):1683–94.
50. Baldassarri SR, Toll BA, Leone FT. A comprehensive approach to tobacco dependence interventions. J Allergy Clin Immunol Pract 2015;3(4):481–8.
51. Stanton A, Grimshaw G. Tobacco cessation interventions for young people. Cochrane Database Syst Rev 2013;(8):CD003289.
52. Moolchan ET, Robinson ML, Ernst M, et al. Safety and efficacy of the nicotine patch and gum for the treatment of adolescent tobacco addiction. Pediatrics 2005;115(4):e407–14.
53. King JL, Pomeranz JL, Merten JW. A systematic review and meta-evaluation of adolescent smoking cessation interventions that utilized nicotine replacement therapy. Add Behav 2015;52:39–45.
54. Bailey SR, Crew EE, Riske EC, et al. Efficacy and tolerability of pharmacotherapies to aid smoking cessation in adolescents. Paediatr Drugs 2012;14(2):91–108.
55. van der Meer RM, Willemsen MC, Smit F, et al. Smoking cessation interventions for smokers with current or past depression. Cochrane Database Syst Rev 2013;(8):CD006102.
56. Brown RA, Ramsey SE, Strong DR, et al. Effects of motivational interviewing on smoking cessation in adolescents with psychiatric disorders. Tob Control 2003;12(Suppl 4):IV3–10.
57. Thurgood SL, McNeill A, Clark-Carter D, et al. A systematic review of smoking cessation interventions for adults in substance abuse treatment or recovery. Nicotine Tob Res 2015. http://dx.doi.org/10.1093/ntr/ntv127.
58. Myers MG, Brown SA. A controlled study of a cigarette smoking cessation intervention for adolescents in substance abuse treatment. Psychol Addict Behav 2005;19(2):230–3.
59. de Dios MA, Vaughan EL, Stanton CA, et al. Adolescent tobacco use and substance abuse treatment outcomes. J Subst Abuse Treat 2009;37(1):17–24.
60. Prochaska JJ, Delucchi K, Hall SM. A meta-analysis of smoking cessation interventions with individuals in substance abuse treatment or recovery. J Consult Clin Psychol 2004;72(6):1144–56.

# Stimulant Use Disorders

Taryn M. Park, MD*, William F. Haning III, MD

## KEYWORDS

- Adolescents • Substance use • Stimulant use disorder • Methamphetamine
- Diagnosis • Assessment

## KEY POINTS

- Compared with other illicit substances, stimulants are not commonly used by adolescents; however, they represent a serious concern regarding substance use among youths.
- Methamphetamine use among adolescents and young adults is a serious health concern with potentially long-term physical, cognitive, and psychiatric consequences.
- Brain development and the effects of misusing stimulants align such that usage in adolescents may be more dangerous than during adulthood.

## INTRODUCTION AND EPIDEMIOLOGY

Stimulants encompass a wide range of substances. Although many stimulants have unique properties, this article focuses on methamphetamine as a model of stimulant use in youths. Some information on cocaine and prescription stimulants is also discussed as they present a pertinent subgroup. Although illicit stimulants are not the most common drug of choice among adolescents, its impact on neurodevelopment, future substance use, and association with other high-risk behaviors make it important to consider. Data from the Substance Abuse and Mental Health Services Administration (SAMHSA) revealed that in 2013 there were 144,000 persons aged 12 years and older who had used methamphetamine for the first time within the past 12 months, with 18.9 years old as the average age of first use. SAMHSA identified 601,000 persons who used cocaine for the first time and 603,000 persons who tried nonprescribed stimulants. Although the trends in usage have remained relatively stable in the past decade, these numbers are still concerning for providers working with youths.[1]

   Data from the Monitoring the Future Study assessed drug use among eighth, tenth, and twelfth graders. Statistics from 2014 indicate that lifetime use of methamphetamines as well as past-year use has declined in eighth and tenth graders. Unfortunately

No conflicts to declare.
Department of Psychiatry, John A. Burns School of Medicine, University of Hawaii, 1356 Lusitana Street, 4th Floor, Honolulu, HI 96813, USA
* Corresponding author.
E-mail address: Taryn.Park@seattlechildrens.org

lifetime use and past-year usage increased from 2013 to 2014 for twelfth graders. With regard to cocaine use, there seems to be an overall downward trend in lifetime and past-year use across all 3 age groups since 2011. There are similar trends for other stimulants, such as cigarettes, smokeless tobacco, and crack cocaine. In reviewing past-year use of amphetamine and dextroamphetamine (Adderall) and methylphenidate hydrochloride (Ritalin), the trends are more variable. Adderall use among eighth graders is lower than it has been in the past 3 years; however, use has increased in tenth graders. For twelfth graders, lifetime Adderall use continues on a downward trend but current lifetime use is still higher than that recorded in 2011. Ritalin use seems to have a more consistent decline across all age groups over the past 3 years.[2]

## BRIEF PHARMACOLOGY OF AMPHETAMINE, METHAMPHETAMINE, PRESCRIPTION STIMULANTS, AND COCAINE
### Amphetamine

The primary pharmacologic use of amphetamine is for its central nervous system effects. It has US Food and Drug Administration approval for treatment of narcolepsy and attention-deficit/hyperactivity disorder (ADHD). Amphetamine acts on the neuronal dopamine transporter (DAT) and the vesicular monoamine transporter 2 (VMAT2), causing release of biogenic amines from their storage in vesicles at nerve terminals, resulting in increased availability. The toxicity of amphetamine is variable. Severe reactions can occur at doses of 30 mg, but doses as large as 400 to 500 mg are not necessarily lethal.[3]

### Methamphetamine

Methamphetamine is closely related to amphetamine and ephedrine and belongs to a class called phenothylamines.[3] It can be produced from readily available over-the-counter cold medications, such as ephedrine and pseudoephedrine.[4] Methamphetamine is a sympathomimetic amine, with stimulant, anorexiant, euphoric, and hallucinogenic effects. It has been used for its stimulant properties to improve alertness and decrease fatigue. Current indications include ADHD, short-term treatment of obesity, and off-label use in the treatment of narcolepsy.[3]

Methamphetamine acts as an indirect agonist, causing the release of catecholamines from presynaptic nerve terminals. Being structurally similar to many monoamines it can act as a substitute at membrane bound transporters, including the DAT, noradrenaline transporter (NET), serotonin transport (SERT), and VMAT2. Methamphetamine reverses the function of VMAT2 and disrupts the natural pH gradient. This disruption releases monoamines from storage vesicles into the cytoplasm. DAT, NET, and SERT on the cell surface are reversed causing dopamine, norepinephrine, and serotonin to be released from the cytosol into the synapse. Methamphetamine also reduces monoamine metabolism by inhibiting monoamine oxidase and inhibits reuptake. Elevated levels of neurotransmitter can activate postsynaptic receptors resulting in adrenergic stimulation.[3,5] Substance use behavior, such as craving and reward, as well as psychiatric symptoms are due to methamphetamine's effects at dopamine receptors.[4]

Methamphetamine is lipophilic and can be administered and absorbed via numerous routes, including oral, pulmonary, nasal, intramuscular, intravenous, rectal, and vaginal.[3,6] Its onset of action varies depending on the route of administration. Effects can occur within seconds if methamphetamine is smoked or injected. If administered intranasally, the onset of action is approximately 5 minutes and if ingested orally about 20 minutes. The plasma half-life of methamphetamine ranges from 12 to 24 hours, whereas its duration of action can persist beyond 24 hours. Methamphetamine is eliminated via hepatic and renal mechanisms.[6]

### Prescription Stimulants

Prescription stimulant medications are quickly absorbed and exhibit rapid extracellular and hepatic metabolism. Doses have a short duration of action, and behavioral effects occur within 30 minutes of administration. Effects reach a peak within 1 to 3 hours and are usually gone by 5 hours. Development of tolerance is rare, and efficacy can be maintained without continued increase in dosage.[7]

### Cocaine

Cocaine and methamphetamine act on similar neurotransmitters, dopamine, norepinephrine, and serotonin. The pharmaceutical form is cocaine hydrochloride, which can be used as a local anesthetic and is the form in which it is abused. Cocaine hydrochloride can be administered via oral, intranasal, or intravenous routes. Cocaine can also be smoked as coca paste, crack, or freebase. Unlike methamphetamine's direct effect on neurotransmitter release, cocaine blocks reuptake. Mechanisms of action include blockade of amine reuptake, sodium channel blockade, and excitatory amino acid stimulation. These mechanisms result in increased amounts of neurotransmitter in the synaptic cleft. The specific action of cocaine at the dopamine transporter is thought to account for its reinforcing effects.[8] Cocaine's effects on norepinephrine mediate physiologic changes in the cardiovascular system.[9] Elevated levels of serotonin account for the euphoric and mood-enhancing effects of cocaine and may also be tied to its addiction potential.[10]

Means of administration impact plasma concentration, onset of action, and duration of effect. Intravenous and smoked forms of cocaine result in rapid absorption and high plasma concentration. The rate of absorption is slower if cocaine is snorted, and the plasma concentration is less. Smoking results in rapid onset and more intense effects in a shorter period of time. The short duration of action, combined with unpleasant posthigh effects, reinforce usage. The high produced by a single dose of intravenous or smoked cocaine lasts for about 30 minutes. It is rapidly metabolized by the liver, producing benzoylecgonine. Benzoylecgonine and cocaine are excreted by the kidney.[9]

## RISK FACTORS AND ASSOCIATED OUTCOMES

Methamphetamine use is related to other problematic behaviors; as the amount of use increases, so do the behaviors.[11] In adolescents, these include risky sexual behavior; adolescent pregnancy; antisocial behaviors; substance use, including alcohol; and having friends who engage in deviant behavior.[11,12] There are important health outcomes to consider with regard to usage of methamphetamine, among them depression, suicidal ideation, and psychosis. Suicide and overdose are significant sources of morbidity and mortality among youths who use methamphetamines. Other mental health and behavioral considerations associated with methamphetamine use include eating disorders, past diagnoses of alcohol or substance use disorders, higher rates of psychotic symptoms, as well as elevated scores on the hypochondriasis and schizophrenia subscales of the Minnesota Multiphasic Personality Inventory.[13] Russell and colleagues[14] compared risk factors of low- and high-risk youths, defining *low risk* as those who did not use illicit drugs and *high risk* as youths who abused drugs other than methamphetamine or were detained in juvenile detention. Factors associated with methamphetamine use among low-risk youths include engagement in high-risk behaviors and history of psychiatric disorder, specifically adjustment disorder, conduct disorder, and ADHD. Among high-risk youths, girls are more likely to use methamphetamines. Unstable family environment, including family history of crime or substance use, and having received treatment of a psychiatric condition were also identified as associated factors.[14] Family history of substance use may be an important factor for adolescents, even more so than in adults. Lyoo and colleagues[15] found a 3-way interaction between cortical thickness of the orbitofrontal cortex, family history of substance use, and methamphetamine use in adolescents. They suggested that premorbid orbitofrontal cortical thickness differences attributable to family history may precede the onset of adolescent methamphetamine dependence.[14,15]

## BRAIN CHANGES: STRUCTURAL AND NEUROTRANSMISSION

Given the maturation process that takes place during adolescence, methamphetamine use during this critical period might impact brain development as well as structure. Compared with adult users, imaging has revealed greater and more widespread gray and white matter alterations in adolescent methamphetamine users. These changes are especially notable in the frontostriatal system. Adolescents also seem more vulnerable to both addiction and brain-induced damage of methamphetamines. Despite the fact that adolescents generally use lower doses of methamphetamine, its effects may be more influential on the developing brain. Smaller doses and shorter duration of methamphetamine exposure can have greater effects as compared with adult usage.[15] Additionally the search for novel stimuli, which is notable in adolescence, shares a common neurobiological substrate with psychostimulants, specifically the reward-related mesolimbic pathway.[16]

Methamphetamine-associated gray and white matter changes are correlated with executive function dysfunction among adolescents. These impairments are greater in adolescent methamphetamine users compared with adults.[15] Additionally normal frontal lobe maturation may be disrupted by methamphetamine use, especially during late adolescence. Specifically the anterior cingulate cortex plays a role in executive functioning and decision-making, and damage to this area may contribute to poorer cognition as this group ages.[11,17] Exposure during adolescence may have an adverse effect on white matter myelination impacting the maturation of tracts in the frontostriatal pathway that play a role in delayed reward.[18,19] Methamphetamine exposure during critical periods in adolescence might contribute to unsuccessful rewiring of these tracts, resulting in prolonged inability to inhibit addictive response.[15]

Repeated exposure to methamphetamine can also result in neurotoxic effects to the dopaminergic and serotonergic systems. Neurotoxicity may also be mediated by the accumulation of reactive oxygen species. Both of which may lead to irreversible loss of nerve terminals and cell bodies, specifically dopaminergic and serotonergic axons and termini.[20,21] Repeated neurotoxic insults can result in cognitive changes, such as memory deficits, impaired coordination, and increased aggression, in accordance with damage to dopamine and serotonin-rich areas.[20] Psychotic symptoms are correlated with neurotoxicity to the striatum, decreased dopamine transporter density in the frontal cortex, and reduced global serotonin receptor density.[22,23] Reduced density of the serotonin receptor transporter can result in elevated levels of aggression, even in currently abstinent methamphetamine users.[24] Despite its impact on brain development, animal studies comparing adolescents with adults suggest that the adolescent brain may be partially protected from the neurotoxic effects of methamphetamine on the dopamine system.[25] Animal models also reveal that the rewarding effects of methamphetamine may be more powerful in adolescence than adulthood.[26] If adolescents experience less aversive properties of methamphetamine use, they may be even more vulnerable to the rewarding effects of use.[16] These findings may help explain the pre-disposition to use and difficulty with relapse that adolescents experience.

## CLINICAL PRESENTATION
### Physiological Symptoms

Patterns of use, such as chronology, route of administration, dose, and potency, can all impact the clinical effects and symptom presentation of methamphetamine intoxication. Smaller doses of methamphetamine have greater central stimulant effects than peripheral.[3] Low to moderate usage results in physiological effects, such as tachycardia, hypertension, pupil dilation, peripheral hyperthermia, and decreased appetite.[20] The clinical picture indicating overdose includes the aforemen-tioned symptoms in addition to agitation, shivering, dyspnea, chest pain, and possibly cardiac, hepatic, and renal failure. Coma and seizure occur less frequently.[27] Both suicide and homicide are significant causes of death associated with methamphet-amine use.[28] With chronic methamphetamine usage, users may appear malnourished. Coronary heart disease and cardiomyopathy can develop.[29] Hypertension and arrhythmia can lead to acute coronary syndrome, acute aortic dissection, and sudden cardiac death.[30–32] Methamphetamine users are at increased risk for ischemic and hemorrhagic stroke. Xerostomia combined with bruxism and jaw clenching can cause dental problems, such as caries, tooth erosion, tooth loss, and tooth fractures.[27]

### Psychiatric and Neurocognitive Symptoms

With acute intoxication, users may experience euphoria, arousal, reduced fatigue, positive mood, increased libido, behavioral disinhibition, and short-term improve-ment in attention and cognition. To a certain extent higher doses correlate with more intense euphoria.[20] Methamphetamines might also cause distressing neuropsy-chiatric symptoms, such as confusion, aggression, anxiety or panic, paranoia, hallu-cinations, suicidal and homicidal tendencies, and delirium. Users may experience immediate onset of neurological effects, such as restlessness, dizziness, tremor, hyperactive reflexes, talkativeness, tenseness, irritability, and weakness.[27] In com-parison with same-age, same-sex peers who do not use methamphetamines, psychi-atric symptoms, such as depression and paranoia, are more common among methamphetamine-using adolescents, especially girls. Greater symptom severity across all measures of the Symptom Checklist-90R, a self-report questionnaire of psychological problems and symptoms of psychopathology, was noted among adolescent users, with female users having the most symptoms. Adolescent users also demonstrate higher cortisol levels to stress testing.[33]

In comparison with nonusing peers, adolescent methamphetamine users exhibit deficits in executive functioning. Specific areas of impairment include abstraction, nonverbal reasoning, conflict resolution, and inhibition. Based on these deficits, meth-amphetamine seems to impair behavioral inhibition and regulation, possibly contrib-uting to impulsivity. Severity of usage impacted the degree of neuropsychological deficit. Some of these deficits may be transient and function can be recovered, as evidenced by improvement in performance with longer duration of abstinence.[34]

With chronic methamphetamine use psychiatric symptoms can become more pro-nounced. Long-time users may present similar to individuals with schizophrenia.[35] Psychotic symptoms induced by methamphetamine use are aptly described as meth-amphetamine psychosis. This psychosis occurs more often in individuals who are methamphetamine dependent. Younger age and longer duration of use are associ-ated with a higher risk of psychosis. The most common psychotic symptoms include hallucinations, suspiciousness, delusions, and odd speech. Of the various types of hallucinations, auditory disturbances are most common. Common delusional themes include persecution, reference, or mind reading. However, the delusion of parasitosis or formication, a phenomenon known as meth mites, might also be present.[35,36] With this symptom, the delusion influences users to repeatedly pick at their skin, which, over time, results in scarring and an increased likelihood of skin infections. Additionally, chronic methamphetamine use can precipitate the development of motor symptoms. Repetitive, non–goal-directed movement known as stereotypy, dyskinesias, or choreoathetoid movements might be present.[37]

Following use, sleep disturbance, depression, anxiety, craving, and cognitive impairment are common features of withdrawal.[38] These symptoms are most likely related to the depletion of presynaptic monoamine stores, downregulation of receptors, and methamphetamine-induced neurotoxicity.[21,38] Physical symptoms of withdrawal include headache, chills, sweating, palpitations, cardiac arrhythmia, angina, changes in blood pressure, dry mouth, taste changes, nausea, vomiting, diarrhea, and abdominal cramping.[3] The *Diagnostic and Statistical Manual of Mental Disorders Fifth Edition* (*DSM-5*) describes specific criteria for the diagnosis of stimulant withdrawal; key symptoms include dysphoric mood, fatigue, vivid unpleasant dreams, sleep disturbance, increased appetite, and psychomotor alterations.[39] Acute withdrawal symptoms last on average for 7 to 10 days, and a subacute withdrawal occurs in the couple weeks that follow. Symptoms peak within 24 hours of last use, are most severe during the acute phase, and improve with continued abstinence. The severity of withdrawal is related to features of use, specifically older age, chronicity, and dependence.[38]

### Cocaine

Cocaine intoxication shares many similar features to that of methamphetamine. Cocaine commonly induces feelings of euphoria; however, other mood states can be heightened as well, among these dysphoria, anger, and irritability. Cocaine can cause inflated self-esteem, increased energy, insomnia, motor excitement, talkativeness, increased libido, anorexia, and disorganized thoughts. The addiction potential of cocaine is influenced by route, frequency, and duration of cocaine use. The psychological and physical effects of the drug, its rapid onset of action, and uncomfortable postuse symptoms all enhance the addiction potential of cocaine.[9]

## DIAGNOSIS

As with other substance use disorders, the *DSM-5* collapsed both abuse and dependence under stimulant use disorder, using severity ratings to represent the varying degrees of use. Severity ratings are also tied to a specific stimulant. The additional changes between the two editions include removal of legal problems[39] and the addition of drug craving[40] to the list of diagnostic criteria. Craving represents an important feature of diagnosis, as it may be a clinical indicator of the underlying pathogenesis of addiction, is related to the vulnerability of relapse, and can predict subsequent use.[20]

## CLINICAL MANAGEMENT
### Acute Management

Supportive measures are the mainstay in managing acute methamphetamine intoxication.[41] Treatment should prioritize the risk of agitation, hypertension, and hyperthermia. Acute agitation in the setting of methamphetamine toxicity can be managed with a benzodiazepine or an antipsychotic agent. In the pediatric population, both benzodiazepines and haloperidol have been used in the setting of methamphetamine toxicity without adverse effects.[42] In cases of methamphetamine-induced hyperthermia, cooling using internal or external means is the primary treatment method.[43] Antihypertensive agents should be used if blood pressure is significantly elevated.[41]

### Long-Term Treatment

Cognitive behavioral therapy, contingency management, and motivational interviewing are the primary treatment modalities.[44] The psychosocial interventions commonly used are moderately effective at reducing use and related harms among stimulant users.[45] Twelve-step programs, such as Narcotics Anonymous, are a common component in treatment.[20] Methamphetamine use is often associated with multiple behavioral problems, so tailoring interventions to target sex- or age-specific behaviors can be beneficial for youths. Specific targets include antisocial activities; risky sex practices; depression; social influences, including peers engaging in antisocial behaviors and drug use; and parenting styles that may favor drug use, poor monitoring, or limit setting. Of all these factors prevention of antisocial behavior, risky sex, and depression may be of highest value regardless of the age or sex of adolescent users.[11] Interventions that address stress-management and prevention of life stressors should be a consideration, especially among female adolescent methamphetamine users who are more susceptible and sensitive to stressful situations. Pharmacologic options that target the hypothalamic-pituitary-adrenal axis or dopaminergic system might also be of help.[33]

There are no specific medications approved by the US Food and Drug Administration for the use of methamphetamine dependence at this time.[20] Medications considered for the treatment of methamphetamine dependence target multiple neurotransmitter pathways, including dopamine, serotonin, $\gamma$-aminobutyric acid, glutamate, and opioid.[46,47] There have been some promising results related to the role of medications, such as methylphenidate, naltrexone, bupropion, mirtazapine, and modafinil, in reducing stimulant use in specific subgroups. However, no specific agent has been proven to be consistently efficacious.[47,48] Similar agents have been investigated for their potential to reduce cravings for methamphetamines, such as dextroamphetamine, rivastigmine, bupropion, nicotine, and naltrexone.[20]

## TREATMENT ISSUES SPECIFIC TO ADOLESCENTS
### Demographic Features

There are some distinctive demographic features among adolescents who use methamphetamines. Numerous studies have shown that adolescent methamphetamine users are more likely to be female, which is unique to this particular substance. Adolescent methamphetamine users may present for treatment with higher levels of dysfunction and higher rates of substance use compared with adolescents who do not use. In comparison with same-age peers in treatment for other drugs of abuse, methamphetamine-using adolescents show increased rates of depression and suicidal ideation and are more likely to have experienced prior substance use treatment.[49,50]

### History of in Utero Exposure

In considering the pediatric population, events that take place in utero are an important part of medical history. The Infant Development, Environment and Lifestyle (IDEAL) study revealed that children exposed to methamphetamines in utero exhibited poorer inhibitory control in childhood compared with their non–methamphetamine-exposed peers.[51] These children may experience more difficulties with inattention and impulsivity and have a higher risk for developing ADHD.[52] Behavioral differences are also noted among in utero cocaine-exposed children. Difficulty with managing impulses, frustration, tension regulation, and arousal were noted in 6 year olds exposed to cocaine.[53] In contrast to the available information on methamphetamine-exposed youths, there are mixed results across the literature regarding the development of children and adolescents who were exposed to cocaine in utero. In those exposed to cocaine, early physiological difficulties may not necessarily lead to behavioral or cognitive deficits in later childhood and adolescence, which is reassuring.[54]

### Misuse and Diversion of Prescription Stimulants

Misuse and diversion of prescribed stimulants is another factor to be considered among adolescents and young adults. In a review of the literature, Wilens and colleagues[55] found that 5% to 9% of grade school–aged and high school–aged and 5% to 35% of college-aged youths reported nonprescribed stimulant use. Monitoring the Future data revealed that tenth and twelfth graders were more likely than eighth graders to use methylphenidate for nonmedical purposes.[56] Rates of diversion, whereby students were asked to give, trade, or sell their medications, range from 16% to 29%.[55] The immediate-release form of methylphenidate was found to be the most often misused or diverted stimulant medication.[57]

Youths with ADHD are more likely to misuse or divert their medications compared with those receiving medications for other conditions. Those who misused their own stimulant prescriptions or skipped doses were more likely to divert their medication.[57] Adolescents who misuse stimulants are more likely to be using other drugs of abuse and carry diagnoses of substance use and conduct disorder compared with their non-using counterparts. They are also more likely to live in metropolitan areas. Adolescents who reported stimulant misuse were also more likely to endorse ADHD-related symptoms, leading to some questions about the possibility of self-medicating undiagnosed ADHD.[55] Adolescents who do not have college plans were more likely to use than their peers who had goals to attend college. However, among college-aged adults, those in college were more likely to misuse stimulant medications than those not attending college. These young adults also reported more negative consequences of their drug and alcohol use compared with the nonmethylphenidate users.[56]

### SUMMARY

Even with the limited focus of this article, it is clear that methamphetamine use among adolescents and young adults is a serious health concern with potentially long-term physical, cognitive, and psychiatric consequences. Although methamphetamine, cocaine, and other illicit stimulants are problematic, providers should be mindful of the growing trend of diversion and misuse of stimulant prescriptions. For children and adolescents using methamphetamines, brain development and drug effects seem to align in a way that may be more deleterious than in adulthood. It seems helpful to keep in mind the differences between adolescents and young adults when implementing interventions. Treatments might be more effective if tailored to the specific substance use difficulties of this population.

### REFERENCES

1. Results from the 2013 national survey on drug use and health: summary of national findings. Available at: http://www.samhsa.gov/data/sites/default/files/NSDUHresultsPDFWHTML2013/Web/NSDUHresults2013.htm#5.8. Accessed October 25, 2015.

2. National Institute on Drug Abuse Monitoring the Future Study: trends in prevalence of various drugs. Available at: http://www.drugabuse.gov/trends-statistics/monitoring-future/monitoring-future-study-trends-in-prevalence-various-drugs Accessed October 25, 2015.

3. Goodman LS, Brunton LL, Gilman A, et al. Goodman & Gilman's the pharmacological basis of therapeutics. 12th edition. New York: McGraw-Hill Medical; 2011. Available at: http://accessmedicine.mhmedical.com/book.aspx?bookId=374 http://www.accesspharmacy.com/resourceToc.aspx?resourceID=28 http://www.accessmedicine.com/resourceTOC.aspx?resourceID=651. This former electronic address redirects to current address when searched on August 25, 2015.

4. Panenka WJ, Procyshyn RM, Lecomte T, et al. Methamphetamine use: a comprehensive review of molecular, preclinical and clinical findings. Drug Alcohol Depend 2013;129(3):167–79.

5. Sulzer D, Sonders MS, Poulsen NW, et al. Mechanisms of neurotransmitter release by amphetamines: a review. Prog Neurobiol 2005;75(6):406–33.

6. Meredith CW, Jaffe C, Ang-Lee K, et al. Implications of chronic methamphetamine use: a literature review. Harv Rev Psychiatry 2005;13(3):141–54.

7. Santosh PJ, Taylor E. Stimulant drugs. Eur Child Adolesc Psychiatry 2000;9(Suppl 1):I27–43.

8. Boghdadi MS, Henning RJ. Cocaine: pathophysiology and clinical toxicology. Heart Lung 1997;26(6):466–83 [quiz: 484–5].

9. Carrera MR, Meijler MM, Janda KD. Cocaine pharmacology and current pharmacotherapies for its abuse. Bioorg Med Chem 2004;12(19):5019–30.

10. Ritz MC, Lamb RJ, Goldberg SR, et al. Cocaine receptors on dopamine transporters are related to self-administration of cocaine. Science 1987;237(4819):1219–23.

11. Embry D, Hankins M, Biglan A, et al. Behavioral and social correlates of methamphetamine use in a population-based sample of early and later adolescents. Addict Behav 2009;34(4):343–51.

12. Zapata LB, Hillis SD, Marchbanks PA, et al. Methamphetamine use is independently associated with recent risky sexual behaviors and adolescent pregnancy. J Sch Health 2008;78(12):641–8.

13. Marshall BD, Werb D. Health outcomes associated with methamphetamine use among young people: a systematic review. Addiction 2010;105(6):991–1002.

14. Russell K, Dryden DM, Liang Y, et al. Risk factors for methamphetamine use in youth: a systematic review. BMC Pediatr 2008;8:48.

15. Lyoo IK, Yoon S, Kim TS, et al. Predisposition to and effects of methamphetamine use on the adolescent brain. Mol Psychiatry 2015;20(12):1516–24.

16. Laviola G, Adriani W, Terranova ML, et al. Psychobiological risk factors for vulnerability to psychostimulants in human adolescents and animal models. Neurosci Biobehav Rev 1999;23(7):993–1010.

17. Goldstein RZ, Volkow ND. Drug addiction and its underlying neurobiological basis: neuroimaging evidence for the involvement of the frontal cortex. Am J Psychiatry 2002;159(10):1642–52.

18. Casey BJ, Jones RM. Neurobiology of the adolescent brain and behavior: implications for substance use disorders. J Am Acad Child Adolesc Psychiatry 2010;49(12):1189–201 [quiz: 1285].

19. Chudasama Y, Robbins TW. Functions of frontostriatal systems in cognition: comparative neuropsychopharmacological studies in rats, monkeys and humans. Biol Psychol 2006;73(1):19–38.

20. Courtney KE, Ray LA. Methamphetamine: an update on epidemiology, pharmacology, clinical phenomenology, and treatment literature. Drug Alcohol Depend 2014;143:11–21.
21. Ricaurte GA, Guillery RW, Seiden LS, et al. Dopamine nerve terminal degeneration produced by high doses of methylamphetamine in the rat brain. Brain Res 1982;235(1):93–103.
22. Sekine Y, Iyo M, Ouchi Y, et al. Methamphetamine-related psychiatric symptoms and reduced brain dopamine transporters studied with PET. Am J Psychiatry 2001;158(8):1206–14.
23. Sekine Y, Minabe Y, Kawai M, et al. Metabolite alterations in basal ganglia associated with methamphetamine-related psychiatric symptoms. A proton MRS study. Neuropsychopharmacology 2002;27(3):453–61.
24. Sekine Y, Ouchi Y, Takei N, et al. Brain serotonin transporter density and aggression in abstinent methamphetamine abusers. Arch Gen Psychiatry 2006;63(1):90–100.
25. Buck JM, Siegel JA. The effects of adolescent methamphetamine exposure. Front Neurosci 2015;9:151.
26. Joca L, Zuloaga DG, Raber J, et al. Long-term effects of early adolescent methamphetamine exposure on depression-like behavior and the hypothalamic vasopressin system in mice. Dev Neurosci 2014;36(2):108–18.
27. Cruickshank CC, Dyer KR. A review of the clinical pharmacology of methamphetamine. Addiction 2009;104(7):1085–99.
28. Logan BK, Fligner CL, Haddix T. Cause and manner of death in fatalities involving methamphetamine. J Forensic Sci 1998;43(1):28–34.
29. Yeo KK, Wijetunga M, Ito H, et al. The association of methamphetamine use and cardiomyopathy in young patients. Am J Med 2007;120(2):165–71.
30. Kaye S, McKetin R, Duflou J, et al. Methamphetamine and cardiovascular pathology: a review of the evidence. Addiction 2007;102(8):1204–11.
31. Turnipseed SD, Richards JR, Kirk JD, et al. Frequency of acute coronary syndrome in patients presenting to the emergency department with chest pain after methamphetamine use. J Emerg Med 2003;24(4):369–73.
32. Swalwell CI, Davis GG. Methamphetamine as a risk factor for acute aortic dissection. J Forensic Sci 1999;44(1):23–6.
33. King G, Alicata D, Cloak C, et al. Psychiatric symptoms and HPA axis function in adolescent methamphetamine users. J Neuroimmune Pharmacol 2010;5(4):582–91.
34. King G, Alicata D, Cloak C, et al. Neuropsychological deficits in adolescent methamphetamine abusers. Psychopharmacology (Berl) 2010;212(2):243–9.
35. Chen CK, Lin SK, Sham PC, et al. Pre-morbid characteristics and co-morbidity of methamphetamine users with and without psychosis. Psychol Med 2003;33(8):1407–14.
36. McKetin R, McLaren J, Lubman DI, et al. The prevalence of psychotic symptoms among methamphetamine users. Addiction 2006;101(10):1473–8.
37. Scott JC, Woods SP, Matt GE, et al. Neurocognitive effects of methamphetamine: a critical review and meta-analysis. Neuropsychol Rev 2007;17(3):275–97.
38. McGregor C, Srisurapanont M, Jittiwutikarn J, et al. The nature, time course and severity of methamphetamine withdrawal. Addiction 2005;100(9):1320–9.
39. American Psychiatric Association, Task Force on DSM-IV. Diagnostic and statistical manual of mental disorders: DSM-IV-TR. 4th edition. Washington, DC: American Psychiatric Association; 2000. Available at: http://www.psychiatryonline.com/resourceTOC.aspx?resourceID=1http://psychiatryonline.com/.

40. American Psychiatric Association, DSM-5 Task Force. Diagnostic and statistical manual of mental disorders: DSM-5. 5th edition. Arlington (VA): American Psychiatric Association; 2013. Available at:http://dsm.psychiatryonline.org/book.aspx?bookid=556.

41. Winslow BT, Voorhees KI, Pehl KA. Methamphetamine abuse. Am Fam Physician 2007;76(8):1169–74.

42. Ruha AM, Yarema MC. Pharmacologic treatment of acute pediatric methamphetamine toxicity. Pediatr Emerg Care 2006;22(12):782–5.

43. Matsumoto RR, Seminerio MJ, Turner RC, et al. Methamphetamine-induced toxicity: an updated review on issues related to hyperthermia. Pharmacol Ther 2014;144(1):28–40.

44. London ED, Kohno M, Morales AM, et al. Chronic methamphetamine abuse and corticostriatal deficits revealed by neuroimaging. Brain Res 2014;1628(Pt A): 174–85.

45. Shearer J. Psychosocial approaches to psychostimulant dependence: a systematic review. J Subst Abuse Treat 2007;32(1):41–52.

46. Vocci FJ, Appel NM. Approaches to the development of medications for the treatment of methamphetamine dependence. Addiction 2007;102(Suppl 1):96–106.

47. Brensilver M, Heinzerling KG, Shoptaw S. Pharmacotherapy of amphetamine-type stimulant dependence: an update. Drug Alcohol Rev 2013;32(5):449–60.

48. McElhiney MC, Rabkin JG, Rabkin R, et al. Provigil (modafinil) plus cognitive behavioral therapy for methamphetamine use in HIV+ gay men: a pilot study. Am J Drug Alcohol Abuse 2009;35(1):34–7.

49. Rawson RA, Gonzales R, Obert JL, et al. Methamphetamine use among treatment-seeking adolescents in Southern California: participant characteristics and treatment response. J Subst Abuse Treat 2005;29(2):67–74.

50. Gonzales R, Ang A, McCann MJ, et al. An emerging problem: methamphetamine abuse among treatment seeking youth. Subst Abus 2008;29(2):71–80.

51. Smith LM, Diaz S, LaGasse LL, et al. Developmental and behavioral consequences of prenatal methamphetamine exposure: a review of the Infant Development, Environment, and Lifestyle (IDEAL) study. Neurotoxicol Teratol 2015;51: 35–44.

52. Kiblawi ZN, Smith LM, LaGasse LL, et al. The effect of prenatal methamphetamine exposure on attention as assessed by continuous performance tests: results from the infant development, environment, and lifestyle study. J Dev Behav Pediatr 2013;34(1):31–7.

53. Chasnoff IJ, Anson A, Hatcher R, et al. Prenatal exposure to cocaine and other drugs. Outcome at four to six years. Ann N Y Acad Sci 1998;846:314–28.

54. Buckingham-Howes S, Berger SS, Scaletti LA, et al. Systematic review of prenatal cocaine exposure and adolescent development. Pediatrics 2013;131(6): e1917–36.

55. Wilens TE, Adler LA, Adams J, et al. Misuse and diversion of stimulants prescribed for ADHD: a systematic review of the literature. J Am Acad Child Adolesc Psychiatry 2008;47(1):21–31.

56. Arria AM, Wish ED. Nonmedical use of prescription stimulants among students. Pediatr Ann 2006;35(8):565–71.

57. Wilens TE, Gignac M, Swezey A, et al. Characteristics of adolescents and young adults with ADHD who divert or misuse their prescribed medications. J Am Acad Child Adolesc Psychiatry 2006;45(4):408–14.

# Opioid Use Disorders

Bikash Sharma, MD[a], Ann Bruner, MD[a,b], Gabrielle Barnett, MA[a],
Marc Fishman, MD[a,c],*

## KEYWORDS

- Opioids • Opioid use disorder • Heroin • Injection • Prescription opioids
- Withdrawal • Overdose

## KEY POINTS

- The current epidemic of opioid use and addiction in adolescents and young adults is worsening, including heroin and nonmedical use of prescription opioids.
- Opioid use has devastating consequences for youth and their families, including: progression to full addiction, severe psychosocial impairment, hepatitis C virus and human immunodeficiency virus transmission with injection use, exacerbation of co-occurring psychiatric disorders, overdose, and death.
- Progression of opioid use disorders (OUDs) in youth often follows a characteristic pattern from use of diverted prescription opioid analgesics to sniffed or smoked heroin to injection heroin.
- Opioid overdose is a life-threatening emergency. Respiratory depression should be treated with naloxone, and respiratory support if necessary. Overdose should always be utilized as an opportunity to initiate addiction treatment.
- Opioid withdrawal management (detoxification) is often a necessary, but never sufficient, component of treatment for OUDs. Medications used in the treatment of withdrawal may include buprenorphine, clonidine, and others for relief of symptoms.
- Treatment for OUDs is effective, but treatment capacity is alarmingly limited and underdeveloped.
- Although there is a limited evidence base for youth-specific treatment, emerging consensus supports the incorporation of relapse prevention medications such as buprenorphine and extended-release naltrexone into comprehensive psychosocial treatment including counseling and family involvement.

## INTRODUCTION/BACKGROUND

The current epidemic of opioid use disorders (both diverted prescription opioids and heroin) in adolescents and young adults is a growing problem with devastating consequences for youth and their families. Progression from initiation to full addiction is

[a] Mountain Manor Treatment Center, Baltimore, MD, USA; [b] Department of Pediatrics, Johns Hopkins University, Baltimore, MD, USA; [c] Department of Psychiatry, Johns Hopkins University, Baltimore, MD, USA
* Corresponding author. 3800 Frederick Avenue, Baltimore, MD 21229.
E-mail address: mjfishman@comcast.net

Child Adolesc Psychiatric Clin N Am 25 (2016) 473–487
http://dx.doi.org/10.1016/j.chc.2016.03.002
1056-4993/16/$ – see front matter © 2016 Elsevier Inc. All rights reserved.

common, and often accelerated compared with other substances. Severe psychosocial impairment includes criminal justice involvement, school dropout, unemployment, and co-occurring psychiatric disorders. Medical morbidity includes the well-known sequelae of injection drug use including hepatitis C virus (HCV), human immunodeficiency virus (HIV), injection site infections, and others. Worst of all is the catastrophic mortality associated with overdose, and nearly every community in the country has now unfortunately experienced this tragic loss of life in a young person with an opioid use disorder (OUD).

The term opioids encompasses a class of a large number of drugs, both natural alkaloid compounds derived directly from the resin of the opium poppy (termed opiates, including morphine and heroin), as well as related synthetic compounds (including oxycodone and hydromorphone.) All members of the opioid drug class share common pharmacologic features as agonists of the *mu* opioid receptor. Opioids are highly addictive, with rapid progression to physiologic dependence with tolerance and withdrawal. There is growing evidence to suggest a relationship between increased nonmedical use of prescription opioids and heroin use in the United States,[1] and a significant proportion of adolescents who start with prescription opioids go on to injection heroin use.[2] The progression of use often follows a pattern that maximizes drug bioavailabilty and effect: oral prescription opioids to inhaled prescription opioids to inhaled heroin to injection heroin. Inhalation can encompass either smoking (heating heroin in foil and inhaling the smoke) and nasal snorting (of the powdered heroin); whether a patient smokes or snorts appears to be mostly influenced by peers and regional variations, but neither method is as potent or efficient as injection, which maximizes bioavailability. This phenomenon is more prominent in adolescent than adult opioid users,[3] and accelerates more quickly with an earlier age of first opioid use. This progression is also related to heroin's lower cost and higher potency, because tolerance to opioids builds up rapidly in adolescents, and prescription opiates become prohibitively expensive with increased requirements for amounts of opioids as addiction advances.[4]

### Etiologic Factors

Though understanding remains limited, there is increasing knowledge of the multiple factors involved in the etiology of opioid use disorders as a particular class of substance use disorders (SUDs). OUDs share many features in common with addiction as a general process and with other SUDs, but there are several features that are specific to OUDs that may interact to influence vulnerability, progression, and course. These factors range over several domains, including pharmacology, genetics, environmental influences, developmental influences, and comorbidities.

Opioids are all enormously reinforcing, 1 feature of their specific pharmacologic properties. Positive reinforcement is largely mediated by the indirect downstream activation of dopamine receptors, one of the main final common pathways of reward. Although opioids produce somewhat less immediate dopamine release than stimulants, they rank high in the hierarchy of rewarding substances and produce higher levels of positive reinforcement in animal and human self-administration models than almost all substances other than stimulants, as a feature of the intrinsic properties of the opioid receptor. Also prominent and perhaps even more clinically significant in chronic OUDs is the typical negative reinforcement produced by opioid withdrawal once physiologic dependence has occurred. Although the onset of withdrawal following opioid discontinuation varies with the half-life of the particular opioid, it produces a characteristic physiologic syndrome with even brief abstinence or even delay of dosing. Steady exposure to opioids can produce this process of neuroadaptation leading to physiologic dependence and withdrawal within as little as 4 to 8 weeks in opioid-naïve individuals, and much faster with reinstatement after relapse in those with prior dependence. Opioid withdrawal includes activation of the locus ceruleus region of the brain with increased systemic sympathetic tone, leading to its characteristic features (including chills, diarrhea, nausea, cramps, and anxiety), accompanied by high intensity cravings.

Approximately 40% to 60% of the vulnerability to any addiction is attributable to genetic factors.[5–7] Broad population twin studies[8] generally suggest that genetic factors have the strongest influence as a common vulnerability to SUDs in general rather than to phenotypic expression of vulnerability to or preference for any specific individual substance. On the other hand, with more advanced genetic techniques, several specific loci have been associated specifically with opioid use and OUDs, with moderate opioid-specific heritable vulnerability. Specific allelic variants have been identified that seem to confer risk, in various genes including those coding for dopamine receptors and the dopamine transporter, opioid receptors, opioid neuropeptides, serotonin receptors and the serotonin transporter, and cannabinoid receptors.[9,10] For example, polymorphisms in the gene for the *mu*-opioid receptor (OPRM1) have been variably linked to differences in binding affinity and signaling efficiency, increased basal cortisol levels and opioid-mediated dynamic cortisol response, and differential analgesic effects of morphine; additionally, some studies have found associations between these allelic variations and rates of opioid dependence, although others have not.[10]

As with genetic factors, environmental factors have strong influence as common factors increasing vulnerability broadly to SUDs. Typical risk factors such as stress, adversity, and exposure to substance use in family and peers tend to increase risk for all substances rather than to opioid use or preference specifically. But, in addition, there are certainly unique environmental influences that differentially increase the risk of OUDs specifically. Such influences include: exposure to opioids as a specific class of substance, most importantly nonmedical use; exposure to medical opioid analgesics; use of opioids by family, peers, and other influential role models; permissive attitudes toward opioid use by influential role models; and access to opioids as a specific substance class.

Access is a particularly important environmental risk factor. The issue of ease of access, both for prescription opioids and for heroin, has been important in the genesis of the current epidemic. With increasing trends in medical prescribing of opioid analgesics over the past 2 decades, the overall US supply of prescription opioids has expanded greatly, with nonmedical diversion an unintended (but perhaps predictable) consequence. From 1999 to 2010, the per capita kilogram sales of prescribed opioid analgesics quadrupled. This trend parallels the concurrent curves of increasing per capita opioid treatment admissions and per capita opioid overdose deaths.[11] And while large increases in prescribing of opioid analgesics have mostly been a phenomenon of adult medical practice, the trend has emerged to a lesser extent in pediatric practice as well.[12] Heroin access has been promoted by increasingly plentiful and cheaper supplies. As with all substances, youth are particularly price-sensitive in their substance use behaviors, often more so than adults.[13,14]

Although prescription opioid use has a 10-fold greater prevalence than heroin among youth, it also fuels heroin use as a gateway of entry. Although the cost of prescription opioids on the street remains high,[15] the cost of heroin has declined,[16] and its purity has increased dramatically in recent years.[17] This makes heroin a more economical alternative to prescription opioids, based both on price and potency (cheaper and better), once opioid addiction has become established.

Increasing purity has also promoted heroin use among youth in another way. Four decades ago, the low purity of available heroin meant that injection use was required to produce meaningful intoxication, and the need for injection has always been a major barrier to initiation of heroin use for youth. But over the past 2 to 3 decades, as heroin purity in street supplies has increased, often exceeding 60% purity, nasal use or smoking is now an efficient route of administration, and a young person can initiate and become addicted to heroin without injection use. Once heroin addiction is established, presumably, the hurdle to injection is less of a barrier.[18]

More recently, efforts to limit the supply of prescription opioids have started to succeed, through various means, including medical education about opioid analgesic prescribing, law enforcement interdiction of pill mills, use of prescription drug monitoring plans, and others. But as the availability of prescription opioids decreases and the street price of pills goes up, there is concern that there may be a corresponding shift toward heroin use. It is hoped that the trend toward less prescription opioid availability will help bring down both initial use of opioids and therefore overall rates of opioid use disorder, but it is also possible that more adolescents may start using heroin earlier after having initiated opioids through prescription opioids, or even using heroin as their first opioid.[19]

Developmental vulnerabilities and comorbid psychiatric disorders are additional factors that confer considerable risk for all SUDs. Examples include problems with affective regulation, depression, anxiety, excitement seeking, extreme extroversion, impulsivity, cognitive impairment, and problems with executive control. As far as anyone knows, like the common environmental and genetic vulnerability factors shared by all SUDs, these tend mostly to increase risk for all substances rather than for opioid use or preference specifically. Both co-occurring psychiatric disorders and deviation from normal developmental trajectory seem to worsen with increasing severity and chronicity of overall SUDs, and vice versa, with reciprocal worsening of course. For some, if unchecked, this progression may lead to opioid addiction. In this context, OUDs may be seen as a more advanced stage of a general progression of SUDs along a continuum. Some have hypothesized that there may be an inexact dose–response relationship for some of these shared factors, making OUDs more likely with increased cumulative risk burden as a more severe form of the more general disorder.

## EPIDEMIOLOGY

The nonmedical use of opioids in the general population is a growing public health and social concern across the entire lifespan.[1] In the United States, the number of people age 12 and older using prescription opioids more than doubled between 1975 and 2008, from 3.5% to over 9%,[2] while the prevalence of marijuana and alcohol abuse decreased or plateaued.[3] In 2009, 2.2 million Americans aged 12 years or older used prescription opioids as their first illicit drug, second only to marijuana.[20] In 2013, there were 169,000 persons aged 12 or older who used heroin for the first time (**Fig. 1**).[21]

### Age

The involvement of youth in the current opioid epidemic is increasing, with alarming impact. In 2011, 8.7% of 12th graders used prescription opioids illegally during the previous year.[22] Another study estimated 13% of high school seniors have a lifetime prevalence of nonmedical use of prescription opioids.[23] In 2009, approximately 250,000 US high school students (1.2%) reported having used heroin at least once,

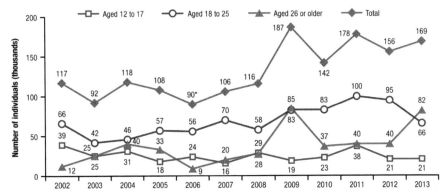

**Fig. 1.** Past-year initiation of heroin among individuals aged 12 or older, by age group: 2002 to 2013. (*From* Lipari RN, Hughes A. The NSDUH report: trends in heroin use in the United States: 2002 to 2013. The CBHSQ Report. Rockville (MD): Substance Abuse and Mental Health Services Administration; Center for Behavioral Health Statistics and Quality; 2015.)

and 77,000 Americans aged 18 to 20 years reported using heroin in the previous year, up from 56,000 in 2008.[20] Across the lifespan, the group with the highest prevalence of both prescription opioid and heroin use, as well as the greatest increases in heroin use, is young adults ages 18 to 25. While the number of users is increasing, the age of first use is decreasing.[24] In 2013, 12.5% of new illegal drug users began with prescription opioids.[25] Although the most recent SAMHSA (Substance Abuse and Mental Health Services Administration) report (2014–2015) shows some encouraging evidence that the rate of prescription opioid use among youths may be declining,[26] other studies have found that more adolescents are starting heroin use at a much younger age.[27]

Age of onset of opioid use is an important clinical epidemiologic indicator and a robust marker of risk and clinical severity. Age of first use is correlated with the lifetime risk of OUDs,[28,29] and earlier age of onset of opioid use is associated with a higher prevalence of dependence, increasing clinical severity, and worsening consequences. Adolescents who are primarily abusing opioids have an earlier age of onset of any substance use compared with those who are currently using marijuana or alcohol (average age 11.7 vs 12.6).[30] The age of onset of opioid use for those who have opioids as their first illicit drug is much earlier compared with those who switch from other substances to opioids.[25,31,32] Heroin users have first substance use much earlier than those who use nonheroin opioids.[33] Adolescents with earlier onset of prescription opioid or heroin use also have a more rapid progression from noninjection to injection heroin use.[15,30,34,35] The strongest predictor for progression to regular heroin use is earlier initial heroin use, while age of initial use of any opioid, and age of regular use of other substances drugs (alcohol, marijuana) are also strong risk factors.[36]

## Gender and Race

Contrary to the popular historic misconception of America's heroin problem being restricted to minorities and the disadvantaged inner city, youth opioid dependence, especially prescription opioid dependence, is a problem of a much broader demographic, including suburbia and higher socioeconomic groups. The prevalence of opioid addiction is highest in white males.[37] The socioeconomic status of youth initiating opioid use has increased over time. More male than female adolescents enter treatment for heroin use, but compared with other SUDs, the representation of females among treatment-seeking youth is much closer to even with males.[15,28,33] Among females seeking treatment for SUDs, there is a higher rate of heroin as their primary substance of use compared with boys.[38] Girls with heroin addiction are more likely to prefer injection use than boys[39] and are also more likely to initiate injection heroin use at a relatively younger age compared with boys. In fact, girls often initiate injection heroin use within a year from their first illicit drug use, a faster rate of progression to injection use than boys.[40] Possible explanations include influence of a romantic partner (often an older male intravenous drug user), having a history of victimization/ongoing victimization, gender-specific personality traits, and a rapid development of tolerance to opioids.

### Injection Use

Injection heroin use is the more advanced and usually later stage of OUDs. Typically, inhaled (smoked or snorted) heroin is a precursor to injection heroin use.[41] There are varying estimates of the proportion of adolescents with any form of opioid addiction who transition to injection heroin use, ranging from 40% to 90%.[2,32] Almost 70% of young heroin users (aged 18–25 years) eventually transition from nasal to injection heroin,[42] and almost half of adolescents with current heroin addiction are injection heroin users.[17,43] Among patients seeking treatment for heroin addiction, the percentage of injection heroin use is even higher (62%–83%).[15,30,33] Sociodemographic factors associated with injection heroin use include poverty or unemployment, homelessness,[37] and history of childhood adversities.[44–47]

### Morbidity and Mortality

Morbidity and mortality related to opioid use have also escalated; in 2013 there were 16,000 deaths from prescription opioids, a 2.5-fold increase since 2001, and there were 8000 deaths from heroin, a 5-fold increase over that same period.[48] One hundred people die from a drug overdose every day in the United States; approximately one half of these are from prescription opioids and approximately one-fifth from heroin. Additionally, drug overdoses have surpassed motor vehicle crashes as the country's leading accidental cause of death.[49] Prescription opioids account for nearly 75% of prescription drug overdoses, and the mortality as a result of opioid overdose has surpassed all other forms of drug poisoning death in the United States.[50,51] From 2004 to 2008, more than half of all drug-related medical emergencies and emergency department (ED) visits were due to heroin and opiates, and during the same period, ED visits involving the nonmedical use of opioids more than doubled.[52] Opioids have been among the most common drugs used in suicide attempts in recent years.[53] The prevalence of HCV in young opioid users is particularly worrisome: in an opioid treatment trial of 16- to 21-year olds, 18% were HCV positive at baseline despite only 1.5 years of opioid dependence, with an additional 5% seroconverted at 12 weeks.[54]

## CLINICAL PRESENTATION AND COURSE

Opioid use disorder in an adolescent presents in many ways: from falling grades and breaking curfew, to legal involvement, to the worst case scenario—near fatal or even fatal overdose. Death does not require dependence: too many families only learn of their child's opioid use when the coroner reports the cause of their child's death, and an adolescent can overdose the very first time he or she tries opioids. One unusual feature of opioids is their ready availability; an adolescent does not need to know a drug dealer. Prescription opiates are easily found in medicine cabinets, on kitchen counters, and in handbags. An adolescent's opioid use may become known after some crisis like arrest, job loss or school expulsion. Most adolescents know about dependence and withdrawal but many falsely believe that prescription opiates are not addictive, often reasoning that a doctor would never prescribe an addictive drug. And among heroin users, there is the myth that only intravenous heroin is addictive, and nasal/smoked heroin is safe. Adolescents who think they are using opioids recreationally are surprised when they experience withdrawal symptoms, and may attribute their opiate withdrawal symptoms to stress, viral illness, or food poisoning. Families may discover their adolescent is opioid dependent when he or she loses access to opioids (being broke, being locked up, or even going on vacation) and goes into withdrawal.

Adolescents can progress from first use to full-blown dependence in months with a course of use that is often shorter than in adults. In general, the development of opioid dependence mirrors other drug dependencies, and possible warning signs may include changes in peer group; decreasing involvement in social/leisure activities; isolation from family/old friends; mood changes such as irritability, depression, anger, and increased frequency of negative behaviors like truancy, lying, running away, stealing, and trouble with the police. As with other SUDs, tolerance develops, and the adolescent needs escalating opioid doses, which increases the risk of overdose and death because of reduced tolerance to respiratory depression.

Addiction to opioids can be conceptualized as the most complex and advanced stage of SUD,[28,34] with the most severe health and social consequences. Adolescents with OUDs generally have higher severity of impairment than those with nonopioid SUDs, including larger amount of substances used, greater number of days of substance use, greater extent of polysubstance use, greater psychopathology and higher rates of co-occurring psychiatric disorders, higher rates of lifetime victimization, and higher rates of criminality.[4,18,27,32,35,40,55,56] And as with adults, youth with heroin use have higher severity than those with prescription opioid use only, including higher rates of high school dropout; more severe psychiatric symptoms including higher rates of depression, suicide attempts, and more history of psychiatric treatment/hospitalizations; more concurrent cocaine use, and more risky sexual behaviors, prostitution, and indiscriminate sex with strangers.[2] Mirroring their rapid development of dependence, adolescents and young adults with opioid addiction often have a more rapid deterioration in life circumstances, which in turn presents extreme barriers to treatment engagement and recovery, entrapping them in a vicious spiral of worsening addiction severity.[39]

## ASSESSMENT AND DIAGNOSIS

A complete assessment for an opioid use disorder requires a thorough medical and social history, in particular gathering information on: education, vocation, family, mental health, living arrangements/family structure and support, social service agency or legal involvement, peers, sex, and use of other drugs. As with other SUDs, opioid use disorder in the Diagnostic and Statistical Manual of Mental Disorders-V (DSM-V) is a diagnosis across a continuum from mild to severe according to the number of diagnostic criteria met. For opioids, withdrawal and cravings are more prominent compared with other substances. Family history of SUDs should look both for family members' past use and how any current use reflects family attitudes and the availability of opioids. The youth's living situation needs careful review of supervision (or the lack of it) and access to opioids (eg, does the adolescent stay on weekends with grandmother who is prescribed pain medications.) There are also high rates of co-occurring mental health disorders, and patients should have a psychiatric assessment, with mood disorders, attention deficit–hyperactivity disorder (ADHD), and conduct disorder commonly seen. Patients with psychiatric illness and addiction are sometimes refused medications until they "get clean," but concurrent treatment of substance abuse and mental health disorders is more effective than trying to treat these conditions serially.[57] High-risk sexual behaviors with sexually transmitted infections (STIs) and pregnancy are common, as is amenorrhea due to the dopaminergic effects of opioids.

Urine drug screens are an essential component of assessment. Most street opioids (heroin, short-acting prescription opioids, crushed long-acting prescription opioid formulations, which then are transformed to short-acting) are detectable in urine for 2 to 3 days after use. Although urine drug screenings are important, they are not sufficient to diagnose OUDs. Patients can time their use, adulterate the specimen, or substitute someone else's urine. It is important to note that certain specific opioids, such as buprenorphine, methadone, or oxycodone, are not detected on many routine drug screens.

Patients describe euphoria, and feeling relaxed and mellow with mild-to-moderate intoxication, while on examination they can be substantially sedated. With higher doses, patients become even drowsier (nodding) and have increasing cognitive impairment. Pupillary constriction is a hallmark sign of opioid intoxication. Itching (from mast-cell histamine release), nausea, constipation, depression, urinary hesitancy, and sexual dysfunction are all common features of opioid use. Signs of injection use may include thrombosed veins (track marks), injection site erythema, bruises, abscesses or cellulitis, or scarring. An adolescent may try to hide visible injection sites with clothing (such as long sleeve shirts.)

### Overdose

Coma, pinpoint pupils, and respiratory depression are the classic triad for opiate overdose. Eventually respiratory depression can lead to full respiratory arrest and death. Youth with OUDs are especially vulnerable to overdose in the context of loss of tolerance following an interruption of opioid use. When they resume use with either a brief lapse or a full relapse, it is easy to miscalculate and use doses that were previously tolerated and seem familiar, but produce overdose due to loss of tolerance. Unfortunately one such vulnerable time is after detoxification, treatment, or other periods of abstinence or partial abstinence, unless patients are protected by relapse prevention medications. It may be that youth are even more vulnerable to this phenomenon than adults, because they are less experienced with drugs and developmentally they are more impulsive and have poor judgment.

Opioid intoxication/overdose should be considered in any emergency in which a young person presents with decreased level of consciousness or obtundation. Many adolescents use multiple drugs, and in an acute/emergent setting blood/urine toxicology screenings for other substances including blood alcohol concentration or breathalyzer should be obtained. In addition, drug use including opioids should be considered in any adolescent involved in a motor vehicle crash or other trauma.

### Withdrawal

Opiate withdrawal is biphasic: an acute phase with marked somatic symptoms and then protracted abstinence with persistent but less severe somatic symptoms accompanied by prominent cravings. Acute withdrawal is not life-threatening but it is extremely uncomfortable, and adolescents who try to quit on their own usually resume use, because they cannot tolerate withdrawal. The half-life of the drug used (for example 4–6 hours for heroin or 1–2 days for methadone) determines the timing of symptom onset. Without the usual exogenous opioids, the opiate receptor is not activated, which causes a rebound increase in central nervous system (CNS) activity. Signs and symptoms of opiate withdrawal include tachycardia, hypertension, mild fever, sweats, rhinorrhea, sneezing, pupillary dilation, anorexia, nausea, vomiting, diarrhea, piloerection, restlessness, irritability, yawning, and insomnia. Patients report severe cravings during acute withdrawal. There are a variety of standardized withdrawal assessment tools such as the Clinical Opioid Withdrawal Scale (COWS) to quantify and track withdrawal severity.[58] Even after acute withdrawal, patients can have ongoing or recurrent complaints (such as malaise, restlessness, insomnia, sweats, anxiety, and irritability). In addition, cravings can persist, and the intensity/frequency of the cravings fluctuates, often elicited or intensified by exposure to triggering cues, either external ("people, places, and things"), or internal ("HALT: being hungry, angry, lonely or tired").

## TREATMENT

There are multiple challenges facing youth with OUDs and their families. Patient engagement is difficult; treatment has to be developmentally appropriate, youth-friendly, and ideally have family involvement. Nationwide, treatment resources for adolescents are scarce, and insurance coverage and other funding varies widely. Outside of major metropolitan areas, there is often limited treatment availability, and what treatment is available may not be affordable. From 2010 to 2013 only 10.9% of those aged 12 or older who needed SUD treatment received treatment at a specialty facility. Unfortunately less than half of patients who felt that they needed help actually made an effort to get treatment.[21] Among adolescent opioid users, from 1998 to 2008 there was a 10-fold increase in admissions to publically funded drug treatment centers for prescription OUDs,[59] but despite this increase, treatment capacity is woefully limited. Detoxification alone is insufficient. The ASAM (American Society of Addiction Medicine) Criteria for adolescents recommends medically monitored inpatient/residential treatment for adolescents needing pharmacologic management for detoxification, followed by intensive outpatient services that slowly taper in frequency and intensity, followed by longitudinal outpatient maintenance and monitoring. There is an increasing treatment role for the medical community given the frequency of comorbid psychiatric disorders, and the increasing knowledge of the benefits of relapse prevention medications. These highly specialized resources are even more limited.

Many people with OUDs are convinced they do not need help and can quit on their own. Youth are even more vulnerable to this idea; developmentally they may believe they are invincible and therefore do not need treatment or medications or any help at all. The first step in treatment is just showing up, and in order to engage youth, treatment programs have to be interesting, relevant, and friendly. The involvement of caring and supportive family/adults is important, and treatment programs need to help families understand what and how much leverage they have and how to best use their influence.

### Detoxification (Withdrawal Management)

Acute opiate withdrawal can be successfully managed with opioid agonists, alpha-2 agonists, nonsteroidal anti-inflammatories, anticholinergics, and antacids. Insomnia and agitation/anxiety should be aggressively managed with agents such as hydroxyzine, diphenhydramine, trazodone, clonidine, or benzodiazepines. Care should be taken when using benzodiazepines in that many patients have often abused them, and benzodiazepines are very reinforcing. Although the alpha-agonist clonidine was long used as the primary detox medication, newer opioid agonists (such as buprenorphine) are now more routinely used, because they are physiologically directed toward the opiate receptor and therefore more effective in alleviating symptoms of acute withdrawal. Buprenorphine, a high affinity partial mu agonist, can be tapered over a period of days or transitioned to a maintenance dose for relapse prevention for medication assisted recovery. Buprenorphine can be used alone but more preferably in combination with naloxone which has poor oral bioavailabilty; when the combination product is given sublingually, there is minimal absorption of naloxone, but if diverted and used intravenously, the naloxone is bioeffective. Because buprenorphine will displace other opioids, the first dose should not be given until the adolescent has moderate withdrawal symptoms to avoid the possibility of precipitated withdrawal.

### Emergency Treatment of Overdose

In an acute overdose setting, patients may need emergency resuscitation including respiratory support. If opiate intoxication/overdose is suspected, the best immediate response is administration of the opiate antagonist naloxone. Naloxone can be administered by multiple routes: intramuscular, intravenous, nasal, subcutaneous, or endotracheal. Naloxone displaces bound opioids from opiate receptors, which reverses the overdose but may precipitate opiate withdrawal. Multiple and/or ongoing naloxone doses may be needed depending on the dose and half-life of the opioid. In response to the national epidemic of opiate abuse, many communities are providing/prescribing naloxone overdose kits to first responders, addicts, and addicts' families, along with appropriate training in an attempt to decrease the number of opiate overdoses and deaths.

### Relapse Prevention Medications

Although there is relatively little information about the use and effectiveness of pharmacotherapies for opioid dependence in adolescents (as opposed to adults in whom they are the clear standard of care), relapse prevention medications are nevertheless gaining more widespread adoption. Without relapse prevention medications, dropout and relapse among youth with OUDs have been the rule, with worse treatment outcomes than nonopioid youth SUDs.[36] Methadone is not easily available for patients under the age of 18, but can be considered when planning aftercare for young adults. Buprenorphine/Naloxone (Bup/Nal) maintenance as a relapse prevention medication has shown promising results in maintaining longer periods of abstinence from opioids, reducing treatment dropout and reducing overdose.[60,61] Another relapse prevention medication for opioid dependence is extended release naltrexone (XR-NTX), which can reduce opioid relapse, improve treatment adherence (including therapy/counseling), and decrease overdose in opioid users,[62] and shows initial promising results in opioid dependent adolescents and young adults.[55] Many adolescents on extended Bup/Nal or XR-NTX treatment still continue to use other nonopioid drugs, relapse on opioids when they discontinue medications, have higher attrition rates compared with older patients, and remain at high risk for overdose, particularly when they drop out of treatment.[63,64] Which of these medications is best for which patient is not yet well understood, but emerging evidence suggests that outcomes are better with medications integrated into comprehensive psychosocial treatment.

### CLINICAL CASES
#### Case 1

SM is a 17-year-old white boy who lives with his parents and 2 younger siblings in a rural town. He was an A/B student in high school, where he played on the varsity team. He began binge drinking and smoking cannabis at parties at age 15, and by 17 was using substances most weekends. During his junior year he broke his ankle, requiring surgery and internal fixation. He was prescribed opioid analgesics perioperatively, continued to have pain and was given repeated prescriptions. Two months postoperatively, he started escalating his use, taking higher doses at shorter frequencies. He started crushing the pills and snorting them. As he ran out of his prescriptions, he took opioids he found at home in the medicine cabinet and then started stealing supplies from friends and neighbors. He progressed to sniffing or smoking heroin when it was difficult to get pills, stealing money from his parents. He became irritable and reclusive, and was failing 2 classes. He tried to stop on multiple occasions, but would get sick, and was afraid to tell anyone. When confronted by his parents about the missing money, he broke down and asked for their help. His parents were devastated; they had never known a drug addict, and brought him to a substance abuse treatment center. During a 3-week inpatient stay, he underwent detoxification and received injectable extended release naltrexone (XR-NTX). He subsequently attended an intensive outpatient program (IOP), where he initially did well but briefly relapsed 6 weeks later after he declined a second dose of XR-NTX and missed sessions of treatment, thinking he could do it on his own. He came back for a brief inpatient treatment episode to restart XR-NTX. He continued in IOP, then stepped down to less intensive outpatient treatment, including monthly doses of XR-NTX with parental monitoring. He has remained abstinent from opioids for 13 months.

## Case 2

KB is a 16-year-old white girl from a suburban area. She was raised by her grandmother after her mother died of a heroin overdose. Her 21-year-old brother is in a methadone treatment program. At age 11, she started using marijuana and cutting school; she has failed seventh grade twice. She smokes 1 pack of cigarettes per day, smokes marijuana daily, and has abused cough syrup, stimulant medications, benzodiazepines, and prescription opiates. Last year she started seeing a 23-year-old man who introduced her to heroin, first nasal then injection. She is absent from her grandmother's house regularly, from overnight to days at a time. She has been on probation for controlled dangerous substances charges, but did not follow through with court-mandated treatment. Her grandmother has had her emergently psychiatrically hospitalized for out-of-control behaviors. Emergency Medical Services were called to her school, because she was unresponsive; she was resuscitated with naloxone. She spent the night in an emergency room and was transferred to inpatient substance treatment. She reported daily injection heroin use. Her laboratory tests showed UDS positive for marijuana and opiates, mildly elevated liver function tests and HCV positivity. She underwent initial detoxification with buprenorphine and then transitioned to ongoing buprenorphine/naloxone as a relapse prevention medication. She was also started on an antidepressant. At grandmother's request, juvenile services placed her in a group home with a GPS electronic monitor. She attends intensive outpatient treatment at a dual diagnosis program where her buprenorphine/naloxone is provided through observed administration several days per week.

## REFERENCES

1. Muhuri PK, Gfroerer JC, Davies C. Associations of Nonmedical Pain Reliever Use and Initiation of Heroin Use in the US. Center for Behavioral Health Statistics and Quality Data Review. SAMHSA; 2013. Available at: http://archive.samhsa.

gov/data/2k13/DataReview/DR006/nonmedical-pain-reliever-use-2013.htm. Accessed October 12, 2015.

2. Subramaniam GA, Stitzer MA. Clinical characteristics of treatment-seeking prescription opioid vs. heroin-using adolescents with opioid use disorder. Drug Alcohol Depend 2009;101:13–9.

3. Subramaniam GA, Stitzer MA, Woody G, et al. Clinical characteristics of treatment seeking adolescents with opioid versus cannabis/alcohol use disorders. Drug Alcohol Depend 2009;99(1–3):141–9.

4. Mills KL, Teesson M, Darke S, et al. Young people with heroin dependence: findings from the Australian Treatment Outcome Study (ATOS). J Subst Abuse Treat 2004;27:67–73.

5. Uhl GR, Grow RW. The burden of complex genetics in brain disorders. Arch Gen Psychiatry 2004;61(3):223–9.

6. Merikangas KR, Stolar M, Stevens DE, et al. Familial transmission of substance use disorders. Arch Gen Psychiatry 1998;55(11):973–9.

7. Tsuang MT, Lyons MJ, Meyer JM, et al. Co-occurrence of abuse of different drugs in men: the role of drug-specific and shared vulnerabilities. Arch Gen Psychiatry 1998;55(11):967–97.

8. Kendler KS, Jacobson KC, Prescott CA, et al. Specificity of genetic and environmental risk factors for use and abuse/dependence of cannabis, cocaine, hallucinogens, sedatives, stimulants, and opiates in male twins. Am J Psychiatry 2003; 160(4):687–95.

9. Nelson EC, Agrawal A, Heath AC, et al. Evidence of CNIH3 involvement in opioid dependence. Mol Psychiatry 2015. [Epub ahead of print].

10. Kreek MJ, Levran O, Reed B, et al. Opiate addiction and cocaine addiction: underlying molecular neurobiology and genetics. J Clin Invest 2012;122(10): 3387–93.

11. Volkow ND, Frieden TR, Hyde PS, et al. Medication-assisted therapies–tackling the opioid-overdose epidemic. N Engl J Med 2014;370(22):2063–6.

12. Fortuna RJ, Robbins BW, Caiola E, et al. Prescribing of controlled medications to adolescents and young adults in the United States. Pediatrics 2010;126:1108–16.

13. Anderson P, Chisholm D, Fuhr DC. Effectiveness and cost-effectiveness of policies and programmes to reduce the harm caused by alcohol. Lancet 2009; 373:2234–46.

14. Chaloupka F, Straif K, Leon ME, et al. Effectiveness of tax and price policies in tobacco control. Tob Control 2011;20:235–8.

15. Kuehn BM. Medication helps make therapy work for teens addicted to prescription opioids. JAMA 2010;303:2343–5.

16. Gordon SM, Mulvaney F, Rowan A. Characteristics of adolescents in residential treatment for heroin dependence. Am J Drug Alcohol Abuse 2004;30:593–603.

17. Werb D, Kerr T, Nosyk B, et al. BMJ Open. The temporal relationship between drug supply indicators: an audit of international government surveillance systems. BMJ Open 2013;3(9):e003077.

18. Hopfer CJ, Khuri E, Crowley TJ, et al. Adolescent heroin use: a review of the descriptive and treatment literature. J Subst Abuse Treat 2002;23:231–7.

19. National Institute on Drug Abuse. Prescription Opioid and Heroin Abuse. Presented by Nora D. Volkow, M.D.House Committee on Energy and Commerce Subcommittee on Oversight and Investigations. Available at: http://www. drugabuse.gov/about-nida/legislative-activities/testimony-to-congress/2015/ prescription-opioid-heroin-abuse. Accessed April 29, 2014.

20. Johnston LD, O'Malley PM, Bachman JG, et al. Monitoring the future National Survey Results On Drug Use, 1975–2010. vol. 1: Secondary school students. Ann Arbor (MI): Institute for Social Research, The University of Michigan; 2011.
21. Substance Abuse and Mental Health Services Administration. Results from the 2013 National Survey on Drug Use and Health: Summary of National Findings, NSDUH Series H-48. HHS Publication No. (SMA) 14–4863. Rockville (MD): Substance Abuse and Mental Health Services Administration; 2014. Available at: http://www.samhsa.gov/data/sites/default/files/NSDUHresultsPDFWHTML2013/Web/NSDUHresults2013.htm.
22. McCabe SE, West BT, Boyd CJ. Motives for medical misuse of prescription opioids among adolescents. J Pain 2013;14(10):1208–16.
23. McCabe SE, West BT, Teter CJ, et al. Medical and nonmedical use of prescription opioids among high school seniors in the United States. Arch Pediatr Adolesc Med 2012;166(9):797–802.
24. Substance Abuse and Mental Health Services Administration; The NSDUH report, State Estimates of Nonmedical Use of Prescription Pain Relievers. Available at: http://archive.samhsa.gov/data/2k12/NSDUH115/sr115-nonmedical-use-pain-relievers.htm. Accessed January 8, 2013.
25. Substance Abuse and Mental Health Services Administration. Results from the 2006 national survey on drug use and health: national findings. Rockville (MD): SAMHSA; 2007. Available at: http://files.eric.ed.gov/fulltext/ED498206.pdf.
26. Substance Abuse and Mental Health Services Administration; Center for Behavioral Health Statistics and Quality, National Survey on Drug Use and Health, 2013 and 2014. Table 1.18A – Nonmedical Use of Pain Relievers in Lifetime, Past Year, and Past Month, by Detailed Age Category: Numbers in Thousands, 2013 and 2014. Available at: http://www.samhsa.gov/data/sites/default/files/NSDUH-DetTabs2014/NSDUH-DetTabs2014.htm#tab1-18b. Accessed October 9, 2015.
27. Branson CE, Clemmey P, Harrell P, et al. Polysubstance use and heroin relapse among adolescents following residential treatment. J Child Adolesc Subst Abuse 2012;21:204–21.
28. Chen CY, Storr CL, Anthony JC. Early-onset drug use and risk for drug dependence problems. Addict Behav 2009;34(3):319–22.
29. Windle M, Windle RC. Early onset problem behaviors and alcohol, tobacco, and other substance use disorders in young adulthood. Drug Alcohol Depend 2012;121(1–2):152–8.
30. Subramaniam GA, Ives ML, Stitzer MA, et al. The added risk of opioid problem use among treatment-seeking youth with marijuana and/or alcohol problem use. Addiction 2010;105:686–98.
31. Barry D, Syed H, Smyth BP. The journey into injecting heroin use. HARCP 2012;14(3):89–100.
32. Chiang S, Chen S, Sun H, et al. Heroin use among youths incarcerated for illicit drug use: psychosocial environment, substance use history, psychiatric comorbidity, and route of administration. Am J Addict 2006;15:233–41.
33. Hopfer CJ, Mikulich SK, Crowley TJ. Heroin use among adolescents in treatment for substance use disorders. J Am Acad Child Adolesc Psychiatry 2000;39:1316–23.
34. Fuller CM, Vlahov D, Ompad DC, et al. High-risk behaviors associated with transition from illicit non-injection to injection drug use among adolescent and young adult drug users: a case-control study. Drug Alcohol Depend 2002;66:189–98.
35. Clemmey P, Payne L, Fishman M. Clinical characteristics and treatment outcomes of adolescent heroin users. J Psychoactive Drugs 2004;36:85–94.

36. Woodcock EA, Lundahl LH, Stoltman JJ, et al. Progression to regular heroin use: examination of patterns, predictors, and consequences. Addict Behav 2015;45: 287–93.

37. Goldsamt LA, Harocopos A, Kobrak P, et al. Circumstances, pedagogy and rationales for injection initiation among new drug injectors. J Community Health 2010; 35(3):258–67.

38. Pugatch D, Strong LL, Has P, et al. Heroin use in adolescents and young adults admitted for drug detoxification. J Subst Abuse 2001;13:337–46.

39. Eaves CS. Heroin use among female adolescents: the role of partner influence in path of initiation and route of administration. Am J Drug Alcohol Abuse 2004;30: 21–38.

40. Doherty MC, Garfein RS, Monterroso E, et al. Gender differences in the initiation of injection drug use among young adults. J Urban Health 2000;77:396–414.

41. Canfield MC, Keller CE, Frydrych LM, et al. Prescription opioid use among patients seeking treatment for opioid dependence. J Addict Med 2010;4:108–13.

42. Gandhi DH, Kavanagh GJ, Jaffe JH. Young heroin users in Baltimore: a qualitative study. Am J Drug Alcohol Abuse 2006;32:177–88.

43. Substance Abuse and Mental Health Services Administration. Treatment Episode Data Set (TEDS). 1999-2009. National Admissions to Substance Abuse Treatment Services, DASIS Series: S-56. HHS Publication No. (SMA) 11-4646. Rockville (MD): Substance Abuse and Mental Health Services Administration; 2011. Available at: http://wwwdasis.samhsa.gov/teds09/TEDS2k9NWeb.pdf.

44. Neaigus A, Miller M, Friedman SR, et al. Potential risk factors for the transition to injecting among non-injecting heroin users: a comparison of former injectors and never injectors. Addiction 2001;96(6):847–60.

45. Neaigus A, Gyarmathy VA, Miller M, et al. Transitions to injecting drug use among noninjecting heroin users: social network influence and individual susceptibility. J Acquir Immune Defic Syndr 2006;41(4):493–503.

46. Hadland SE, Werb D, Kerr T, et al. Childhood sexual abuse and risk for initiating injection drug use: a prospective cohort study. Prev Med 2012;55(5):500–4.

47. Ompad DC, Ikeda RM, Shah N, et al. Childhood sexual abuse and age at initiation of injection drug use. Am J Public Health 2005;95(4):703–9.

48. National Institute on Drug Abuse. Overdose Death Rates. Available at: http://www.drugabuse.gov/related-topics/trends-statistics/overdose-death-rates. Accessed September 21, 2015.

49. Centers for Disease Control and Prevention. Vital signs: overdoses of prescription opioid pain relievers—United States, 1999-2008. MMWR Morb Mortal Wkly Rep 2011;60:1487–92. Available at: http://www.cdc.gov/vitalsigns/PainkillerOverdoses/index.html.

50. Rudd RA, Paulozzi LJ, Bauer MJ, et al, Centers for Disease Control and Prevention. Increases in heroin overdose deaths 28 States, 2010 to 2012. MMWR Morb Mortal Wkly Rep 2014;63(39):849–54. Atlanta, GA: Centers for Disease Control and Prevention.

51. Chen LH, Hedegaard H, Warner M. Drug-poisoning deaths involving opioid analgesics: United States, 1999-2011. NCHS Data Brief 2014;(166):1–8.

52. Substance Abuse and Mental Health Services Administration. Drug Abuse Warning Network report: trends in emergency visits involving nonmedical use of narcotic pain relievers, 2010. Available at: http://www.samhsa.gov/data/sites/default/files/DAWN096/DAWN096/SR096EDHighlights2010.htm. Accessed October 9, 2015.

53. Substance Abuse and Mental Health Services Administration. Drug Abuse Warning Network, 2011: National Estimates of Drug-Related Emergency Department Visits. HHS Publication No. (SMA) 13–4760, DAWN Series D-39. Rockville (MD): Substance Abuse and Mental Health Services Administration; 2013. Available at: http://www.samhsa.gov/data/sites/default/files/DAWN2k11ED/DAWN2k11ED/DAWN2k11ED.pdf.
54. Subramaniam GA, Fishman MJ, Woody G. Treatment of opioid-dependent adolescents and young adults with buprenorphine. Curr Psychiatry Rep 2009; 11(5):360–3.
55. Fishman MJ, Winstanley EL, Curran E, et al. Treatment of opioid dependence in adolescents and young adults with extended release naltrexone: preliminary case-series and feasibility. Addiction 2010;105:1669–76.
56. Wu L, Woody GE, Yang C, et al. How do prescription opioid users differ from users of heroin or other drugs in psychopathology? Results from the National Epidemiological Survey on Alcohol and Related Conditions. J Addict Med 2011;5:28–35.
57. Riggs PD, Mikulich SK, Davies RD, et al. A randomized controlled trial of fluoxetine and cognitive behavioral therapy in adolescents with major depression, behavior problems, and substance use disorders. Arch Pediatr Adolesc Med 2007;161:1026–34.
58. Wesson DR, Ling W. The Clinical Opiate Withdrawal Scale (COWS). J Psychoactive Drugs 2003;35(2):253–9. Available at: https://www.drugabuse.gov/sites/default/files/files/ClinicalOpiateWithdrawalScale.pdf.
59. Substance Abuse and Mental Health Services Administration, Center for Behavioral Health Statistics and Quality. Treatment Episode Data Set (TEDS): 1998-2008. State Admissions to Substance Abuse Treatment Services, DASIS Series: S-55, HHS Publication No. (SMA) 10-4613. Rockville (MD): 2010. Available at: http://wwwdasis.samhsa.gov/teds08/TEDS2k8Sweb.pdf. Accessed October 12, 2015.
60. Warden D, Subramaniam GA, Carmody T, et al. Predictors of attrition with buprenorphine/naloxone treatment in opioid dependent youth. Addict Behav 2012; 37(9):1046–53.
61. Woody GE, Poole SA, Subramaniam G, et al. Extended vs short term buprenorphine- naloxone for treatment of opioid- addicted youth: a randomized trial. JAMA 2008;300:2003–20.
62. Krupitsky E, Nunes EV, Ling W, et al. Injectable extended-release naltrexone for opioid dependence: a double-blind, placebo-controlled, multicentre randomised trial. Lancet 2011;377(9776):1506–13.
63. Schuman-Olivier Z, Weiss RD, Hoeppner BB, et al. Emerging adult age status predicts poor buprenorphine treatment retention. J Subst Abuse Treat 2014; 47(3):202–12.
64. Dreifuss JA, Griffin ML, Frost K, et al. Patient characteristics associated with buprenorphine/naloxone treatment outcome for prescription opioid dependence: results from a multisite study. Drug Alcohol Depend 2013;131(1–2):112–8.

# Hallucinogen Use Disorders

Rashad Hardaway, MD[a],*, Jason Schweitzer, MD[b], Joji Suzuki, MD[c]

## KEYWORDS

- Hallucinogen • LSD • MDMA • Psilocybin • PCP • Adolescent • Treatment

## KEY POINTS

- Perceptions among adolescents regarding hallucinogens use are changing. Current trends show there are increasing emergency department presentations from use of these drugs.
- Use of novel hallucinogens, such as 25I-NBOMe, is gaining popularity and can have serious medical complications.
- Hallucinogen use may result in psychiatric disorders that may occur at time of use or afterward and may cause secondary psychotic, mood, or anxiety disorders. Limited data exist regarding treatment of these psychiatric disorders in adolescents, and evidence is extrapolated from adult studies. Benzodiazepines and behavioral techniques are recommended first-line treatments. Certain antipsychotics may worsen hallucinogen disorders and should be used with caution.

## INTRODUCTION/BACKGROUND

Hallucinogens have been used throughout history to serve various functions in different cultures. For example, native populations have incorporated use of hallucinogens into cultural practices over centuries.[1] Hallucinogens may be found in nature, but over the past century, novel agents have been synthesized, creating a wide array of effects, and manufactured in different preparations and formulations.[2,3]

Today, these psychotomimetic substances are gaining popularity among US youth as club drugs because they induce "trips" and other experiences for its users that are often pleasurable. Although banned by US federal law for use among the general public, certain native groups are protected by the American Indian Religious Freedom Act, enacted in 1994 by the government, for use in religious ceremonies and centuries-old rituals.

[a] Department of Psychiatry and Behavioral Medicine, Seattle Children's Hospital, 4800 Sand Point Way NE, Seattle, WA 98105, USA; [b] Department of Child and Adolescent Psychiatry, Rady Children's Hospital, 3665 Kearny Villa Road, San Diego, CA 92123, USA; [c] Department of Psychiatry, Brigham and Women's Hospital, 75 Francis Street, Boston, MA 02115, USA
* Corresponding author.
*E-mail address:* Rashad.Hardaway@seattlechildrens.org

Child Adolesc Psychiatric Clin N Am 25 (2016) 489–496
http://dx.doi.org/10.1016/j.chc.2016.03.006
1056-4993/16/$ – see front matter © 2016 Elsevier Inc. All rights reserved.

childpsych.theclinics.com

The classical definition of a hallucinogen, as defined by Hollister in 1968, states that the substances predominantly cause changes in thought, perception, and mood with minimal intellectual or memory impairment. In addition, hallucinogens should induce minimal craving.[4] The members of this drug class have been shown to be agonists at the same receptor class in the brain. Common classical hallucinogens include lysergic acid diethylamide (LSD), psilocybin (mushrooms or "shrooms"), and mescaline/peyote. Other popular drugs that produce similar effects to classical hallucinogens act via other receptors and mechanisms. Among these are phencyclidine (PCP) and 3,4-methylene-dioxy-methamphetamine (MDMA), a street drug that has gained popularity among today's youth and is increasingly recognized for its hallucinogenic properties.[5]

The Drug Abuse Warning Network (DAWN) monitors presentations to emergency rooms secondary to substance use. Over nearly the past decade, intoxications secondary to hallucinogens, and specifically use of PCP by adolescents, that have reached the attention of an emergency room clinician have been on the increase. Perceptions about hallucinogens among youth are changing. The current trends in hallucinogen use now raise clinical concern and make recognition and treatment of the clinical effects of these drugs more essential.

Efforts have been made to ascertain the public health impact of hallucinogens and have typically targeted use of LSD, psilocybin, and mescaline in data reporting.[6–9] The Diagnostic and Statistical Manual of Mental Disorders, fifth edition (DSM-5), published by the American Psychiatric Association categorizes hallucinogens into 2 categories: those related to PCP use and those related to use of other hallucinogens.[10] For the purpose of this review, the aforementioned substances are included in addition to MDMA, given its popularity of use and impact on the adolescent population.

## EPIDEMIOLOGY

Governmental organizations and academic groups, such as DAWN, monitor the use of substances by adolescents in the United States. These data have been reported in the National Survey on Drug Use and Health (NSDUH) and the Monitoring the Future study (MTF) among others. Over the past decade, there has been a declining rate in general substance use among adolescents. In 2011, up to 1 in 4 adolescents have been noted to use alcohol and 1 in 5 adolescents have used an illicit drug. It is also notable that rates of illicit drug use and misuse and abuse of pharmaceuticals have remained stable over the period of 2004 to 2011.[6]

The MTF study is an annual survey of 8th, 10th, and 12th graders among whom striking trends for LSD use have been noted. Since the late 1990s, adolescents have reported decreasing use of this substance. Adolescents perceived that LSD is less available and reported decreasing use during this period. At the same time, adolescents perceive LSD use to be less risky than prior years, and rates of disapproval of its use are decreasing.[11] The NSDUH, produced by the Substance Abuse and Mental Health Services Administration, monitors trends in alcohol, tobacco, and illicit substance use among individuals 12 and older. This study shows similar trends regarding LSD particularly in reported prevalence and perceptions of use[6] (**Fig. 1**).

It has been argued that MDMA use has decreased across the United States since the early 2000s. However, the DAWN report found that Emergency Room visits involving MDMA in patients younger than 21 more than doubled, from 460 visits in 2005 to 10,176 visits in 2011. It is also of note that from 1999 to 2008 it was more likely to be used by girls than by boys.[12] Another study found that 4.4% of high school seniors across the United States have tried MDMA within the past year.[13] These data underscore the clinical relevance of this drug.

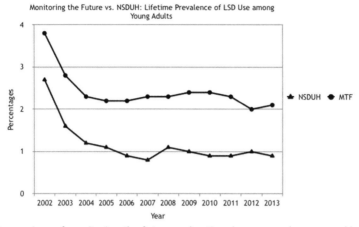

**Fig. 1.** Comparison of monitoring the future and national survey on drug use and health LSD lifetime prevalence of use data (2002–2013) for young adults aged 12–17. (*Data from* Substance Abuse and Mental Health Services Administration. Results from the 2013 National Survey on Drug Use and Health: summary of national findings. NSDUH Series H-48, HHS Publication No. (SMA) 14-4863. Rockville (MD): Substance Abuse and Mental Health Services Administration; 2014. p. 1–143.)

Native American adolescents are a vulnerable population for hallucinogen use. A study of these youth, who were admitted to a residential substance abuse treatment facility, found notable characteristics for these users. Almost 11% used peyote illicitly and 9% met DSM-IV criteria for hallucinogen abuse. The median number of substances used was almost 5.5, and the median number of substance use disorders was about 3. This finding emphasizes that hallucinogen use is a pervasive problem that reaches many demographic groups and communities.[14]

## CLINICAL PRESENTATION

Hallucinogens may cause a variety of physical and psychological effects for the user. The DSM-5 describes some of the experienced symptoms as it defines an intoxicated state with a hallucinogen substance. These effects may be observed in the autonomic, neurologic, and gastrointestinal systems. Psychological signs and symptoms might include change or intensification of affective states, perceptual disturbances, derealization and depersonalization, paranoia, or even suicidal ideation. **Table 1** lists the common effects of hallucinogens for users.

When ingested, MDMA increases levels of serotonin, norepinephrine, and dopamine in the central nervous system, leading to subjective mood changes, euphoria, and alterations in perception of time. Common objective findings can include ataxia, agitation, bruxism, and vital sign abnormalities, such as hypertension, tachycardia, and hyperthermia. Severe adverse effects are uncommon, but have been noted in the literature, including hepatotoxicity, hyponatremia, and serotonin syndrome. Although milder side effects should resolve within hours, more serious effects require emergent management of acute poisoning, and subsequent management of sequelae on inpatient basis.

There are several comorbidities associated with long-term use of MDMA among adolescents. These comorbidities include an increase in depressive symptoms,[15] possible long-term effects on memory,[16] and increased risk of hallucinogen use

**Table 1**
**Selected hallucinogenic effects of indolealkylamine and phenylalkylamine hallucinogens (including lysergic acid diethylamide, psilocybin, and peyote)**

| Hallucinogen Effects | |
| --- | --- |
| Physical Effects | Psychological Effects |
| Regular (mild to very mild): Tachycardia, Palpitations, Hypertension/hypotension, Diaphoresis, Hyperthermia, Motor incoordination, Tremors, Hyperreflexia, Altered neuroendocrine functioning | Intensification/lability of affectivity with euphoria |
| | Acute neuropsychological/cognitive impairments |
| Regular (mild to strong): mydriasis, arousal, insomnia | Anxiety |
| | Depression |
| Occasional: nausea/vomiting, diarrhea, blurred vision, salivation | Illusions/pseudo-hallucinations/hallucinations/synesthesias |
| | Megalomania |
| | Derealization/depersonalization |
| | Paranoid/suicidal ideation |

*Adapted from* Suzuki J, Halpern JH, Passie T, et al. Hallucinogens. In: Cohen LM, Collins FL, Young AM, et al, editors. Pharmacology and treatment of substance abuse: evidence- and outcome-based perspectives. New York; Hove (East Sussex): Routledge; 2009. p. 403.

disorder. A study among adolescents from 12 to 17 years of age with lifetime MDMA use found the rate of suicide attempts was almost double that of matched adolescents who used drugs other than MDMA, and almost 9 times non-drug-using controls.[17]

25I-NBOMe is a designer hallucinogen with high affinity for or potency at 5HT-2a receptor, leading to its hallucinogenic properties. It additionally acts as an agonist on $\alpha$-adrenergic receptors, causing sympathomimetic effects. It is available in preparations such as a vapor, intravenous, pill, and blotter. Duration of its effects may last 3 to 13 hours, whereas its toxicity may last for days. In **Box 1**, intoxication with 25I-NBOMe resembles that of LSD and psilocybin.

## DIAGNOSIS

The DSM-5 organizes hallucinogen-related disorders by time of exposure and subsequent effects. The subsequent effects range from acute intoxication and use disorder to persistence of symptoms and psychiatric disorders occurring secondary to hallucinogen use. Further categorization makes the distinction between PCP use disorders and other hallucinogen use disorders. Although PCP is an anesthetic with hallucinogenic properties and is not considered a classical hallucinogen, the DSM includes it in this category of substances. Compared with DSM-IV text revision (TR), DSM-5 defines use disorder as medical (craving, tolerance) and psychosocial effects. As compared with DSM-IV-TR, the use of "abuse" and "dependence" has been eliminated. Use disorders are characterized by severity (mild = 2–3 symptoms; moderate = 4–5; severe = 6 or more).

Intoxication of PCP may have other effects from classical hallucinogens. PCP was formerly used as an anesthetic before its popularity as a street drug. In differentiating this from other hallucinogens, PCP intoxication may produce nystagmus, hypoesthesia, hyperacusis, or even coma with significant amounts of ingestion. Adrenergic symptoms occur in intoxication with PCP as well as other hallucinogens; however, the latter may involve other physical signs such as pupillary dilation, vision disturbance, diaphoresis, and tremors. Significant behavioral changes are noticed with intoxication and the signs and symptoms of intoxication are not secondary to another cause.[10]

| Box 1 |
| --- |
| **Effects of ingestion of 25I-NBOMe** |
| *Adverse Effects of 25I-NBOMe Intoxication* |
| Delirium |
| Agitation/aggression |
| Paranoia |
| Dysphoria |
| Self-harm |
| Hyperthermia |
| Seizures |
| Fever |
| Tachycardia |
| Hypertension |
| Mydriasis |
| Hyperreflexia |
| *Data from* Suzuki J, Dekker M, Valenti ES, et al. Toxicities associated with NBOMe ingestion—a novel class of potent hallucinogens: a review of the literature. Psychosomatics 2015;56(2):129–39. |

Differing from PCP intoxication, DSM-5 describes intoxication with other hallucinogens as causing significant behavioral or psychological changes. Such changes may include anxiety or depression, ideas of reference, paranoid ideation, and altered judgment that occur shortly after the ingestion period. Perceptual changes typically occur while alert and may include enhancement of perceptions, depersonalization, derealization, and hallucinations. Physical signs that accompany intoxication may include autonomic signs (eg, tachycardia) or sweating. Other observed signs may include palpitations, vision changes (eg, blurring), and neurologic changes like poor coordination.

Some users of hallucinogens may experience other or persistent neuropsychiatric sequelae after episodes of ingestion. Hallucinogen persisting perception disorder (HPPD) is a syndrome in which users will have continued perceptual symptoms that occurred during intoxication, and these symptoms lead to significant distress or impairment. Others may develop psychiatric disorders such as mood disturbance, anxiety, or psychosis, secondary to their hallucinogen use. In these instances, there are no other medical or psychiatric conditions that would better account for the symptoms.

## BRIEF SUMMARY OF CLINICAL MANAGEMENT

Specific studies regarding the management of hallucinogen use and its sequelae in adolescents have not been performed recently. Most of the literature that exists to date pertains to the management of adult psychiatric disorders from hallucinogen use. This data have been extrapolated for treatment of adolescents in medical centers.

### Hallucinogen Intoxication

Among the interventions used for intoxication with these substances, behavioral and supportive interventions yield the best effect, as seen in **Table 2**.[18,19]

**Table 2**
**Recommended behavioral interventions for treating hallucinogen intoxication**

| | |
|---|---|
| Reality testing The "Talkdown" | Describes this as guiding the patient through their experience and using simple statements to aid in reality testing. Stating the patient's name or even labeling objects in the environment may provide reassurance. |
| Observation | A clinician or staff person should remain with the patient until the patient has "come down" from their "trip." |
| Environment | Creating a low stimulus environment–although too little stimulation might exacerbate the patient's distressed state. |
| Support | Offering emotional support and constant monitoring are also helpful for management. |
| Acuity | Hospitalization for psychotic or mood symptoms persisting longer than 24 h. |

Pharmacologic approaches for agitation and anxiety include use of benzodiazepines and use of haloperidol if benzodiazepines are not sufficient. Intramuscular midazolam and diazepam may be considered in the absence of sufficient intravenous access for use of lorazepam.[20,21] Given the $\alpha$-2 antagonist properties and potential to lower the seizure threshold, use of some antipsychotics (eg, chlorpromazine) should be carefully considered. It is recommended to also remain cognizant of the patient's underlying medical comorbidities and presentation with medication management.[22]

Measures that have not been demonstrated to be effective or are recommended against include

- Gastric lavage has not been demonstrated to be effective given the rapid gastrointestinal absorption of these substances.
- Caution should be given to the use of neuroleptic agents, including chlorpromazine, phenothiazines, and 5HT-2a antagonists such as risperidone. These agents may have a paradoxic effect or worsen HPPD symptoms.[23–27]

### Hallucinogen Persisting Perception Disorder

Strong evidence for use of various treatment modalities for flashbacks and persistent perceptual disturbances is minimal. **Table 3** reviews examples of treatments that have yielded positive and negative effects on these symptoms.[24,28,29] As stated above, phenothiazines, chlorpromazine, and 5HT-2a antagonists may worsen HPPD.

**Table 3**
**Useful and adverse treatment of hallucinogen persisting perception disorder**

| Recommended Treatments for HPPD | |
|---|---|
| Positive Effects | Adverse Effects |
| Haloperidol | Risperidone |
| Benzodiazepines | Phenothiazines |
| Psychotherapy | Hallucinogens |
| Behavioral modification | Marijuana/substance use |
| Clonidine | Selective serotonin reuptakes |
| Sunglasses | — |
| Carbamazepine | — |

## Hallucinogen Use and Related Disorders

For hallucinogen use disorder and substance-induced psychosis, no controlled trials for treatment have been performed. No established pharmacologic treatments to decrease use of hallucinogens currently exist. It is recommended that adolescents with regular use be referred to a mental health specialist for treatment. A general approach for treatment of substance use should be applied.[30] Motivational interviewing and referral to self-help groups (eg, Narcotics Anonymous) may be helpful. Given the prevalence of comorbid psychiatric and substance use disorders, evaluation and appropriate treatment of these should occur. As with hallucinogen intoxication, the acute treatment recommendation for psychosis induced by hallucinogens may apply.

Should use of hallucinogens become more popular among adolescents, more data and evidence-based treatments may arise to provide effective treatments for this population.

## REFERENCES

1. Carod-Artal F. Alucinógenos en las culturas precolombinas mesoamericanas. Neurologia 2015;30:42–9.
2. King LA, Kicman AT. A brief history of "new psychoactive substances". Drug Test Anal 2011;3(7–8):401–3.
3. Weaver MF, Hopper JA, Gunderson EW. Designer drugs 2015: assessment and management. Addict Sci Clin Pract 2015;10(1):8.
4. Glennon RA. Neurobiology of hallucinogens. In: Galanter M, Kleber H, editors. The American psychiatric publishing textbook of substance abuse treatment. 4th edition. Washington, DC: APPI; 2008. p. 181–9.
5. National Institute on Drug Abuse. MDMA (Ecstasy or Molly). 2013. Available at: http://www.drugabuse.gov/publications/drugfacts/mdma-ecstasy-or-molly. Accessed September 24, 2015.
6. Substance Abuse and Mental Health Services Administration. Results from the 2013 National Survey on drug use and health: summary of national findings. NSDUH Series H-48, HHS Publication No. (SMA) 14–4863. Rockville (MD): Substance Abuse and Mental Health Services Administration; 2014. p. 1–143.
7. Substance Abuse and Mental Health Services Administration, Center for Behavioral Health Statistics and Quality. The CBHSQ Report: a day in the life of young adults: substance use facts. Rockville (MD): 2014. p. 1–7.
8. Substance Abuse and Mental Health Services Administration, Center for Behavioral Health Statistics and Quality. The DAWN report: emergency department visits involving phencyclidine (PCP). Rockville (MD): 2013.
9. Substance Abuse and Mental Health Services Administration, Center for Behavioral Health Statistics and Quality. The DAWN report: ecstasy-related emergency department visits by young people increased between 2005 and 2011; Alcohol involvement remains a concern. Rockville (MD): 2013.
10. American Psychiatric Association. Diagnostic criteria from DSM-5. Washington, DC: American Psychiatric Publishing; 2013.
11. Johnston LD, Miech RA, O'Malley PM, et al. Use of alcohol, cigarettes, and number of illicit drugs declines among U.S. teens. Ann Arbor (MI): University of Michigan News Service; 2014. Available at: http://www.monitoringthefuture.org.
12. Wu P, Liu X, Hoang TP, et al. Ecstasy use among U.S. adolescents from 1999 to 2008. Drug Alcohol Depend 2010;112(1–2):33–8.

13. Palamar JJ, Kamboukos D. An examination of sociodemographic correlates of ecstasy use among high school seniors in the United States. Subst Use Misuse 2014;49(13):1774.

14. Novins DK, Fickenscher A, Manson SM. American Indian adolescents in substance abuse treatment: diagnostic status. J Subst Abuse Treat 2006;30(4): 275–84.

15. Brière FN, Fallu J-S, Janosz M, et al. Prospective associations between meth/amphetamine (speed) and MDMA (ecstasy) use and depressive symptoms in secondary school students. J Epidemiol Community Health 2012;66(11):990–4.

16. Wright NE, Strong JA, Gilbart ER, et al. 5-HTTLPR genotype moderates the effects of past ecstasy use on verbal memory performance in adolescent and emerging adults: a pilot study. PLoS One 2015;10(7):e0134708.

17. Kim J, Fan B, Liu X, et al. Ecstasy use and suicidal behavior among adolescents: Findings from a national survey. Suicide Life Threat Behav 2011;41(4):435–44.

18. Strassman RJ. Hallucinogenic drugs in psychiatric research and treatment: perspectives and prospects. J Nerv Ment Dis 1995;183:127–38.

19. Taylor RL, Maurer JI, Tinklenberg JR. Management of "bad trips" in an evolving drug scene. J Am Med Assoc 1970;213:422–5.

20. Abraham HD, McCann UD, Ricaurte GA. Psychedelic drugs. In: Davis KL, Charney D, Coyle JT, et al, editors. Neuropsychopharmacology: the fifth generation of progress. Philadelphia: Lippincott Williams & Wilkins; 2002. p. 1545–56.

21. D'Orazio JL, Bassett R, Boroughf WL. Hallucinogen toxicity. 2015. Available at: http://emedicine.medscape.com/article/814848. Accessed October 8, 2015.

22. Tacke U, Ebert MH. Hallucinogens and phencyclidine. In: Kranzler HR, Ciraulo DA, editors. Clinical manual of addiction psychopharmacology. Washington, DC: American Psychiatric; 2005. p. 211–41.

23. Abraham HD. Visual phenomenology of the LSD flashback. Arch Gen Psychiatry 1983;40:884–9.

24. Abraham HD, Mamen A. LSD-like panic from risperidone in post-LSD visual disorder. J Clin Psychopharmacol 1996;16:228–31.

25. Morehead DB. Exacerbation of hallucinogen-persisting perception disorder with risperidone. J Clin Psychopharmacol 1997;17:327–8.

26. Schwarz CJ. e complications of LSD: a review of the literature. J Nerv Ment Dis 1968;146:174–86.

27. Strassman RJ. Adverse reactions for psychedelic drugs: a review of the literature. J Nerv Ment Dis 1984;172:577–95.

28. Halpern JH, Pope HG Jr. Hallucinogen persisting perception disorder: what do we know after 50 years? Drug Alcohol Depend 2003;69:109–19.

29. Markel H, Lee A, Holmes RD, et al. LSD flashback syndrome exacerbated by selective serotonin reuptake inhibitor antidepressants in adolescents. J Pediatr 1994;125:817–9.

30. El-Mallakh RS, Halpern JH, Abraham HD. Substance abuse: hallucinogen- and MDMA-related disorders (chapter 60). In: Tasman A, Maj M, First MB, et al, editors. Psychiatry. 3rd edition. London: John Wiley & Sons; 2008. p. 1100–26.

# Inhalant Abuse and Dextromethorphan

Michael Storck, MD[a],*, Laura Black, MD[b], Morgan Liddell, MD[a]

## KEYWORDS

- Inhalant abuse • Epidemiology • Detection

## KEY POINTS

- Inhalant abuse is difficult to detect and crosses demographic variables.
- Inhalant abuse is associated with significant morbidity.
- Abuse occurs with readily available household substances.
- Inhalant abuse is mostly associated with younger populations and generally fades out by the end of high school.
- "Over-the-counter" products such as dextromethorphan are sought by youth for abuse purposes.

## INTRODUCTION

Compared with alcohol, marijuana, and virtually every other abused substance, inhalant use is a low-frequency occurrence for youth. Nonetheless, it poses a disproportionately serious health problem for this patient population. The relatively heightened concern for inhalant abuse rests, in part, on the socially isolative, hidden nature of its use. Along with inhalants (which primarily are legal substances found in households), dextromethorphan (DM), an ingredient in nonprescription cold remedies, is likely the most commonly used dissociative agent among youth. To appreciate the range of health risks of these substances, consider these 5 brief clinical vignettes:

- An 8-year-old boy is brought to his pediatrician after being found at home unconscious. A syncope evaluation was negative; however, a toluene-based solvent was found open in his bedroom.
- A 12-year-old girl raises concerns at school when her teacher notes a perioral rash, tell-tale stigmata of "bagging," inhaling paint or other volatile fumes from a plastic bag.

Disclosure Statement: The authors have no conflicts of interest.
<sup>a</sup> Department of Child Psychiatry, Seattle Children's Hospital, 4800 Sand Point Way NE, Seattle, WA 98105, USA; <sup>b</sup> New York University, Department of Psychiatry, One Park Avenue, 8 th floor, New York, NY 10016, USA
* Corresponding author.
*E-mail address:* storck@uw.edu

Child Adolesc Psychiatric Clin N Am 25 (2016) 497–508
http://dx.doi.org/10.1016/j.chc.2016.03.007
1056-4993/16/$ – see front matter © 2016 Elsevier Inc. All rights reserved.

childpsych.theclinics.com

- A 14-year-old boy, coming in from the barn, is noted by his grandfather to have clothing that smells like gasoline (unclear if he was alone or with friends).
- A young coworker has had a decline in productivity and has quit socializing after work. She takes frequent breaks during the day and seems irritable and anxious. She was observed purchasing a large quantity of aerosolized computer duster spray.
- A 15-year-old boy is brought to the emergency room from school, actively hallucinating. Physical examination was pertinent for significant hypertension, and in his pants pocket, multiple empty bubble pill sheets of Coricidin were found.

The rate of inhalant abuse among children and young adults has sustained a very promising decline in the last 2 decades. In the US National Institutes of Health (NIH) National Youth Risk Behavior Survey (YRBS) for high school students, student reporting of using an inhalant to get 'high" at least one time in their life decreased from 20.3% in 1995 to 8.9% in 2013.[1] Nonetheless, inhalant use remains a very dangerous activity affecting a surprisingly young demographic. It is a daunting task for counselors, teachers, families, and health care practitioners to stay alert to the risks of inhalant abuse given the broad and ever-evolving array of household substances that are often used surreptitiously.

## TYPES OF SUBSTANCES AND PRODUCTS ABUSED

The term "inhalant" encompasses a wide range of pharmacologically diverse substances that readily vaporize. More than 200 different inhalant product categories were reported to US poison control centers in 1993 to 2008.[2] Inhalants can be divided into 3 groups (**Table 1**) based on pharmacologic effects. The most commonly abused inhalants are group I, aliphatic, aromatic, or halogenated hydrocarbons (including propellants). Group II are gases (including those typically used in medical settings) and other aerosols. Group III alkyl nitrites have dropped considerably in popularity. Of the above-mentioned inhalants, only propellants (most commonly now is computer duster spray) have shown a substantial increase in abuse since the early 2000s. In contrast, gasoline and paint inhalation have significantly declined, but are still responsible for greater than 50% of inhalant-related poison control cases in children 6 to 7 years old.[2] Overall, patterns of inhalant use vary widely across the middle childhood

| Table 1 Pharmacologic classification of inhalants: chemical content of product examples | |
|---|---|
| Group I | Volatile solvents, fuels, and anesthetics<br>• Solvents: toluene, acetone, methylene chloride, ethyl acetate, trichloroethane, tetrachloroethylene, hexane, hydrocarbons (eg, paint thinner, polish remover, correction fluid, felt-tip markers, glues, cleaning fluids, spray paint, hairspray, computer/electronics cleaning [duster] spray)<br>• Fuels: butane or propane lighters or pressurized fuel tanks, gasoline, racing car octane boosters, refrigerants<br>• Anesthetics: ether, halothane, enflurane, ethyl chloride |
| Group II | Nitrous oxide: diverted medical anesthetic, whipped-cream dispenser charger (whippets), whipping-cream aerosol |
| Group III | Volatile alkyl nitrites: chlorohexyl nitrite (eg, liquid aroma/liquid incense air fresheners or room odorizers), isobutyl or butyl nitrite, isopropyl nitrite |

*Adapted from* Williams JF, Storck M. Inhalant abuse. Pediatrics 2007;119(5):1010; with permission.

and adolescent years, varying from community to community and also based on environmental or occupational risk factors.

Although nicotine and alcohol are not classified as inhalants, the recent trend of inhaling alcohol and nicotine vapors ("vaping") is a related emerging serious public health issue. Now that the prevalence of vaping of nicotine has surpassed smoking cigarettes in many schools,[3] vaping nicotine may emerge as a factor in the gateway to other inhalant abuse by youth.

DM and chlorpheniramine maleate are common ingredients in more than 140 over-the-counter (OTC) products, including Coricidin and Robitussin, liquid and pill versions. When used at recommended doses, DM is an effective and safe antitussive agent with minimal side effects. However, DM is increasingly abused by young people and is hypothesized to be the most commonly used dissociative.[4] Street names for Coricidin HBP and specifically the DM component include Triple C, Red Devils, Red Hots, poor man's PCP, Skittles, and Robo (from Robatussin), giving rise to terms used for illicit use, including skittling and robo-tripping. Increasing recognition of the potential for abuse by adolescents has led to state bans, first in California and then adopted in numerous other states, on the sale of DM to adolescents.

## Epidemiology

Inhalant abuse occurs across all geographic and socioeconomic zones. Among pediatric populations in the United States, inhalant use has shown a promising overall decline in the last 20 years, as evidenced in the NIH's databases from periodic surveys of middle and high school youth: the National Survey on Drug Use and Health (NSDUH),[5] the Monitoring the Future Program (MTF),[6] and the YRBS.[1] However, it is worth noting that these surveys do not reach school dropouts or children younger than 13; therefore, the trends may not be quite as promising.

The peak age of inhalant abuse in the United States is 14 to 15 years, with onset in children as young as 5 or 6 years of age.[7] Most initiation has occurred by the end of ninth grade,[6] and poison control data suggest that nearly 25% of users initiate their inhalant abuse between ages 6 and 12.[1] According to MTF survey results:

- For eighth graders, inhalants rank second only to marijuana among illicit drugs.
- Eleven percent of eighth graders report trying inhalants; 2.3% reported inhalant use in the month before the survey.
- Inhalants are the only class of drug for which use decreases during adolescence: use typically declines by 10th grade but can continue into adulthood.
- Gender gaps in inhalant use differ from nearly all other types of substance use: eighth-grade girls have a greater 30-day and lifetime prevalence of inhalant use than do eighth-grade boys, but the reverse is true for 10th and 12th graders.
- Marsolek and colleagues[1] reported 15 years of data collection (between 1993 and 2008) by the National Poison Data System (NPDS) of calls to poison control centers regarding inhalant exposure. NPDS data show an overall substantial decline of inhalant use among all ages. In contrast with a lack of gender disparity with inhalant use rates, though, NPDS data show that for youth between 12 and 17, boys accounted for 73% of the known cases of suspected inhalant toxicity.
- There are significant ethnic and geographic differences in inhalant use
  - Hispanic and non-Hispanic Caucasians are more likely to use than African Americans.
  - Rural and remote areas show overall higher rates of inhalant abuse. This rate may reflect increased use among Caucasian youths in the southeast United States.

Inhalant abuse in the United States steadily increased from the 1970s into the early 1990s, after which use declined and is now, for eighth and 10th graders, at the lowest point in the history of the MTF study and near the lowest point for 12th graders. However, it is worth noting that this decline in the mid-1990s coincided with an active public health campaign, the 1995 Partnership for a Drug-Free America. Since the late 1990s, perceived risk for inhalant use has been steadily falling; this portends some risk for a resurgence in inhalant use.

DM abuse rates increased substantially in the early 2000s, but they have also had a slight decline recently. Poison control center data indicate an increasing rate of DM abuse among adolescents in the early 2000s.[8–10] Between 2001 and 2006, Coricidin exposures reported to the poison control doubled in Illinois with more than 80% of total exposures reported involving children 18 years old or younger.[8] The California Poison Control System noted a 10-fold increase, in the early 2000s, in DM exposures with, three-fourths of the total cases involving children 9 to 17 years of age.[11] However, recent MTF data note that DM use has steadily decreased from 2012 to 2015.

In terms of social prestige, inhalants are typically viewed by adolescents as a "younger," less socially appealing drug.[12] Nonetheless, the experience of using together and "shared hallucinations" are cited as a means of social bonding,[13] and teens report peer influence and desire to join a social group as motivators to use. Users are characterized by higher levels of sensation seeking[14]; most have already tried alcohol and marijuana by the time they initiate use,[15] and 94% cite "experimentation" as their reason for first use.[16] Others cite escapism from a negative emotional state.[12,13,17] Of note, inhalant users have a substantially higher lifetime prevalence of mood (48%), anxiety (36%), and personality (45%) disorders[18] as well as disordered eating.[19] In female users, there is a predominance of mood disorders, whereas in male users, antisocial personality disorder is more frequent. Hopelessness, suicidality, and frequency of suicide attempts are also increased among users.[12,15,20,21] Longitudinal surveys show that adolescents who use inhalants are at elevated risk for subsequent cocaine (40%) and injectable drug use (9%) as adults[15]; those who use both inhalants and marijuana were nearly 3 times as likely to eventually use heroin and other intravenous drugs.[18] Adolescent users were also more likely to engage in high-risk behaviors as adults, such as damaging property and selling drugs.[15]

Miller and colleagues[22] proposed that adolescents gravitate toward using DM as it is the "SMART" (acronym) choice:

- Stigma: unlike illicit street drugs, there is no negative connotation when purchasing OTC preparations with this drug
- Money: it is a relatively inexpensive OTC drug (although anecdotally, some practitioners have asserted that most adolescents steal this medication from stores rather than purchasing it)
- Access: it is OTC and found in many home medicine cabinets
- Risks: DM is available from respectable medical companies with strict quality control
- Testing: routine drug tests do not test for DM.

Inhalant abuse is often thought of as occurring more in impoverished and/or isolated communities. An example of a generational story line from a cultural perspective can be found in North American Indian and Alaska Native child health. Some rural Native American communities have historically borne a greater burden of inhalant use; in some communities, practices such as "bagging" gasoline have been endemic, and children younger than 12 were frequently found using together in groups.[7] Many come from families with a history of substance abuse and domestic violence; 80%

of First Nations youths in Canada's residential treatment centers for inhalant use reported a history of childhood sexual abuse.[7] However, in the last 20 years, there has been a sustained drop off in the proportion of Native youth using inhalants; the current rate is slightly lower than that of non-Native youth.[23] This change has been attributed to community mobilization and an effort to create substance abuse treatment approaches that focus on the intersection between positive psychology and components of indigenous culture.[24]

International trends in inhalant use are diverse, and these patterns may be of special interest to physicians treating immigrant populations. In terms of prevalence, most South American countries report a much lower past-year prevalence of inhalant use among secondary school students than in the United States, ranging from 1.11% to 3.60%.[25] Of note, Brazil is an exception, with a high prevalence similar to the United States, and a predominance of the substance *lança* or *loló* (chloroform ether, traditionally used during Carnaval), particularly among older high school students and those of higher socioeconomic status (odds ratio 0.2 for lowest socioeconomic status compared with highest).[26] In contrast, many studies show increased inhalant use among the most socioeconomically deprived global populations, such as indigenous and homeless youths. A survey of Indian street children found that 35% were using whitener (containing toluene), with a mean age of initiation of 10.3 years old.[27] In Upper Egypt, a survey of street children found 91% were using volatile substances, primarily a glue called Kolla. Children reported a desire for comfort, escape from problems, and assertion of one's manhood.[28] In a survey of the Roma community of Eastern Slovakia, chronic toluene users were overwhelmingly male (90%) children, with 15% being younger than the age of 10.[29]

## CLINICAL PRESENTATION
### *Methods of Inhalation and Absorption and Mechanisms of Action*

Inhalant abusers use volatile products that are capable of producing a quick and generally initially pleasurable sensory experience, or "high," with rapid dissipation and minimal "hangover" symptoms. Inhaled substances are widely available, convenient, inexpensive, easily concealed, and legal for specific intended uses but are intentionally misused by abusers. Many of these qualities are important factors that promote use in a young age group, because children have less sophisticated resources for acquiring alternative substances of abuse. Inhalant abuse, here, is distinct from toxic hydrocarbon exposures that can occur through unintentional ingestions and occupational exposures, although certainly the health risks certainly overlap.

Inhalants are abused through a variety of methods, and many "street" terms for this activity have been generated (**Table 2**). Innocent-looking containers are often used to conceal inhalant abuse (eg, inhaling spray paint fumes from a soft drink can or nitrous oxide–filled balloons). Volatile substances may also be applied to fingernails or a shirt collar to be inhaled, or substances may be chewed (eg, mothballs).

Inhalants are absorbed through the lungs and then rapidly metabolized through the cytochrome P450 system of the liver. Inhalants, except nitrites, are central nervous system (CNS) depressants.[30,31] Nitrous oxide likely acts through opiate and $\gamma$-aminobutyric acid (GABA) receptors[30]; volatile hydrocarbons have GABAergic effects and also likely inhibit $N$-methyl-$_D$-aspartate (NMDA) receptors.[32] Immediate effects often include an initial stimulating "rush" followed by light-headedness, disinhibition, and impulsivity. Intoxication lasts minutes but can be extended for hours by inhaling repeatedly. Slurred speech, dizziness, diplopia, ataxia, and disorientation occur as the inhalant dose increases. Euphoria is followed by drowsiness, lingering headache, and sleep, particularly after repeated cycles of inhalation. With prolonged use, visual

**Table 2**
**"Street" terms for methods used to abuse inhalants**

| Term | Mode of Delivery |
| --- | --- |
| Sniffing, snorting | Inhale through nose from original container |
| Huffing | Inhale through mouth from original container, or inhale from chemical-saturated rag held to face or mouth |
| Glading | Inhalation of air freshener |
| Dusting | Inhalation of aerosol computer dusting spray via mouth or nose |
| Bagging | Paper or plastic bag containing inhalant is held over mouth and nose or over the head; more commonly related to intentional self-harm or suicidal behavior |
| Ocean water | Combined alcohol and inhalant use, or combined water or mouthwash with hairspray[27] |
| Snotballs | Ball of rubber cement; heated before inhaling |

Additional contemporary street terms listed at http://www.inhalant.org/inhalant-abuse/slang-terms-in-use/.

hallucinations and marked time distortion occur; these are cited as a motivator for continued use.[13] Low-frequency users report more pleasurable experiences, whereas chronic users have mixed pleasurable and unpleasant/noxious experiences.[33]

DM is a synthetic opioid and is the dextro-isomer of the codeine analogue levorphanol. It was patented in the United States as an antitussive agent made from a morphinelike base by Hoffmann-La Roche in 1954. It has specific serotonergic and σ-1 opioidergic properties. DM is metabolized in the liver by CYP2D6 to Dextrorphan, which acts as a strong noncompetitive NMDA receptor antagonist, an $\alpha3/\beta4$ nicotinic receptors antagonist, and an agonist at the opioid σ1 and 2 receptors, and inhibits the reuptake of serotonin. It acts as a cough suppressant by inhibiting the medullary cough centers to nearly the same extent that opiate alkaloids (including codeine) do, but with less opioid effects, such as analgesia, CNS depression, and respiratory suppression.[22] However, it is likely the effect at the NMDA receptors contribute to DM's acute and long-term abuse potential and neuropsychiatric manifestations.[34]

### Warning signs and adverse effects
Inhalants, as a group, have a greater hazard index and fatality rate than any other pharmaceutical and nonpharmaceutical agent. Observers may notice a particular constellation of warning signs that a young person may be exposed or experimenting with inhalants (**Box 1**). Of the inhalants, butane has the highest hazard index and fatality rate. The prevalence of cases of suspected propellant hydrocarbon toxicity (principally due to "dusters") doubled from 2003 to 2008, whereas rates were declining for nearly all other inhalant categories.

Reported toxic effects of inhalants include the following (**Box 1**)[31,35]:

- Mucous membrane irritation: rhinorrhea, epistaxis, sneezing, coughing, excess salivation, conjunctival injection, dyspnea, wheezing
- A variety of cardiac arrhythmias and electrical changes
- Gastrointestinal: nausea, vomiting, diarrhea, abdominal cramps
- Renal: metabolic alkalosis, specific autoimmune responses
- Dermatologic: perioral rash, frostbitelike injury from computer duster spray
- CNS: drowsiness and eventual coma, cerebellar dysfunction with gait disturbance,[36–38] chronic encephalopathy, mood changes, and dementia[35–39]

---

**Box 1**
**Warning signs of inhalant abuse**

*General*

- Appearance of poor hygiene and grooming, stained clothing, chemical or sweet solvent odor on breath (may persist for hours after using)
- Appetite changes, weight loss, chronic malaise and fatigue, gastrointestinal complaints and headache

*Behavioral*

- Hoarding or hiding products (eg, cans of computer duster spray under bed)
- Social withdrawal or significant shift in family and peer relationships and activities, drop in grades
- Somatization
- Chronic neuropsychiatric changes, including confusion, poor concentration, depression, irritability, hostility, or paranoia

*Dermatologic*

- Chronic rhinitis, conjunctivitis, recurrent epistaxis, oral or nasal ulcerations
- "Huffer's rash": classically a perioral or perinasal dermatitis with pyoderma
- Frostbite on the face or oral/nasal cavity (caused by refrigerants and chlorofluorohydrocarbon propellants in computer duster spray)[50]
- Dermatitis of the face or hands (may look like nonspecific contact dermatitis or perioral eczema, or may have a yellow crust if caused by nitrites)

---

- Peripheral nervous system: muscle weakness, tremor, peripheral neuropathy, spasticity[35–39]
- Tolerance, dependence, and withdrawal symptoms[40–43]
- Teratogenicity: toluene embryopathy, neonatal withdrawal[40–42]
- Death: "sudden sniffing death syndrome," suffocation, or aspiration, accidental injury

Morbidity and mortality generally increase as frequency of inhalant use increases, with the important exceptional concern about "sudden sniffing death syndrome" (**Box 2**). First-time inhalant abusers may be particularly at risk for sudden death.

---

**Box 2**
**Causes of death from inhalant abuse**

*Acute*

- Direct causes, (such as sudden sniffing death syndrome)
- Indirect causes, (such as asphyxiation)

*Delayed*

- Cardiomyopathy
- Central nervous system toxicity: toluene dementia and brainstem dysfunction
- Hematologic: aplastic anemia, leukemia
- Hepatocellular carcinoma
- Renal toxicity: nephritis, nephrosis, tubular necrosis

Sudden sniffing death syndrome is the leading cause of fatality related to inhalant abuse.[32] Bass[44] in the 1970s hypothesized that hydrocarbons and other inhalants such as toluene "sensitize" the myocardium to epinephrine, and in sudden stress or fright, an epinephrine surge can cause coronary artery spasm or a fatal cardiac arrhythmia. Slow dissipation of the substance in lipid-rich membranes sets the individual at risk for several hours after inhalation.[45] This vulnerability to adrenergic activation is an important factor to keep in mind in acute treatment environments. This type of sudden death leaves no specific macroscopic or microscopic postmortem features, so often a cause cannot be identified at autopsy.

Given the younger age of initiation of inhalant use, sometimes as early as 5 to 6 years old, as well as the difficulty detecting inhaled substances, the toxic effects of inhalant abuse may go unrecognized in patients seen for injuries and medical problems, such as syncope, headaches, and rashes. The diversity of inhalant substances that can be abused corresponds to a diversity of possible sequelae. For most organs, if chronic solvent abuse is terminated, there is remarkable reversibility of many of the pathologic effects. Compared with other organ systems, the nervous system has less regenerative capacity, and damage often has a more pervasive impact. Of all biological membranes, myelin has the highest fat content at 75%, and neuronal membranes may contain up to 45% lipid. Frequent and longer-term inhalant use leads to nervous system absorption of these highly lipophilic substances (**Box 3**).[35–39] Chronic hydrocarbon exposure is implicated in impairments in memory, attention, processing speed, and visual-spatial conceptualization.[46] Computed tomography has demonstrated a loss of brain mass, and particularly in the thalamus, basal ganglia, pons, and cerebellum.[47] Chronic exposure may also cause toxicity to the hippocampus and basal ganglia and impair executive functioning and processing speed.[48]

Adverse effects and toxicities of DM:

- For individuals with genetic polymorphisms of CYP2D6 causing them to be rapid metabolizers of DM, they are more prone to neuropsychiatric manifestations. When it binds to NMDA receptors, it produces euphoria, dissociation, hyperactivity and psychosis, bidirectional nystagmus, and extrapyramidal neuromuscular effects.[34]
- Other signs and symptoms can include tachycardia, hypertension, chest pain, lethargy/somnolence, mydriasis, nystagmus, agitation, ataxia, dizziness, disorientation, slurred speech, vomiting, hallucinations, tremor, headache, syncope, and seizure.[9,10]
- Toxic effects of other substances in OTC preparations containing DM (eg, acetaminophen causing liver toxicity, antihistaminergic agents causing

---

**Box 3**
**Major neurotoxic consequences of inhalant abuse**

- Cerebellar ataxia
- Cranial neuropathy: usually cranial nerves V and VII
- Encephalopathy: acute or chronic
- Multifocal: both cortical and subcortical central nervous system damage, both central nervous system and peripheral nerve effects
- Parkinsonism
- Peripheral neuropathy

anticholinergic toxicity). These other substances, especially acetaminophen, can be the most toxic and life-threatening variables in OTC substance ingestions.

## SUMMARY: PROVIDER AND PARENT/CLINICIAN GUIDANCE

In summary, inhalants and OTC cold remedies represent a relatively small proportion of the youth problems with substance abuse. The age group demographics and the surreptitious nature of acquisition and exposure, though, make for some very worrisome risks and clinical problems, which may appear unsuspected in the clinic, the school, the home, and the work place. Treatment challenges are posed by the diversity of abused inhalants and user populations, comorbid psychopathology, psychosocial problems, polydrug use, and the physiologic and neurologic effects of inhalant abuse.

Risk reduction recommendations
- Parents and providers: be aware that inhalant abuse occurs in all patient populations. Maintain a broad "index of suspicion" given surreptitious use and experimentation in younger children. Reduce access to means and be aware of the ubiquity of household agents abused (encourage families to know where their household supplies are, clean up the garage, shed, paints).
- Public education: social media and the Internet may include risk-reduction strategies as well as enticements targeting youth and discussion of newer patterns of substance use including computer duster, "vaping" of electronic cigarettes, and alcohol.
- Look for updates on marketing changes and regulation of products (nitrate, correction fluid, OTC cough syrup). Check the National Inhalant Prevention Coalition, www.inhalants.com, an information and referral clearinghouse. Be knowledgeable of local and regional trends; the local poison control center may be the best place to start.
- There is very limited research concerning specific rehabilitation treatment needs and successful treatment modalities specific to inhalant users. Pharmacotherapy is usually not useful in the treatment of inhalant abusers except to address comorbid conditions.
- In an effort to harness youths' own risk awareness, openness, motivations, and values, motivational interviewing techniques[49] are quite helpful for rapport building and the clinical relationship.
- Clinicians treating immigrant and refugee populations should be aware of global trends in inhalant use that may affect their patients.
- Increasing personal and ethnic self-identity through role modeling has been helpful in treating some groups of inhalant abusers, and positive cultural identification has been shown to be important in prevention.

## REFERENCES

1. Kann L, Kinchen S, Shanklin SL, et al. Youth risk behavior surveillance—United States, 2013. MMWR Suppl 2014;63(4):1–168.
2. Marsolek MR, White NC, Litovitz TL. Inhalant abuse: monitoring trends by using poison control data, 1993-2008. Pediatrics 2010;125(5):906–13.
3. Durmowicz E. The impact of electronic cigarettes on the paediatric population. Tob Control 2014;23:ii41–56.
4. Miller S. Dextromethorphan psychosis, dependence and physical withdrawal. Addict Biol 2005;10(4):325–7.

5. National survey on drug use and health 2014. Survey results. Available at: https://nsduhweb.rti.org; http://www.samhsa.gov/data/sites/default/files/NSDUH-FRR1-2014/NSDUH-FRR1-2014.pdf. Accessed September 25, 2015.
6. Johnston LD, O'Malley PM, Miech RA, et al. Monitoring the future: national survey results on drug use 1975-2015. Ann Arbor (MI): Institute for Social Research; The University of Michigan; 2016. Available at: http://www.monitoringthefuture.org/pubs/monographs/mtf-overview2015.pdf.
7. Eggertson L. Children as young as six sniffing gas in Pikangikum. CMAJ 2014; 186(3):171–2.
8. Yin S, Wahl M. Intentional Coricidin product exposures among Illinois adolescents. Am J Drug Alcohol Abuse 2011;37(6):509–14.
9. Baerji S, Anderson IB. Abuse of Coricidin HBP cough and cold tablets: episodes recorded by a poison center. Am J Health Syst Pharm 2001;58(19):1811–4.
10. Baker SD, Borys DJ. A possible trend suggesting increased abuse from Coricidin exposures reported to the Texas poison network: comparing 1998 to 1999. Vet Hum Toxicol 2002;44(3):169–71.
11. Bryner J, Wang U, Hui J, et al. Dextromethorphan abuse in adolescence: an increasing trend: 1999-2004. Arch Pediatr Adolesc Med 2006;160(12):1217–22.
12. Siegel JT, Alvaro EM, Patel N, et al. "...you would probably want to do it. Cause that's what made them popular": exploring perceptions of inhalant utility among young adolescent nonusers and occasional users. Subst Use Misuse 2009; 44(5):597–615.
13. Cruz SL, Dominguez M. Misusing volatile substances for their hallucinatory effects: a qualitative pilot study with mexican teenagers and a pharmacological discussion of their hallucinations. Subst Use Misuse 2011;46(Suppl 1):84–94.
14. Nonnemaker JM, Crankshaw EC, Shive DR, et al. Inhalant use initiation among U.S. adolescents: evidence from the national survey of parents and youth using discrete-time survival analysis. Addict Behav 2011;36(8):878–81.
15. Shamblen SR, Miller T. Inhalant initiation and the relationship of inhalant use to the use of other substances. J Drug Educ 2012;42(3):327–46.
16. Verma R, Balhara YP, Deshpande SN. Inhalant abuse: a study from a tertiary care de-addiction clinic. East Asian Arch Psychiatry 2011;21(4):157–63.
17. Perron BE, Howard MO, Maitra S, et al. Prevalence, timing, and predictors of transitions from inhalant use to inhalant use disorders. Drug Alcohol Depend 2009; 100(3):277–84.
18. Wu LT, Howard MO. Is inhalant use a risk factor for heroin and injection drug use among adolescents in the United States? Addict Behav 2007;32(2):265–81.
19. Pisetsky EM, Chao YM, Dierker LC, et al. Disordered eating and substance use in high-school students: results from the youth risk behavior surveillance system. Int J Eat Disord 2008;41(5):464–70.
20. Zubaran C, Foresti K, Thorell MR, et al. Anxiety symptoms in crack cocaine and inhalant users admitted to a psychiatric hospital in southern Brazil. Rev Assoc Med Bras 2013;59(4):360–7.
21. Freedenthal S, Vaughn MG, Jenson JM, et al. Inhalant use and suicidality among incarcerated youth. Drug Alcohol Depend 2007;90(1):81–8.
22. Miller SC. Coricidin HBP cough and cold addiction. J Am Acad Child Adolesc Psychiatry 2006;44(6):509.
23. Miller KA, Beauvais F, Burnside M, et al. A comparison of American Indian and non-Indian fourth to sixth graders' rates of drug use. J Ethn Subst Abuse 2008; 7(3):258–67.

24. Dell D, Hopkins C. Residential volatile substance misuse treatment for indigenous youth in Canada. Subst Use Misuse 2011;46(Suppl 1):107–13.
25. Hynes-Dowell M, Mateu-Gelabert P, Barros HM, et al. Volatile substance misuse among high school students in South America. Subst Use Misuse 2011;46(Suppl 1):27–34.
26. Sanchez ZM, Ribeiro LA, Moura YG, et al. Inhalants as intermediate drugs between legal and illegal drugs among middle and high school students. J Addict Dis 2013;32(2):217–26.
27. Praveen D, Maulik PK, Raghavendra B, et al. Determinants of inhalant (whitener) use among street children in a south Indian city. Subst Use Misuse 2012;47(10):1143–50.
28. Elkoussi A, Bakheet S. Volatile substance misuse among street children in Upper Egypt. Subst Use Misuse 2011;46(Suppl 1):35–9.
29. Vazan P, Khan MR, Poduska O, et al. Chronic toluene misuse among Roma youth in Eastern Slovakia. Subst Use Misuse 2011;46(Suppl 1):57–61.
30. Balster RL. Neural basis of inhalant abuse. Drug Alcohol Depend 1998;51:207–14.
31. Lorenc JD. Inhalant abuse in the pediatric population: a persistent challenge. Curr Opin Pediatr 2003;15:204–9.
32. Tormoehlen LM, Tekulve KJ, Nanagas KA. Hydrocarbon toxicity: a review. Clin Toxicol (Phila) 2014;52(5):479–89.
33. Garland EL, Howard MO. Phenomenology of adolescent inhalant intoxication. Exp Clin Psychopharmacol 2010;18(6):498–509.
34. Bobo WV, Fulton RB. Commentary on: severe manifestations of Coricidin intoxication. Am J Emerg Med 2004;22(7):624–5.
35. Brouette T, Anton R. Clinical review of inhalants. Am J Addict 2001;10:79–94.
36. Meadows R, Verghese A. Medical complications of glue sniffing. South Med J 1996;89:455–62.
37. Maruff P, Burns CB, Tyler P, et al. Neurological and cognitive abnormalities associated with chronic petrol sniffing. Brain 1998;121:1903–17.
38. Tenenbein M, deGroot W, Rajani KR. Peripheral neuropathy following intentional inhalation of naphtha fumes. Can Med Assoc J 1984;131:1077–9.
39. Lolin Y. Chronic neurological toxicity associated with exposure to volatile substances. Hum Toxicol 1989;8:293–300.
40. Keriotis AA, Upadhyaya HP. Inhalant dependence and withdrawal symptoms. J Am Acad Child Adolesc Psychiatry 2000;39:679–80.
41. Pearson MA, Hoyme HE, Seaver LH, et al. Toluene embryopathy: delineation of the phenotype and comparison with fetal alcohol syndrome. Pediatrics 1994;93:211–5.
42. Arnold GL, Kirby RS, Langendoerfer S, et al. Toluene embryopathy: clinical delineation and developmental follow-up. Pediatrics 1994;93:216–20.
43. Tenenbein M, Casiro OG, Seshia MM, et al. Neonatal withdrawal from maternal volatile substance abuse. Arch Dis Child Fetal Neonatal Ed 1996;74:F204–7.
44. Bass M. Sudden sniffing death. JAMA 1970;212:2075–9.
45. Shepherd RT. Mechanism of sudden death associated with volatile substance abuse. Hum Toxicol 1989;8:287–91.
46. Meyer-Baron M, Blaszkewicz M, Henke H. The impact of solvent mixtures of neurobehavioral performance: conclusions from epidemiological data. Neurotoxicology 2008;29(3):349–60.

47. Rosenberg NL, Grigsby J, Dreisbach J, et al. Neuropsychologic impairment and MRI abnormalities associated with chronic solvent abuse. J Toxicol Clin Toxicol 2002;40:21–34.
48. Scott KD, Scott AA. An examination of information-processing skills among inhalant-using adolescents. Child Care Health Dev 2012;38(3):412–9.
49. Tevyaw TO, Monti PM. Motivational enhancement and other brief interventions for adolescent substance abuse: foundations, applications and evaluations [Review]. Addiction 2004;99(Suppl 2):63–75.
50. Moreno C, Bejerle EA. Hydrofluoric acid burn in a child from a compressed air duster. J Burn Care Res 2007;28(6):909–12.

# Internet Addiction and Other Behavioral Addictions

Alicia Grattan Jorgenson, MD[a], Ray Chih-Jui Hsiao, MD[a],
Cheng-Fang Yen, MD, PhD[b],*

## KEYWORDS

- Internet addiction • Internet gaming disorder • Compulsive internet use
- Behavioral addiction • Adolescence

## KEY POINTS

- Teens are spending increasing amounts of time online. Although there are many benefits, there are also risks related to excessive use.
- Internet addiction is a type of behavioral addiction. Precise definitions vary and establishing clear diagnostic criteria is needed.
- It is important to recognize signs and symptoms of problematic Internet use and addiction including compulsive use, withdrawal, tolerance, and adverse consequences.
- Internet addiction is highly associated with depression, attention deficit hyperactivity disorder, and other substance use disorders. Treatment involves identifying and treating these comorbid conditions.
- More research is needed on targeted treatments for Internet addiction.

## INTRODUCTION
### Behavioral Addiction

Certain behaviors can produce short-term rewards or "highs." When this leads to diminished control over the behavior despite adverse consequences, the behavior itself can become the source of addiction rather than a psychoactive substance.[1–3]

Pathologic gambling is the best characterized behavioral addiction,[2,4] making a debut in the fifth version of the *Diagnostic and Statistical Manual of Mental Health Disorders* (DSM-5) under substance-related and addictive disorders.[5] Other behaviors that can produce similar short-term rewards include compulsive buying, sexual addiction, and excessive use of the Internet.[3,6,7] There is debate about which behaviors to include as behavioral addictions, because some may be better classified as impulse

[a] Seattle Children's Hospital, 4800 Sand Point Way NE, Mailstop OA.5.154, Seattle, WA 98105, USA; [b] Department of Psychiatry, Kaohsiung Medical University Hospital, School of Medicine, College of Medicine, Kaohsiung Medical University, Kaohsiung, Taiwan, China
* Corresponding author.
*E-mail address:* chfaye@cc.kmu.edu.tw

Child Adolesc Psychiatric Clin N Am 25 (2016) 509–520
http://dx.doi.org/10.1016/j.chc.2016.03.004
1056-4993/16/$ – see front matter © 2016 Elsevier Inc. All rights reserved.

childpsych.theclinics.com

| Abbreviations | |
|---|---|
| ADHD | Attention deficit hyperactivity disorder |
| CBT | Cognitive–behavioral therapy |
| DSM | *Diagnostic and Statistical Manual of Mental Health Disorders* |
| IA | Internet addiction |

control disorders.[2,3] Growing evidence suggests that problematic Internet use should be conceptualized as a behavioral addiction.[8–12] Internet gaming disorder was identified in Section III of the DSM-5 as an area of future research[5] and is the next most likely candidate to join pathologic gambling as a behavioral addiction.

Behavioral addictions resemble substance use disorders in terms of phenomenology, natural history, and neurobiology.[3,13,14] The typical onset of behavioral addiction occurs in adolescence and young adulthood and follows a chronic course with remissions and exacerbations.[3] Adolescence is a developmentally vulnerable period for the initiation of addictive behavior, a time when social demands (increasingly online) are high, risk-taking behavior is expected, and novel situations are encouraged.[14]

### Increasing Use and Misuse of the Internet

The influence of the Internet is undeniable, particularly in the lives of young people. It is not surprising that time spent online is increasing. According to the most recent 2013 Youth Risk Behavior Survey, 41.3% of adolescents in the United States spent more than 3 hours online on school days for something that was not school work, increasing from 22% in 2003.[15] Online gaming is increasingly popular, notably massively multiplayer role-playing games or MMORGs.[16] Just as overall Internet use is increasing, problematic Internet use has become clinically concerning. There are a number of reports highlighting the negative consequences of overuse including problems with sleep, mood, and interpersonal relationships.[9,17–20] In some Asian countries, Internet addiction (IA) is considered a major public health issue.[21]

Many terms have been applied to this problem, including Internet gaming disorder, excessive Internet use, compulsive Internet use, problematic Internet usage, and pathologic Internet usage. For the purpose of this article, Internet Addiction (IA) will be used.

### Aims

The purpose of this paper is to review the current literature on the neurobiological underpinnings, epidemiology, clinical presentation, diagnosis, and treatment of IA in adolescence.

## NEUROBIOLOGY

The addictive process involves problems with aberrant reward systems and impulsivity.[14,22] Past research suggests that neural circuits in the brain involving reward get hijacked and rewired during the process of addiction.[14,23] Specifically, mesolimbic dopaminergic projections to the nucleus accumbens from the ventral tegmental area have been implicated.[14] Dopamine increases in the nucleus accumbens with the administration of drugs of abuse or certain behaviors (gaming, gambling, sexual behavior).[14] It has also been recognized that use of dopaminergic medication in Parkinson's patients can lead to pathologic gambling and other addictive behaviors such as binge eating and hypersexuality.[24]

Like other addictions, the development of behavioral addiction, including IA, is associated with an overall reward deficiency and involvement of these dopaminergic pathways.[13,14] A PET study found striatal dopamine release in healthy volunteers during video game play.[25] Striatal dopamine receptor levels were reduced in men with IA compared with controls.[26] Kühn and colleagues[27] conducted an imaging study on 154 adolescents, comparing frequent and infrequent video game users. This study found higher volumes in left ventral striatum associated with frequent video game playing, which is consistent with findings of enhanced dopamine release during video game playing. A functional MRI study of addicted Internet gamers found that presenting cues of gaming elicited activation of right orbitofrontal cortex, right nucleus accumbens, right dorsolateral prefrontal cortex, and right caudate nucleus in contrast with the control group.[28] These findings support a similar neurobiological process to drug cravings for substance use disorders. Small gray matter structural changes in these pathways have also been implicated in adolescents with IA.[29,30] IA is also characterized by reward deficiency, specifically with diminished activity of ventral medial prefrontal cortex and involvement of dopaminergic mesolimbic pathways.[31]

Substance use disorders are known to run in families, with genes and temperament as well as early life experiences being important mediators.[14] Dopamine polymorphisms have previously been implicated in alcoholism and pathologic gambling. Han and colleagues[32] identified 2 genetic polymorphisms in dopamine genes that were more likely to be present in adolescents who were excessive video gamers compared with age-matched control subjects. Adolescents diagnosed with problematic Internet use in South Korea (compared with healthy control subjects) were found to be more likely to have anomalies in serotonin transporter genes.[33]

Poor behavioral inhibition or impulsivity leads to an emphasis on short-term consequences without consideration for longer term consequences. In IA, there is a tendency to discount rewards rapidly and perform poorly on decision making tests.[34–36] Individuals with IA are more likely to have high trait impulsivity.[35,37] Functional MRI studies on inhibitory tasks suggest impaired recruitment of frontal cortical projections.[38]

## PREVALENCE

Prevalence estimates of IA vary owing to methodologic differences and a lack of consensus diagnostically as well as the contribution of regional/cultural differences. Surveys in the United States and European countries suggest a range of prevalence between 1.5% and 8.2%.[11] The incidence of problematic Internet use in a large young European sample (11,356 adolescents in 11 European countries) found a prevalence of 4.4%, which was higher in males who preferred online gaming than females who preferred social networking.[39] Siomos and colleagues[40] found 8.2% of Greek adolescents to have IA whereas Bakken and colleagues[41] found the prevalence of IA to be 1% across the lifespan, with 3% to 4% prevalence rates in young men in Norway. Data from Germany suggest a prevalence of 1.5% to 3.5% of IA in adolescents.[42]

The prevalence of IA seems to be higher in Asian countries (specifically China, Taiwan, and South Korea), but it is unclear why. Yen and colleagues[43] identified the rate of IA to be 17.9% in Chinese high schoolers and 12.3% in college students.[44] The largest study in Taiwan (n = 9405) found that 18.8% of teenagers met IA criteria using Chen Internet Addiction Scale.[45] In a subsequent study by Ko and colleagues[46] in Taiwan, a lower rate of 10.8% was identified. Lam and colleagues[47] found that 10.8% of 13- to 18–year-olds in China were severely addicted to the Internet using the Internet Addiction Test. Park and colleagues[48] found that 10.7% of adolescents in Korea had IA. Ni and colleagues[49] identified a rate of 6.4% first year college students in China. In Hong Kong, the prevalence was identified to be 6.7% using Young's criteria and clinical interviews.[50]

## Risk Factors

Studies consistently show that males are more likely to become Internet addicted than females.[7,33,37,39,40,43,46] Online gaming is the most common source of IA.[40,51] However, both online gaming and use of social networking sites have been associated with increased risk for IA.[52,53]

In a recent study comparing problematic Internet use between gamers and non-gamers among high school students, there were some notable differences: gamers with problematic Internet use were more likely to be male and have peer relation problems, whereas female Internet users were more likely to be nongamers.[54] There was a higher risk of depression in the non-gamers. Both groups showed elevated levels of psychopathology (depression, conduct disorder, attention deficit hyperactivity disorder [ADHD]) and more self-harming behavior compared with typical Internet users.[54]

Environmental risk factors include access to computer availability with Internet capability. Increasing time spent online is correlated with development of IA.[9,50,52,55] Family dysfunction and conflict as well as low family monitoring are frequently cited as contributors for IA.[48,56,57] Female adolescents may be at greater risk for the contribution of family factors to the development of IA.[56]

Various studies have identified several personality risk factors for IA. These factors include high exploratory excitability, low reward dependence, sensation seeking, and hostility, as well as low self-esteem and loneliness.[3,37,43,52,58,59]

One large survey based study in South Korea suggests that substance abuse often precedes IA, specifically smoking and drug use.[33] There is also some evidence to suggest that those with preexisting mental health conditions are more vulnerable to IA. In a prospective study, hostility in males and ADHD in females were the most significant predictors of development of IA.[46]

Little is known about prognosis in IA. In a 1-year prospective study, low hostility and low interpersonal sensitivity predicted remission of IA.[60]

## Comorbidity

High rates of psychiatric comorbidity can make it difficult to tease out the contribution of IA from other psychiatric conditions. Depression and ADHD are the most commonly cited comorbidities throughout the literature.[11,61–67] Social anxiety has also been reported.[43,61–63,65] Yen and associates[65] found that more severe psychiatric symptoms were associated with IA compared with other substance use disorders. A variety of substance use disorders have been associated with IA, including harmful alcohol use.[57,68] Other psychiatric disorders like bipolar disorder and various personality disorders have been reported in association with IA in adults.[61]

## CLINICAL PRESENTATION

CLINICAL VIGNETTE

*James is a 16-year-old boy who spends most of his time online. He struggles to make it to school and has missed many days. He has a tendency to procrastinate and supposedly does "homework" online while actually gaming instead. He spends more than 5 hours online on school nights and goes to bed around 2 AM. This has led to increasing conflict at home. Of note, James has been diagnosed with major depression and social anxiety disorder.*

Compulsive use, tolerance, withdrawal, and diminished control despite adverse consequences currently define addictive disorders in DSM-5.[5] In keeping with this definition of addiction, there are several key features of IA.

1. The first is preoccupation with the Internet. More than 20 hours a week is consistent with prolonged Internet use.[9,69,70]
2. Next is spending time for longer amounts than originally intended and needing more time to achieve satisfaction (tolerance).
3. Some teens may develop mood symptoms (agitation/irritability/depression) when limits are set on use of the Internet, consistent with withdrawal.
4. It becomes difficult to manage the amount of time spent online (diminished control).

In addition, there must be evidence of functional impairment or adverse consequences as a result of excessive Internet use. Normal obligations are neglected. Commonly, this manifests as sleep deprivation with excessive daytime sleepiness,[17] school or work avoidance, worsening depression, social isolation, and family conflict.[8,9,11] It is extremely worrisome when time spent on the Internet interferes with food and water intake or neglect of hygiene.[9] Hand and wrist pain as well as back and eye strain may also develop as a result of IA.[9]

Some research suggests that those with IA are more likely to develop depression later in life.[71] IA has also been associated with aggression, suicidal ideation, and self-harm.[45,63,66,67] Full psychiatric diagnostic assessment is important, because comorbid depressive and anxiety disorders are common, as well as ADHD.[63] The differential diagnoses include mood disorders, anxiety disorders, and ADHD as the primary drivers of excessive Internet use, rather than a separate addictive disorder. It is also important to distinguish IA from normal Internet use.

## ASSESSMENT

Young was the first to define IA in clinical terms, developing the Young Diagnostic Questionnaire and the Internet Addiction Test.[11] Young defines IA by the presence of 5 or more items out of 8 endorsed regarding Internet use: preoccupation, tolerance, withdrawal, failure to control, more use than intended, functional impairment, lying about use, and use to escape a dysphoric mood.[11] The Internet Addiction Test consists of 20 questions about Internet use that are answered on a 5-point scale, ranging from rarely to often. A score of 80 or greater is clinically significant for problematic Internet use.[11] The Internet Addiction Test has been well-validated.[8,72,73] The Chen Internet Addiction Scale is another tool for IA and is a self-report measure consisting of 26 questions with ratings on a 4-point Likert scale with a cutoff score of 64 or more suggestive of problematic Internet use. The Chen Internet Addiction Scale assesses for compulsive use, withdrawal, tolerance, and negative adverse consequences of use and also has been well-validated.[8,73]

## DIAGNOSIS

The proposed criteria for Internet gaming disorder in DSM-5 include:

a. Preoccupation with Internet games (individual thinks about previous gaming activity or anticipates playing the next game; Internet gaming becomes the predominant activity in daily life);
b. Withdrawal symptoms when the Internet is taken away (typically irritability, anxiety, sadness);

c. Tolerance (the need to spend increasing amounts of time on Internet games to achieve the same "high");
d. Unsuccessful attempts to control or cut down the participation in Internet games;
e. Loss of interest in previously enjoyable activities with the exception of Internet gaming;
f. Continued excessive use despite knowledge of negative psychosocial problems;
g. Has deceived family members, therapists, or others regarding time spent on gaming;
h. Use of Internet games to escape or improve dysphoric mood; and
i. Jeopardized or lost relationships, jobs, educational opportunities because of Internet use.

The presence of 5 or more of these symptoms in the past 12 months in combination with persistent, maladaptive, and recurrent use of the Internet is required.[5]

However, Internet gaming disorder does not encompass all forms of problematic Internet use. Other online activities have a similar addictive potential. In a longitudinal study of 447 heavy Internet users, online gaming and sexual activities were most highly associated with problematic Internet use.[51] Other studies suggest that social media interfaces are also important sources of IA, particularly in females.[53,54,74]

Although controversy remains on this topic, there is some evidence that the same criteria for addiction can be applied to other uses of the Internet.[31,53,54] Specific diagnostic criteria of IA in adolescence was explored by Ko and colleagues[69] who proposed that there are 9 characteristic symptoms: preoccupation, uncontrolled impulse, more use than intended, tolerance, withdrawal, impairment of control, excessive time and effort spent online, and impaired decision making. Next, there must be evidence of functional impairment, namely, failure to fulfill role obligations at school and home and/or impaired social relationships.[69,70] Other definitions draw from pathologic gambling criteria and/or substance dependence criteria.[11] Unfortunately, more nosologic precision is needed.

## CLINICAL MANAGEMENT

There is growing demand for evidence-based recommendations for the treatment of IA. Treatment for IA is currently largely based on interventions and strategies used in substance use disorders. The goal in any addiction treatment is to modify neurobiological as well as psychosocial risk factors in combination with limiting exposure or access to a substance or behavior.[3,11,14]

### Comorbidity

The first step in clinical management of IA is a careful assessment of comorbid psychiatric disorders. Comorbid disorders should be treated to prevent their deteriorating effect on the prognosis of IA. In particular, effective evaluation and treatment of ADHD and depression is imperative.[46,60,75] Ongoing attention to hostility and aggression, especially in males, is relevant given the association with IA.[43] Prevention of IA in turn may improve treatment of preexisting depression, which can be exacerbated by spending excessive time online.[71]

### Prevention

Early screening and prevention of IA could be effective but has not been tested.[71] Some practical tips for parents include:

1. Encourage other interests and activities that do not involve the Internet. Team sports and after school clubs can promote healthy face-to-face peer interactions.

2. Set clear limits on time spent online (<2 hours per night). Restrict use of the computer to a common area so you can monitor online activity. Consider various apps to help limit use of the Internet through smartphones (limiting data usage, restricting texting and web browsing to certain times of day). Model appropriate use of the Internet yourself.
3. Talk to your teen about stressors in their life. Consider the role of anxiety or depression. Seek professional help if there are concerns about mood.

### Psychosocial Interventions

Winkler and colleagues[76] conducted a metaanalysis of IA treatment in 2013. This study suggests effective psychological interventions exist in targeting IA directly (effect size = 1.61), as well as decreasing time spent online (effect size = 0.94), depression (effect size = 0.90), and anxiety (effect size = 1.25). These results need to remain preliminary owing to the number of studies and methodologic limitations. Another review of treatment of IA by King and colleagues[77] was less optimistic about recommending treatment owing to a lack of diagnostic and methodologic consistency (absence of controls and objective outcomes) throughout studies.

Several studies suggest that cognitive–behavioral therapy (CBT) and other psychosocial interventions can be effective at reducing time spent online and reducing depressive symptoms.[8,14,42,76–79] CBT-IA has been created by Young[78] to target IA specifically and preliminary results in adults are encouraging. The intervention focuses on monitoring of behavior (keeping a log of Internet activity), teaching time management skills, goal setting, and restructuring cognitive distortions. One small pilot study of online pornography addiction with acceptance commitment therapy showed promising results.[80] Teaching coping skills around distress tolerance (or frustration intolerance) may be useful, but targeted studies are lacking.[81]

Other psychosocial treatments include 12-step self-help approaches and motivational enhancement.[7] These interventions rely on a relapse prevention model to reduce IA, including avoiding or coping with high-risk situations.[7,10,11] Support groups are not well-defined for IA compared with other addictions, particularly not support groups found online.[8] Motivation to change addictive behaviors is often low in adolescents and parents may be the ones presenting with concerns. However, certain motivational enhancement strategies can be useful, for example, helping teens to recognize what important activities or values are being neglected because of time spent online and careful consideration of the pros and cons of online use.[46] A multilevel counseling center in Hong Kong (incorporating elements of motivational enhancement, CBT, and family interventions) was effective in reducing IA symptoms in a group of 59 individuals, mainly adolescents.[82] Orzack and colleagues[83] combined features of CBT and motivation enhancement in a 16 week group treatment of cybersex IA for adults, which resulted in reduced depressive symptoms and improved quality of life but no change in sexual behavior.

A family-based approach makes sense in light of the familial risk factors associated with IA. Specifically, Ko and colleagues[56] found that reducing interparental conflict and promoting family function and Internet regulation were helpful in preventing IA. Reducing family conflict and improving communication are natural targets of treatment.[84] Furthermore, families play an important role in limiting access to excessive Internet usage.[46]

### Pharmacotherapy

No medications have been approved for treatment of behavioral addictions, but some show promise for IA like bupropion and methylphenidate.[76] Bupropion was helpful in reducing cravings and severity of IA in a small study of 11 men and also modified cue-induced brain activity.[85] Another study by Han and colleagues[86] showed that treatment with methylphenidate in drug-naïve ADHD kids helped to reduce time spent on the Internet. Escitalopram has been studied in a small open label trial of 19 subjects, with no significant difference reported.[87]

## SUMMARY

Although the Internet remains a powerful and positive force in the lives of many, a minority of users may become addicted. This is of particular concern for adolescents, because they are spending increasing amounts of time online and they are uniquely vulnerable to the development of addictive behavior.

IA is a type of behavioral addiction that resembles substance use disorders in phenomenology and neurobiology. Although this disorder has received attention from both scientists and the media, formal consensus on diagnostic criteria for IA is lacking. The repercussions of excessive Internet use are clear and impairing, ranging from sleep deprivation to worsening depression to school avoidance to family conflict. There are high rates of comorbid depression, anxiety, ADHD, and other substance use disorders. Other risk factors include various personality traits (notably impulsivity, hostility, sensation seeking), family conflict, low parental monitoring, and male gender. At this point, clinical management of IA includes treatment of comorbid conditions, CBT, motivational enhancement, family work, and some very preliminary pharmacologic studies. Further research is certainly indicated to better clarify formal diagnosis and treatment.

## REFERENCES

1. Holden C. Behavioral addictions debut in proposed DSM-V. Science 2010;327(5968):935.
2. Potenza MN. Should addictive disorders include non-substance-related conditions? Addiction 2006;101(1):142–51.
3. Grant JE, Potenza MN, Weinstein A, et al. Introduction to behavioral addictions. Am J Drug Alcohol Abuse 2010;36(5):233–41.
4. Clark L, Limbrick-Olfield EH. Disordered gambling: a behavioral addiction. Curr Opin Neurobiol 2013;23(4):655–9.
5. American Psychiatric Association. Diagnostic and statistical manual of mental disorders. 5th edition. Washington, DC: American Psychiatric Association; 2013.
6. Robbins TW, Clark L. Behavioral addictions. Curr Opin Neurobiol 2015;30:66–72.
7. Brezing C, Derevensky JL, Potenza MN. Non-substance addictive behaviors in youth: pathological gambling and problematic internet use. Child Adolesc Psychiatr Clin N Am 2010;19(3):625–41.
8. Aboujaoude E. Problematic internet use: an overview. World Psychiatry 2010;9(2):85–90.
9. Young KS. Internet addiction: the emergence of a new clinical disorder. Cyberpsychol Behav 1998;1(3):237–44.
10. Shaw M, Black DW. Internet addiction: definition, assessment, epidemiology and clinical management. CNS Drugs 2008;22(5):353–65.
11. Weinstein A, Lejoyeux M. Internet addiction or excessive internet use. Am J Drug Alcohol Abuse 2010;36(5):277–83.
12. Spada MM. An overview of problematic internet use. Addict Behav 2014;39(1):3–6.

13. Kuss DJ, Griffiths MD. Internet and gaming addiction: a systematic literature review of neuroimaging studies. Brain Sci 2012;2(3):347–74.
14. Hammond CJ, Mayes LC, Potenza MN. Neurobiology of adolescent substance use and addictive behaviors: prevention and treatment implications. Adolesc Med State Art Rev 2014;25(1):15–32.
15. Kann L, Kinchen S, Shanklin SL, et al. Youth risk behavior surveillance—United States, 2013. MMWR Surveill Summ 2014;63(4):1–168.
16. Kuss DJ, Louws J, Wiers RW. Online gaming addiction? Motives predict addictive play behavior in massively multiplayer online role-playing games. Cyberpsychol Behav Soc Netw 2012;15(9):480–5.
17. Choi K, Son H, Park M, et al. Internet overuse and excessive daytime sleepiness in adolescents. Psychiatry Clin Neuroci 2009;23(4):455–62.
18. Milani L, Osualdella D, Di Blasio P. Quality of interpersonal relationships and problematic internet use in adolescents. Cyberpsychol Behav 2009;12(6):681–4.
19. Nalwa K, Anand AP. Internet addiction in students: a cause for concern. Cyberpsychol Behav 2003;6(6):653–6.
20. Christakis DA, Moreno MA. Trapped in the net: will internet addiction become a 21st century epidemic? Arch Pediatr Adolesc Med 2009;163(10):959–60.
21. Stewart CS. Obsessed with the internet: a tale from China. 2010. Available at: http://www.wired.com/2010/01/ff_Internetaddiction/. Accessed October 18, 2015.
22. Goodman A. Neurobiology of addiction: an integrative review. Biochem Pharmacol 2008;75(1):266–322.
23. Joffe ME, Greuter CA, Grueter BA. Biological substrates of addiction. Wiley Interdiscip Rev Cogn Sci 2014;5(2):151–71.
24. Dagher A, Robbins TW. Personality, addiction, dopamine: insights from Parkinson's disease. Neuron 2009;61:502–10.
25. Koepp MJ, Gunn RN, Lawrence AD, et al. Evidence for striatal dopamine release during a video game. Nature 1998;393(6682):266–8.
26. Kim SH, Baik SH, Park CS, et al. Reduced striatal dopamine D2 receptors in people with internet addiction. Neuroreport 2011;22(8):407–11.
27. Kühn S, Romanowski A, Schilling C, et al. The neural basis of video gaming. Transl Psychiatry 2011;1:e53.
28. Ko CH, Lin GC, Hsiao S, et al. Brain activities associated with gaming urge of online gaming addiction. J Psychiatr Res 2009;43(7):739–47.
29. Yuan K, Qin W, Wang G, et al. Microstructure abnormalities in adolescents with internet addiction disorder. PLoS One 2011;6(6):e20708.
30. Zhou Y, Lin FC, Du YS, et al. Gray matter abnormalities in internet addiction: a voxel based morphometry study. Eur J Radiol 2011;79(1):92–5.
31. Brand M, Young KS, Laier C. Prefrontal control and internet addiction: a theoretical model and review of neuropsychological and neuroimaging findings. Front Hum Neurosci 2014;8:375.
32. Han DH, Lee YS, Yang KC, et al. Dopamine genes and reward dependence in adolescents with excessive internet video game play. J Addict Med 2007;1(3):133–8.
33. Lee YS, Han DH, Kim SM, et al. Substance abuse precedes internet addiction. Addict Behav 2013;38(4):2022–5.
34. Irvine MA, Worbe Y, Bolton S, et al. Impaired decisional impulsivity in pathological videogamers. PLoS One 2013;8(10):e75914.
35. Little M, van den Berg I, Luijten M, et al. Error processing and response inhibition in excessive computer game players: an event-related potential study. Addict Biol 2012;17(5):934–47.

36. Sun DL, Chen ZJ, Ma N, et al. Decision making and prepotent response inhibition functions in excessive internet users. CNS Spectr 2009;14(2):75–81.

37. Munno D, Saoldi M, Bechon E, et al. Addictive behaviors and personality traits in adolescents. CNS Spectr 2015;13:1–7.

38. Dong G, Hu Y, Lin X, et al. What makes internet addicts continue playing online even when faced by severe negative consequences? Possible explanations from an fMRI study. Biol Psychol 2013;94(2):282–9.

39. Durkee T, Kaess M, Carli V, et al. Prevalence of pathological internet use among adolescents in Europe: demographic and social factors. Addiction 2012;107(12): 2210–22.

40. Siomos KE, Dafouli ED, Braimiotis DA, et al. Internet addiction among Greek adolescent students. Cyberpsychol Behav 2008;11(6):653–7.

41. Bakken IJ, Wenzel HG, Gotestam KG, et al. Internet addiction among Norwegian adults: a stratified probability sample study. Scand J Psychol 2009;50(2):121–7.

42. Peukert P, Sieslack S, Barth G, et al. Internet and computer game addiction: phenomenology, comorbidity, etiology, diagnostics and therapeutic implications for the addicts and their relatives. Psychiatr Prax 2010;37(5):219–24.

43. Yen JY, Ko CH, Yen CF, et al. The comorbid psychiatric symptoms of internet addiction: attention deficit and hyperactivity disorder (ADHD), depression, social phobia, and hostility. J Adolesc Health 2007;41(1):93–8.

44. Yen JY, Yen CF, Chen CS, et al. The association between adult ADHD symptoms and internet addiction among college students: the gender difference. Cyberpsychol Behav 2009;12(2):187–91.

45. Ko CH, Yen JY, Liu SC, et al. The associations between aggressive behaviors and internet addiction and online activities in adolescents. J Adolesc Health 2009; 44(6):598–605.

46. Ko CH, Yen JJ, Chen CS, et al. Predictive values of psychiatric symptoms for internet addiction in adolescents: a 2 year prospective study. Arch Pediatr Adolesc Med 2009;163(10):937–43.

47. Lam LT, Peng ZW, Mai JC, et al. Factors associated with internet addiction among adolescents. Cyberpsychol Behav 2009;12(5):551–5.

48. Park SK, Kim JY, Cho CB. Prevalence of internet addiction and correlations with family factors among South Korean adolescents. Adolescence 2008;43(172): 895–909.

49. Ni X, Yan H, Chen S, et al. Factors influencing internet addiction in a sample of Freshman University students in China. Cyberpsychol Behav 2009;12(3):327–30.

50. Fu KW, Chan WS, Wong PW, et al. Internet addiction: prevalence, discriminant validity and correlates among adolescents in Hong Kong. Br J Psychiatry 2010;196(6):486–92.

51. Meerkerk GJ, Van Den Eijnden RJ, Garretsen HF. Predicting compulsive internet use: it's all about sex! Cyberpsychol Behav 2006;9(1):95–103.

52. Kuss DJ, Griffiths MD, Binder JF. Internet addiction in students: prevalence and risk factors. Comput Hum Behav 2013;29(3):959–66.

53. Kuss DJ, Griffiths MD. Online social networking and addiction – a review of the psychological literature. Int J Environ Res Public Health 2011;8(9):3528–52.

54. Strittmater E, Kaess M, Parzer P, et al. Pathological internet use among adolescents: comparing gamers and non-gamers. Psychiatry Res 2015;228(1):128–35.

55. Chou WJ, Liu TL, Yang P, et al. Multi-dimensional correlates of internet addiction symptoms in adolescents with attention-deficit/hyperactivity disorder. Psychiatry Res 2015;225(1–2):122–8.

56. Ko CH, Wang PW, Liu TL, et al. Bidirectional associations between family factors and internet addiction among adolescents in a prospective investigation. Psychiatry Clin Neurosci 2015;69(4):192–200.

57. Lam LT. Risk factors of internet addiction and the health effect of internet addiction on adolescents: a systematic review of longitudinal and prospective studies. Curr Psychiatry Rep 2014;16(11):508.

58. Gentile D. Pathological video game use among youths: a two-year longitudinal study. Pediatrics 2011;127(2):319–29.

59. Mehroof M, Griffiths MD. Online gaming addiction: the role of sensation seeking, self-control, neuroticism, aggression, state anxiety, and trait anxiety. Cyberpsychol Behav 2010;13(3):313–6.

60. Ko CH, Yen JY, Yen CF, et al. Factors predictive for incidence and remission of internet addiction in young adolescents: a prospective study. Cyberpsychol Behav 2007;10(4):545–51.

61. Bernardi S, Pallanti S. Internet addiction: a descriptive clinical study focusing on comorbidities and dissosociative symptoms. Compr Psychiatry 2009;50(6):510–6.

62. Carli V, Durkee T, Wasserman D, et al. The association between pathological internet use and comorbid psychopathology: a systematic review. Psychopathology 2013;46(1):1–13.

63. Ko CH, Yen JY, Yen CF, et al. The association between internet addiction and psychiatric disorders: a review of the literature. Eur Psychiatry 2012;27(1):1–8.

64. Yen JY, Ko CH, Yen CF, et al. Psychiatric symptoms in adolescents with internet addiction: comparison with substance use. Psychiatry Clin Neurosci 2008;62(1):9–16.

65. Yen CF, Chou WJ, Liu TL, et al. The association of internet addiction symptoms with anxiety, depression and self-esteem among adolescents with attention-deficit/hyperactivity disorder. Compr Psychiatry 2014;55(7):1601–8.

66. Lin IH, Ko CH, Chang YP, et al. The association between suicidality and internet addiction and activities in Taiwanese adolescents. Compr Psychiatry 2014;55(3):504–10.

67. Kim K, Ryu E, Chon MY, et al. Internet addiction in Korean adolescents and its relation to depression and suicidal ideation: a questionnaire survey. Int J Nurs Stud 2006;43(2):185–92.

68. Yen JY, Ko CH, Yen CF, et al. The association between harmful alcohol use and internet addiction among college students: comparison of personality. Psychiatry Clin Neurosci 2009;63(2):218–97.

69. Ko CH, Yen JY, Chen CC, et al. Proposed diagnostic criteria of internet addiction for adolescents. J Nerv Ment Dis 2005;193:728–33.

70. Ko CH, Yen JY, Chen SH, et al. Proposed diagnostic criteria and the screening and diagnosing tool of internet addiction in college students. Compr Psychiatry 2009;50(4):378–84.

71. Lam LT, Peng ZW. Effect of pathological use of the internet on adolescent mental health: a prospective study. Arch Pediatr Adolesc Med 2010;164(10):901–90.

72. Widyanto L, Griffiths MD, Brunsden V. A psychometric comparison of the internet addiction test, the internet-related problem scale, and self-diagnosis. Cyberpsychol Behav Soc Netw 2011;14(3):141–9.

73. Beard KW. Internet addiction: a review of current assessment techniques and potential assessment questions. Cyberpsychol Behav 2005;8(1):7–14.

74. Van Rooij AJ, Schoenmakers TM, van de Eijnden RJ, et al. Compulsive internet use: the role of online gaming and other internet applications. J Adolesc Health 2010;47(1):51–7.

75. Ko CH, Liu TL, Wang PW, et al. The exacerbation of depression, hostility, and social anxiety in the course of internet addiction among adolescents: a prospective study. Compr Psychiatry 2014;55(6):1377–84.

76. Winkler A, Dorsey B, Rief W, et al. Treatment of internet addiction: a meta-analysis. Clin Psychol Rev 2013;33(2):317–29.

77. King DL, Delfabbro PH, Griffiths MD, et al. Assessing clinical trials of internet addiction treatment: a systematic review and CONSORT evaluation. Clin Psychol Rev 2011;31(7):1110–6.

78. Young KS. Cognitive behavior therapy with internet addicts: treatment outcomes and implications. Cyberpsychol Behav 2007;10(5):671–9.

79. Du YS, Jiang W, Vance A. Longer term effect of randomized, controlled group cognitive behavioural therapy for internet addiction in adolescent students in Shanghai. Aust N Z J Psychiatry 2010;44(2):129–34.

80. Twohig MP, Crosby JM. Acceptance and commitment therapy as a treatment for problematic internet pornography viewing. Behav Ther 2010;41(3):285–95.

81. Ko CH, Yen JY, Yen CF, et al. The association between internet addiction and belief of frustration intolerance: the gender difference. Cyberpsychol Behav 2008;11(3):273–8.

82. Shek DT, Tang VM, Lo CY. Evaluation of an internet addiction treatment program for Chinese adolescents in Hong Kong. Adolescence 2009;44(174):359–73.

83. Orzack MH, Voluse AC, Wolf D, et al. An ongoing study of group treatment for men involved in problematic internet-enabled sexual behavior. Cyberpsychol Behav 2006;9(3):348–60.

84. Yen JY, Yen CF, Chen CC, et al. Family factors of internet addiction and substance use experience in Taiwanese adolescents. Cyberpsychol Behav 2007;10(3):323–9.

85. Han DH, Hwang JW, Renshaw PF. Bupropion sustained release treatment decreases craving for video games and cue-induced brain activity in patients with internet video game addiction. Exp Clin Psychopharmacol 2010;18(4):297–304.

86. Han DH, Lee YS, Na C, et al. The effect of methylphenidate on internet video game play in children with attention-deficit/hyperactivity disorder. Compr Psychiatry 2009;50(3):251–6.

87. Hadley SJ, Baker BR, Hollander E. Efficacy of escitalopram in the treatment of compulsive-impulsive computer use disorder. Biol Psychiatry 2006;69(3):452–6.

# Psychiatric Comorbidity and Complications

Michael J. Mason, PhD*, Alexis Aplasca, MD, Rosa Morales-Theodore, MD, Nikola Zaharakis, PhD, Julie Linker, PhD

## KEYWORDS

- Co-occurring disorder • Substance use disorder • Psychiatric comorbidity
- Dual diagnosis • Treatment • Adolescents

## KEY POINTS

- Among adolescents, 1.4% meet criteria for both a comorbid psychiatric and a substance use disorder (SUD), yet more than half of adolescents in SUD treatment have a comorbid psychiatric diagnosis.
- Adolescents should be routinely screened for adolescent substance use and mental health disorders, which can include brief clinical interviews, screening measures, and structured diagnostic assessments or rating scales.
- Evidence-based individual and family-focused psychosocial interventions for the treatment of comorbid psychiatric and SUDs are available, with many rooted in cognitive behavioral therapy, motivational interviewing, and family therapy.
- Although limited medications exist to treat SUDs in adolescents, guidelines are available for treating adolescents with comorbid diagnoses that draw on relevant evidence from the adult literature.
- Addressing barriers and obstacles to treatment, such as financial issues, access problems, and diversion of medication with abuse-potential, is important in facilitating the most positive outcomes for adolescents with comorbid diagnoses.

## INTRODUCTION

Individuals with co-occurring substance use and mental health disorders can be identified as having a comorbid disorder. The term co-occurring disorder for this article broadly refers to the co-occurrence of a substance use disorder (SUD) and psychiatric illness, although several may be present. Recent psychiatric epidemiology estimates indicate that 1.4% of the US adolescents aged 12 to 17 (359,000 adolescents) had both a substance use and a mental health disorder during the past year.[1] Addressing both disorders requires understanding the cause, severity, and course of these

Department of Psychiatry, Commonwealth Institute for Child & Family Studies, Virginia Commonwealth University, 515 North 10th Street, P.O.Box 980489, Richmond, VA 23298-0489, USA
* Corresponding author.
E-mail address: mjmason@vcu.edu

Child Adolesc Psychiatric Clin N Am 25 (2016) 521–532
http://dx.doi.org/10.1016/j.chc.2016.02.007
1056-4993/16/$ – see front matter © 2016 Elsevier Inc. All rights reserved.
childpsych.theclinics.com

dynamic, interactive psychiatric conditions. The goal of this article is to provide an overview of the prevalence of co-occurring disorders in youth, screening and assessment strategies, treatment approaches, and barriers to care.

## COMORBID SUBSTANCE ABUSE AND MENTAL HEALTH DISORDERS

Most youth with a SUD have a comorbid mental health diagnosis. Community samples estimate comorbidity at 60%,[2] with rates increasing with the severity of the substance abuse, with those with greater severity having higher rates of psychiatric diagnoses compared with those with less severity. The national comorbidity study found that adolescents with an SUD are at 3-fold risk for depression.[3] Clinical samples have even higher comorbidity, because youth in substance use treatment settings are more likely to have greater severity of psychiatric impairment, and higher numbers of disorders.

### Adolescents with Substance Use Disorders

Studies of adolescents presenting for substance use treatment reveal that between 55% and 88% of youth meet criteria for a co-occurring psychiatric problem.[4–7] The most common co-occurring problems among this population are externalizing disorders, such as conduct disorder, with reported rates ranging from 50% to 80%,[8–10] and attention deficit hyperactivity disorder (ADHD), with rates ranging from 13% to 77%[4,5,8]; however, internalizing disorders are also quite common. Rates of depression range from 14% to 50%[5,8,11] and rates of anxiety disorders range from 7% to 40%.[4,8,12,13]

### Adolescents with Mental Health Disorders

Conversely, adolescents with mental health disorders have higher rates of SUDs, with rates varying according to the type of mental health diagnosis.[2] Depression has been the most frequently studied, providing a wide range of estimates. However, most studies have suggested a range of 20% to 30% comorbidity of SUDs and depression. Anxiety has the smallest and least consistent comorbidity (estimated at 16.2%). Some anxiety disorders may be protective for SUDs, perhaps because of the avoidance that is the hallmark of those disorders. However, there are gender differences, because girls with anxiety disorders have more comorbidity than boys.

The disruptive behavior disorders (conduct disorder, oppositional defiant disorder, and ADHD) have the highest co-occurrence with SUDs, with a median prevalence of 46%. Within this set of disorders, ADHD is an outlier, with much lower comorbidity (median 12.3%). In addition to this much lower prevalence of SUDs, there appears to be a different developmental relationship between SUDs and ADHD than with other behavioral disorders.

### Developmental Psychopathology

There is not a clear directional pattern indicating whether psychiatric disorders or SUDs come first. At least for some of the disorders, psychiatric symptoms (without meeting the threshold for diagnosis) precede onset of substance use.[14] Earlier onset of substance abuse tends to have worse outcomes. It has been reported that half of all lifetime mental disorders begin by age 14 years and three-quarters begin by age 24 years, indicating that childhood psychiatric illnesses must be fully evaluated and addressed, because the presence of these disorders further complicate and worsen outcomes when not addressed. Furthermore, improvement of any domain of adolescent functioning positively affects a child's developmental trajectory. There are several possible developmental pathways that explain the presence of comorbidity, and several mechanisms may be occurring at once.[15]

---

**Developmental Pathways of Comorbidity:**

- Comorbidity as a marker for the severity of relatively undifferentiated symptoms of 2 or more disorders
- One disorder is a manifestation of the other
- One disorder causes the other
- There is a shared common cause for both (ie, early child abuse, parental psychopathology, negative family life events, peer affiliations)
- Comorbidity is a marker for a unique disorder subtype

---

## COMORBIDITY AND SUICIDE

Comorbidity often represents a profile of higher impairment. For example, compared with those who only had one of the disorders, those with both major depressive disorder and alcohol use disorder had higher risk of severe alcohol use disorder, higher rates of suicide attempts, lower levels of global functioning, and less life satisfaction.[15] Increased suicidality in individuals with comorbidity is well established. Comorbidity is also associated with more behavior problems and functional impairment.[16]

### Assessment

Routine screening for psychiatric and SUDs by pediatricians and other medical professionals has been recommended by several expert groups in the field, including the American Academy of Pediatricians[17] and the National Institute on Drug Abuse[18] as a best practice guideline when working with adolescents. At a minimum, screening for SUD is recommended during psychiatric evaluation. As part of a comprehensive evaluation of any adolescent presenting with problems in at least one functional domain, screening for psychiatric and substance use problems is warranted. Brief screenings offer early identification and treatment of potentially significant illnesses. Many clinicians working with adolescents cite lack of knowledge of appropriate assessment and referral practices for identifying and treating psychiatric and SUDs. Practitioners also have concerns for when to involve parents in this discussion and when to respect an adolescent's privacy. Finally, there is often a lack of time to address SUD and psychiatric illness in the context of a busy clinical practice.

However, assessing for psychiatric and SUDs does not require extensive time and training on the part of the clinician. Recommendations for assessment of comorbid psychiatric and SUD include clinical interview, screening measures, and comprehensive assessment with structured diagnostic assessments or rating scales. See Kaminer and Winters[19] and Winters and Kaminer[20] for lists of some of the most widely used instruments.

### Recommendations for assessment

**Brief clinical interview** A good starting point may be to inquire directly about the adolescent's substance use and psychiatric symptoms. This method often yields the best results when a clinician has already established a working relationship and good rapport with an adolescent. Clinicians may begin by posing a few open-ended questions nonjudgmentally (eg, Tell me about your use of any alcohol or marijuana).

**Brief screening measures** Many well-validated brief screening tools exist that take only a few minutes to complete and offer immediate reliable feedback. To increase reliability, providing privacy for completing these measures is important. These measures, such as the CRAFFT,[21] can efficiently be completed by patients in the waiting room before their visit, offering an easy opportunity to screen all incoming patients for SUD problems and potentially reducing the stigma associated with substance use and mental health treatment need.[18] Alternatively, a screener may be administered after a positive response to an initial brief interview.

**Comprehensive assessment** A more comprehensive evaluation should occur after a positive result on one of the brief screening tools. Several semistructured interviews are available, such as the Adolescent Diagnostic Interview,[22] the Global Assessment of Individual Needs,[23] and the Kiddie Schedule for Affective Disorders and Schizophrenia (K-SADS).[24] Comprehensive rating scales, such as the Child Behavior Checklist[25] and the Behavior Assessment Scales for Children,[26] can also provide valuable information when evaluating. These assessments may require various levels of training, but can be especially useful in probing for information from an adolescent resistant to sharing with the clinician. Several of these interviews, including the KSADS and the GAIN (Gain Appraisal of Individual Needs), now meet DSM-5 (Diagnostic Statistical Manual of Mental Disorders-5) diagnostic criteria for SUD.

### Privacy and confidentiality

Medical professionals are encouraged to gather this information in a private setting without parents present, in order to encourage honest answers, informing parents only when there is a clear safety risk to the adolescent or others.[27] When there is a need to refer an adolescent to treatment for psychiatric or SUD, the medical professional should involve the parent as appropriate to increase the likelihood that an adolescent will engage in treatment. The provider needs to consider the risks carefully between breaking confidentiality with the adolescent and potentially losing the therapeutic alliance developed, on the one hand, with the risks of maintaining confidentiality and potentially permitting the adolescent to continue engagement in maladaptive behavior, on the other hand.[27] Medical professionals should familiarize themselves with state laws in their geographical area of practice, because regulations in some states permit an adolescent to enter SUD treatment without parent consent.

### Utilizing assessment results

An integrated treatment plan takes into account results of the assessment and the medical professional's clinical judgment. Assessment results should determine which areas the adolescent is functioning most poorly in and should create a hierarchical problem list. Clinical targets can then be generated based on the objective assessment. Clinicians are encouraged to offer treatment referral when necessary, and of course, when referrals are available. One strategy is to partner with their adolescent patients' primary care provider through the sharing of assessment results and treatment plans. This partnership can begin a more comprehensive and coordinated treatment approach through tracking the adolescent's progress and coordinating ongoing care[27] as needed.

### Approaches to Treatment

### Psychosocial treatments

Relapse rates are high for adolescents who receive substance abuse treatment (35%–75% at 1 year) and are worse for those with Axis I comorbidity. Youth with externalizing disorders most rapidly return to substance use.[28] Youth with comorbidity are difficult to work with because of their combination of internalizing and externalizing symptoms, higher impairment, multiple risk factors (including impaired family functioning and relationships), and poor insight and motivation.[29]

| Psychosocial interventions focus on the following: |
| --- |
| • Psychoeducation |
| • Problem solving |
| • Decreased avoidance/increased positive social engagement |
| • Motivation |
| • Family communication and problem solving. |

Treatment for comorbidity is often impeded by separate systems for treatment of SUDs and mental health disorders. There are frequently disparate conceptualizations and treatment philosophies for these 2 types of disorders, separate funding and administrative streams, and separate training and licensing pathways for treatment providers. These barriers can lead to treatment efforts that lack effective coordination and collaboration between the multiple systems that provide services to youth with comorbid disorders. Integrated treatment is the "gold standard" for treatment of co-occurring disorders and involves a single treatment plan that addresses both mental health and SUDs. Most integrated practices focus on treatment planning and care coordination and center on the needs of the individual adolescent and family. Therefore, intensive case management and wraparound services are necessary to coordinate the interventions needed in these complex cases.

### Community and cognitive-behavioral treatments

Treatments that target substance abuse problems can be effective with youth with co-occurring disorders, but may need to include features that respond to mental health treatment needs, such as an emphasis on medication management and compliance. For example, a large trial of the Adolescent Community Reinforcement Approach, which emphasizes using the adolescent's "community" to gain positive reinforcement, has been shown to be even more effective with youth with both internalizing and externalizing difficulties than with SUDs alone.[30]

Most psychosocial treatments that target both psychiatric and SUDs use cognitive behavioral therapy (CBT) approaches, often integrated with motivational interviewing (MI), enhancement approaches, and family therapy. CBT treatments conceptualize both mental health and substance use symptoms as learned behavior. These behaviors reinforce and maintain cognitive processes and environmental responses. Dialectic behavior therapy is useful with this population and includes elements of CBT with a focus on emotional validation, acceptance, and self-regulation skills. MI strategies help counter resistance and increase readiness and motivation for change, although MI alone is unlikely to produce sustained change (**Table 1**).

### Family-based interventions

Family-based interventions tend to have better outcomes than more individually focused interventions, perhaps because of impacting contextual factors and stronger treatment engagement (**Table 2**). Whether treatment is focused on the individual teen or the family system, treatment that is individualized and culturally attuned is needed for successful engagement and positive outcomes.

| Family-based interventions focus on the following: |
| :--- |
| • Viewing adolescent problem behavior within the context of family and community, |
| • The important role of parents/caregivers in treatment outcomes, |
| • Use of engagement and communication with the family. |

### Pharmacotherapy

It is important that when a diagnosis of a co-occurring disorder is established, that both therapeutic and pharmacologic interventions be selected to provide for the best treatment of these disorders. Pharmacologic interventions for SUD can be in the form of direct and indirect treatments. Direct treatments include those medications addressing cravings, aversion, reduction, substitution, and detoxification. As implied, the indirect treatments address underlying psychiatric disorders. As such, this article explores the evidence and provides possible options for pharmacologic treatments that may improve outcomes in the treatment of SUDs.

**Medication considerations** Co-occurring SUDs and psychiatric illness in adolescents present an additional scope of management that is imperative to address. There is limited available literature of controlled studies regarding the use of pharmacotherapy in adolescents with co-occurring disorders as compared with adults. Of those studied, mood disorders (ie, major depression and bipolar disorder) and ADHD have the largest body of research. The typical current system of treatment frequently fails to address these conditions concurrently, often requiring individuals to enroll in substance abuse treatment programs before addressing psychiatric illness. Although there are few pharmacologic agents approved for the treatment of SUDs in adolescents, there are several approved for psychiatric illness, which should be considered in the treatment plan.

**Recommendations** The American Academy of Child and Adolescent Psychiatry provides evidence-based guidelines for the primary treatment of psychiatric illness and children, and many take into consideration the presence of a SUD. The overall effectiveness of pharmacotherapy for psychiatric illness in the setting of active substance use is often difficult to assess. There is some research to support that treating the psychiatric illness results in decreased substance use. A recent systematic review and meta-analysis by Zhou and colleagues[31] examined the efficacy and tolerability of antidepressants in the treatment of adolescents and young adults with substance use. A

| Table 1 | | |
| :--- | :--- | :--- |
| **An overview of individual interventions** | | |
| **Cognitive Behavioral Therapy** | **Dialectic Behavior Therapy** | **Motivational Inteviewing** |
| • Present-focused | • Focused on mood dysregu- | • Increasing treatment |
| • Goal-directed | lation that frequently oc- | engagement and reten- |
| • Identify and challenge | curs in youth with | tion, motivation to change |
| maladaptive beliefs | comorbid diagnoses | • Goal setting |
| • Cognitive restructuring | • Emotional validation and | • Empathetic nonjudgment |
| • Increased self-monitoring | acceptance | • Developing discrepancy |
| • Improved coping skills (ie, | • Skills training | • Avoiding argumentation |
| communication and con- | • Self-regulation | • Rolling with resistance |
| flict resolution) | | • Supporting self-efficacy |
| • Relapse prevention | | |

**Table 2**
**An overview of family-based interventions**

| Family Behavior Therapy | Multidimensional Family Therapy | Multisystemic Therapy |
|---|---|---|
| • Community reinforcement theory<br>• Behavioral contracting<br>• Stimulus control<br>• Urge control<br>• Communication skills training | • Targets multiple domains of risk, resilience, and functioning in child, family, and community<br>• Focus on goals of the adolescent<br>• Parenting issues<br>• Parenting and family relationships<br>• Influences outside the family | • Family and community based for SUDs and antisocial behavior<br>• Social ecology theory<br>• Restructures environment to promote healthy behaviors<br>• Draws from CBT, behavioral, and family therapy approaches, applied outside of traditional care settings (home, school, and community) |

small overall effect in reducing depression was found; however, such treatment did not improve substance use outcomes. In the case of ADHD, some studies have more positive outcomes on ADHD and the SUD, suggesting that pharmacologic treatment of ADHD may lower rates of substance use.[32]

Although there are no medications with US Food and Drug Administration approval for the treatment of SUDs in children and adolescents, evidence extrapolated from adult studies has been used in practice. These medications target the range of physiologic and psychological symptoms that contribute to addiction, including acute intoxication and withdrawal states, craving, maintenance, and aversion therapies. However, more data are needed to formulate treatment parameters. Pharmacologic treatment is a key component in the comprehensive treatment of SUDs in adolescents, and as the research in the neurobiology of addiction has become more robust, biologic treatments are gaining support.

**Barriers/obstacles to treatment**

**Treatment integration** The treatment of SUD is central to improving the quality of life and future of patients. The ideal treatments would integrate interventions in a variety of arenas (school, primary care, specialty care) of the child's life, and outreach programs and access to treatment would be readily obtained. Access to treatment from multiple avenues will improve likelihood of engagement and benefits to the patients and families. However, the reality of access is very different from the aforementioned. The leading reason for individuals not receiving treatment is concerns about health insurance coverage and the cost of treatment.[1]

**Patient characteristics** Along with financial and access challenges, the patient's interest and personal motivation are key to improved outcomes. There are various patient characteristics identified to impact progress as it relates to substance use. Among these are patients with externalizing and internalizing problems.[33] These patients often receive services from multiple systems, have severe symptoms, and have overwhelming psychosocial and family issues. A multifaceted approach to SUDs continues to show positive outcomes.

**Differing outcomes by diagnoses** Outcomes are also influenced by the comorbid diagnosis. Those patients with anxiety and mood disorders are more likely to perceive need for and seek treatment for SUD. In contrast, patients with ADHD have more negative associations with treatment. Identification of SUD before comorbid disorders showed higher rates of treatment engagement than those diagnosed with other non-substance use mental health disorders first. It is clear that more research is needed to improve the substance use treatment.

### Safety and diversion issues

**Safety issues** Treating SUDs can become more complex when other psychiatric co-occurring disorders are present. Specifically, there is concern for worsening substance use or initiating cross-addiction to other substances. As such, there has been more recent focus on exploring ways to reduce this potential risk. There is evidence to support that treating comorbid psychiatric illness helps improve outcomes when this is done concomitantly with substance use treatment.[34] There are some controversial findings that have not shown any significant improvement in substance use outcomes when treating depression. However, the overwhelming evidence states the contrary. It is important to avoid initiating treatment with addictive substances if other options are available. A good example of this would be the use of serotonin reuptake inhibitors instead of benzodiazepines (addictive agent) in the treatment of anxiety. One exception to this rule would be the treatment of ADHD. The literature suggests that initiating treatment for substance use before treating ADHD may yield better outcomes. Research supports the treatment of ADHD with stimulants early in life to prevent later development of SUDs. It has in fact been shown that treatment decreases risk of later substance use.[35,36] However, other research[37] has recommended that clinicians consider nonstimulants, such as atomoxetine, as initial or first-line agents for the treatment of ADHD in patients with comorbid substance use.

**Diversion issues** Drug diversion is the transfer of prescribed medication from the individual for whom it was prescribed to another person for any illicit use. Diversion behaviors are more prevalent in people who have been diagnosed with ADHD[38–40] and in people who screen positive for ADHD.[41,42] Nonetheless, diversion continues to be a problem for certain psychotropics with addictive potential. Among those agents are primarily stimulants. Opioids and benzodiazepines are also misused, but this tends to show up in different populations, such as young adults.[43] About one-third of college students reported misusing prescription medications in their lifetime in a study looking at attitudes of college students toward psychotropics, with approximately 15% to 17% using these in the last year.[43] Moreover, this study noted that those with positive attitudes toward psychotropics were most likely to misuse them, and those misusing them were more likely to have symptoms of alcohol/drug abuse.

## PREVENTION

One way to improve outcomes is to focus on preventive health care practices. Health care has long focused on the prevention of physical illness and has sought ways to improve outcome by understanding trends and applying evidence-based interventions to halt the progression of illness. This same preventive and early intervention effort toward psychiatric and SUDs would yield substantial benefits by reducing the burden on patients, families, and society. In order to provide the best care and work toward the wellness, the clinician should have a clear picture of the premorbid function and risks for the patient. Several clinical approaches have emerged to help decipher the complexities of co-occurring disorders. Among these is the recognition that sub-diagnostic substance use may predict future SUD, and thus, should be addressed. Looking at the common factors for genetic vulnerability, either secondary substance use or mental illness and bidirectional (pre-existing mental illness or SUD) approach can help the clinician to maintain awareness of challenges and pitfalls in the treatment of patients with SUDs.

## SUMMARY

This article sought to highlight the prevalence of co-occurring disorders among adolescents and to underscore the complexity and opportunities of treating these patients in a systematic, comprehensive approach. As evidenced by this review, the need exists to develop and test models of care that integrate co-occurring disorders into both psychiatric and substance abuse treatment settings. The challenge for pediatric practitioners is to provide detailed assessments linked to evidence-based treatment plans to account for the variations in adolescent development and the unique risk factor profile of each patient. Clearly, the issues related to comorbidity are vast and continue to grow with a rapidly increasing research literature. Although these challenges may at first appear overwhelming, at the most basic level co-occurring disorders represent the interaction among risk factors. Applying known clinical and descriptive research methods in order to identify the timing of the expressions of these risk factors is an important first step. Distilling this complex clinical area into manageable components may be a starting point for practitioners charged with understanding the developmental psychopathology of high-risk youth.

The challenge continues to provide adequate care for youth with co-occurring disorders. The national comorbidity study of adolescents shows that even among those youth with 3 or more disorders, fewer than half had recently received any specialty mental health care.[44] Clearly, the health care system in the United States needs to develop creative approaches in order to address this issue for the most vulnerable in our society. This nexus of need and challenge is a logical point for clinical research to begin to develop translational studies of treatment within real-world settings. This type of informative research initiative requires funding, leadership, and public support.

## REFERENCES

1. Substance Abuse and Mental Health Services Administration. Results from the 2012 National Survey on Drug Use and Health: Summary of National Findings, NSDUH Series H-46, HHS Publication No. (SMA) 13-4795. Rockville, MD: Substance Abuse and Mental Health Services Administration; 2013.
2. Armstrong TD, Costello EJ. Community studies on adolescent substance use, abuse, or dependence and psychiatric comorbidity. J Consult Clin Psychol 2002;70(6):1224–39.
3. Avenevoli S, Swendsen J, He J-P, et al. Major depression in the national comorbidity survey–adolescent supplement: prevalence, correlates, and treatment. J Am Acad Child Adolesc Psychiatry 2015;54(1):37–44.e2.
4. Chan YF, Dennis ML, Funk RR. Prevalence and comorbidity of major internalizing and externalizing problems among adolescents and adults presenting to substance abuse treatment. J Subst Abuse Treat 2008;34(1):14–24.
5. Grella CE, Hser Y-I, Joshi V, et al. Drug treatment outcomes for adolescents with comorbid mental and substance use disorders. J Nerv Ment Dis 2001;189(6): 384–92.
6. Grella CE, Joshi V, Hser Y-I. Effects of comorbidity on treatment processes and outcomes among adolescents in drug treatment programs. J Child Adoles Subst Abuse 2004;13(4):13–31.

7. Sterling S, Weisner C. Chemical dependency and psychiatric services for adolescents in private managed care: implications for outcomes. Alcohol Clin Exp Res 2005;29(5):801–9.

8. Diamond G, Panichelli-Mindel SM, Shera D, et al. Psychiatric syndromes in adolescents with marijuana abuse and dependency in outpatient treatment. J Child Adoles Subst Abuse 2006;15(4):37–54.

9. Hser Y-I, Grella CE, Collins C, et al. Drug-use initiation and conduct disorder among adolescents in drug treatment. J Adolesc 2003;26(3):331–45.

10. Kaminer Y, Burleson JA, Goldberger R. Cognitive-behavioral coping skills and psychoeducation therapies for adolescent substance abuse. J Nerv Ment Dis 2002;190(11):737–45.

11. Bukstein OG, Glancy LJ, Kaminer Y. Patterns of affective comorbidity in a clinical population of dually diagnosed adolescent substance abusers. J Am Acad Child Adolesc Psychiatry 1992;31(6):1041–5.

12. Clark LA, Watson D, Reynolds S. Diagnosis and classification of psychopathology: challenges to the current system and future directions. Annu Rev Psychol 1995;46(1):121–53.

13. Kaminer Y. Adolescent substance abuse and suicidal behavior. Child Adolesc Psychiatr Clin N Am 1996;5(1):59–71.

14. Costello E, Angold A. Epidemiology of psychiatric disorder in childhood and adolescence. In: Gelder M, Andersen N, Lopez-Ibor J, et al, editors. New Oxford textbook of psychiatry, vol. 2. Oxford (United Kingdom): Oxford University Press; 2009. p. 1594–9.

15. Brière FN, Rohde P, Seeley JR, et al. Comorbidity between major depression and alcohol use disorder from adolescence to adulthood. Compr Psychiatry 2014; 55(3):526–33.

16. King RD, Gaines LS, Lambert EW, et al. The co-occurrence of psychiatric and substance use diagnoses in adolescents in different service systems: frequency, recognition, cost, and outcomes. J Behav Health Serv Res 2000;27(4):417–30.

17. Levy SJL, Kokotailo PK. Substance use screening, brief intervention, and referral to treatment for pediatricians. Pediatrics 2011;128(5):e1330–40.

18. U.S. Department of Health and Human Services; National Institutes of Health, National Institute on Drug Abuse. Screening for drug use in general medical settings: Resource Guide; 2014. Available at: https://www.drugabuse.gov/sites/default/files/resource_guide.pdf.

19. Kaminer Y, Winters K. Clinical manual of adolescent substance abuse treatment. Arlington (VA): American Psychiatric Publishing; 2011.

20. Winters KC, Kaminer Y. Screening and assessing adolescent substance use disorders in clinical populations. J Am Acad Child Adolesc Psychiatry 2008;47(7): 740–4.

21. Knight JR, Shrier LA, Bravender TD, et al. A new brief screen for adolescent substance abuse. Arch Pediatr Adolesc Med 1999;153(6):591.

22. Winters K, Henley G. Adolescent diagnostic interview (ADI) manual. Los Angeles (CA): Western Psychological Services; 1993.

23. Dennis M. Gain appraisal of individual needs (GAIN): administration guide for the GAIN and related measures. Bloomington (IL): Chestnut Health Systems; 1999.

24. Kaufman J, Birmaher B, Brent D, et al. Schedule for affective disorders and schizophrenia for school-age children-present and lifetime version (K-SADS-PL): initial reliability and validity data. J Am Acad Child Adolesc Psychiatry 1997;36(7):980–8.

25. Achenbach T. Manual for the child behavior checklist and 1991 profile. Burlington (VT): University of Vermont Department of Psychiatry; 1991.

26. Reynolds CR, Kamphaus RW. Behavior assessment system for children. 2nd edition. Circle Pines (MN): AGS Publishing; 2006.

27. Levy S, Winters KC, Knight JR. Screening and brief interventions for adolescent substance use in the general office setting. In: Kaminer Y, Winters KC, editors. Clinical manual of adolescent substance abuse treatment. Arlington (VA): American Psychiatric Publishing; 2011. p. 65–81.

28. Tomlinson KL, Brown SA, Abrantes A. Psychiatric comorbidity and substance use treatment outcomes of adolescents. Psychol Addict Behav 2004;18(2):160–9.

29. Bukstein OG, Horner MS. Management of the adolescent with substance use disorders and comorbid psychopathology. Child Adolesc Psychiatr Clin N Am 2010; 19(3):609–23.

30. Godley MD, Godley SH, Dennis ML, et al. A randomized trial of assertive continuing care and contingency management for adolescents with substance use disorders. J Consult Clin Psychol 2014;82(1):40–51.

31. Zhou X, Qin B, Del Giovane C, et al. Efficacy and tolerability of antidepressants in the treatment of adolescents and young adults with depression and substance use disorders: a systematic review and meta-analysis. Addiction 2015;110(1): 38–48.

32. Steinhausen H-C, Bisgaard C. Substance use disorders in association with attention-deficit/hyperactivity disorder, co-morbid mental disorders, and medication in a nationwide sample. Eur Neuropsychopharmacol 2014;24(2):232–41.

33. Hendriks V, van der Schee E, Blanken P. Matching adolescents with a cannabis use disorder to multidimensional family therapy or cognitive behavioral therapy: treatment effect moderators in a randomized controlled trial. Drug Alcohol Depend 2012;125(1):119–26.

34. Riggs PD. Treating adolescents for substance abuse and comorbid psychiatric disorders. Sci Pract Perspect 2003;2(1):18–29.

35. Dalsgaard S, Mortensen PB, Frydenberg M, et al. ADHD, stimulant treatment in childhood and subsequent substance abuse in adulthood—a naturalistic long-term follow-up study. Addict Behav 2014;39(1):325–8.

36. Groenman AP, Oosterlaan J, Rommelse NNJ, et al. Stimulant treatment for attention-deficit hyperactivity disorder and risk of developing substance use disorder. Br J Psychol 2013;203(2):112–9.

37. Kollins SH. A qualitative review of issues arising in the use of psycho-stimulant medications in patients with ADHD and co-morbid substance use disorders. Curr Med Res Opin 2008;24(5):1345–57.

38. Harstad E, Levy S. Attention-deficit/hyperactivity disorder and substance abuse. Pediatrics 2014;134(1):e293–301.

39. Wilens TE, Gignac M, Swezey A, et al. Characteristics of adolescents and young adults with ADHD who divert or misuse their prescribed medications. J Am Acad Child Adolesc Psychiatry 2006;45(4):408–14.

40. Wilens TE, Adler LA, Adams J, et al. Misuse and diversion of stimulants prescribed for ADHD: a systematic review of the literature. J Am Acad Child Adolesc Psychiatry 2008;47(1):21–31.

41. Upadhyaya HP, Rose K, Wang W, et al. Attention-deficit/hyperactivity disorder, medication treatment, and substance use patterns among adolescents and young adults. J Child Adolesc Psychopharmacol 2005;15(5):799–809.

42. Poulin C. From attention-deficit/hyperactivity disorder to medical stimulant use to the diversion of prescribed stimulants to non-medical stimulant use: connecting the dots. Addiction 2007;102(5):740–51.
43. Stone AM, Merlo LJ. Attitudes of college students toward mental illness stigma and the misuse of psychiatric medications. J Clin Psychol 2011;72(2):134–9.
44. Costello EJ, He JP, Sampson NA, et al. Services for adolescents with psychiatric disorders: 12-month data from the National comorbidity survey–adolescent. Psychiatr Serv 2014;65(3):359–66.

# Medical Comorbidity and Complications

Scott E. Hadland, MD, MPH[a,b,c,*], Leslie Renee Walker, MD[d,e]

## KEYWORDS

- Adolescents • Chronic disease • Substance-related disorders • Ethanol
- Street drugs • Tobacco products • Electronic cigarettes

## KEY POINTS

- A substantial proportion of youth with chronic medical conditions (YCMC) use substances, including cigarettes (traditional and smokeless products such as e-cigarettes), alcohol, and illicit drugs, and also may engage in nonmedical use of prescription drugs.
- Substance use has direct harms for all youth, but YCMC may be at even higher risk for harm owing to clinically significant disease-substance interactions as well as medication nonadherence and poor disease management in the setting of substance use.
- It is incumbent on all clinicians, primary care providers, specialty providers, and behavioral health specialists, to screen for substance use, briefly intervene, and refer to treatment as appropriate.

To date, the wealth of observational studies on youth substance use has focused on the general adolescent population, which comprises predominantly healthy youth. As established in previous articles, alcohol use and drug use are associated with a wide range of adverse health effects and neurocognitive changes for all adolescents. Less studied, however, are the *additional* potential consequences for youth with chronic medical conditions (YCMC) who use substances. There has been almost no

Dr S.E. Hadland is supported by the Division of Adolescent and Young Adult Medicine at Boston Children's Hospital, the Leadership Education in Adolescent Health Training Program T71 MC00009 (MCH/HRSA) and a National Research Service Award 1R03DA037770-01, 1T32HD075727-01 (NIH/NICHD).
Conflict of Interest Statement: The authors have no conflicts of interest to disclose.
[a] Division of Adolescent/Young Adult Medicine, Department of Medicine, Boston Children's Hospital, 300 Longwood Avenue, Boston, MA 02115, USA; [b] Department of Health Policy and Management, Harvard T. H. Chan School of Public Health, Kresge Building, 677 Huntington Avenue, Boston, MA 02115, USA; [c] Department of Pediatrics, Harvard Medical School, 25 Shattuck Street, Boston, MA 02115, USA; [d] Division of Adolescent Medicine, Seattle Children's Hospital, 4800 Sand Point Way Northeast, Seattle, WA 98105, USA; [e] Department of Pediatrics, University of Washington, 1959 Northeast Pacific Street, Box 356320, Seattle, WA 98195, USA
* Corresponding author. Division of Adolescent/Young Adult Medicine, Department of Medicine, 300 Longwood Avenue, Boston, MA 02115.
*E-mail address:* scott.hadland@childrens.harvard.edu

Child Adolesc Psychiatric Clin N Am 25 (2016) 533–548
http://dx.doi.org/10.1016/j.chc.2016.02.006

systematic epidemiologic examination of substance use among YCMC, thus consti-
tuting an enormous knowledge gap. Because alcohol and drugs have widespread
and potentially harmful physiologic effects throughout the body, the potential for organ
systems to sustain a "double hit, both from chronic illness and from substance use, is
high.

This article reviews (1) the epidemiology of substance use among YCMC, (2) mechanisms whereby substances might alter the course of illness for YCMC, and (3) recommendations for routine health care and medical screening for all adolescents who use
substances, with special consideration for YCMC. Using case examples, some
special considerations are also presented for YCMC with regard to the substances
they use and potential disease-specific concerns (**Boxes 1–3**).

## EPIDEMIOLOGY OF SUBSTANCE USE AMONG YOUTH WITH CHRONIC MEDICAL CONDITIONS

Despite readily available information on drug and alcohol use among the general
adolescent population (eg, Refs.[1–3]), there have been no similarly rigorous, large-
scale, systematic epidemiologic studies of substance use among YCMC. Because
at least 1 in 10 of adolescents lives with identified chronic conditions, there is urgent
need for further study.[4,5] Data on substance use are available from smaller samples of
YCMC, but data are increasingly outdated and do not capture more recent trends
(eg, the emergence of e-cigarette use and of synthetic cannabinoids[1]).

Fortunately, data from small studies are available from multiple settings worldwide,
but findings from one country do not necessarily generalize to other locations. In addition, there has been no systematic comparison across different illnesses: for example,
comparing youth with asthma to youth with type 1 diabetes mellitus (T1DM) or to youth
with inflammatory bowel disease (IBD), to help understand the interplay between
different illness experiences and substance use. Finally, most samples are clinic-
based, which exclude YCMC who are not actively receiving medical care and may
have poorer disease control; although this has not been studied, these same youth
may be more likely to use substances and experience related harm.

Many studies conducted to date have demonstrated comparable or even slightly
*lower* prevalence of lifetime or recent drug, alcohol, or tobacco use among
YCMC.[6–9] However, as outlined in later discussion, there have also been documented
notable exceptions to this, particularly among adolescents with asthma,[10–12] suggesting that there may be critical differences among different chronic medical conditions.
In addition, what is clear from studies to date is that even when the prevalence of substance use is lower among YCMC, there remains a substantial number of youth who
do use substances, thus necessitating careful screening by all health care providers
for alcohol, tobacco, and drug use, and their associated harms.

### Asthma

No large-scale epidemiologic studies provide stable estimates of the proportion of
youth with asthma who smoke cigarettes or use alcohol or other drugs, although
several studies have suggested that cigarette smoking and other substance use
may be higher among youth with asthma than without.[10–12] Reasons for this remain
unclear. One national survey of adolescents recruited from schools (rather than
from clinics) demonstrated that adolescents with asthma were significantly more likely
to smoke cigarettes daily and smoked more cigarettes per day on average.[11] However, the investigators also found that adolescents with asthma were more likely to
have started smoking at a younger age, which raises the question of whether their

**Box 1**
**Case example 1: asthma**

J.V. is a 15-year-old male adolescent with moderate persistent asthma and near-daily use of cigarettes and marijuana. In the last 2 years, J.V. has been hospitalized 3 times for status asthmaticus, including a recent admission to the intensive care unit (ICU) requiring intravenous magnesium sulfate and continuous albuterol.

A careful history by the ICU clinician reveals that J.V. began smoking e-cigarettes (ie, "vaping") with friends when he was 14 years old, and then shortly thereafter, began smoking combustible (ie, traditional) cigarettes. J.V. currently smokes 3 to 4 cigarettes per day with friends before and after school and occasionally vapes at home in the evenings. He also has been smoking marijuana blunts more days than not, sometimes with friends, and sometimes alone in his backyard. He does not drink alcohol. Although J.V.'s mother, with whom he lives, wants him to quit marijuana and cigarettes, J.V. reports that he is not interested in cutting back or quitting. In fact, J.V. feels as though smoking marijuana actually helps him breathe easier, but his mother has noted that he seems to cough more when she has caught him using it.

*Considerations*

- The prevalence of cigarette smoking is elevated among youth who present to clinical attention with an asthma exacerbation,[76] so all patients with asthma should be screened to assess for history of smoking.
- Cigarette smoke (both firsthand and secondhand) is a well-established trigger for asthma,[13,77] and indeed, may be a risk factor for development of a new diagnosis of asthma.[78]
- Similarly, although smoking marijuana may cause bronchorelaxation,[37] it is also associated with worsened airway inflammation, mucous production, cough, and wheeze,[37] and youth with asthma should be counseled regarding the possibility for worsening asthma symptoms with marijuana use.
- E-cigarette use is an increasingly recognized risk factor for transition to smoking combustible cigarettes,[79,80] and their role as a cessation aid (ie, using nicotine-containing e-cigarettes as a replacement for combustible cigarettes among cigarette smokers) is not well established.[81]
- Furthermore, the potential harms of e-cigarette use among youth (including those with asthma) are not well studied,[82] so all adolescents should be counseled regarding their as-yet unknown potential harms.
- Adolescents with asthma who use substances are less likely to adhere to their medications than those who do not use substances[9,11]; medication adherence should be carefully assessment among youth with asthma who use substances.
- The prevalence of cigarette smoking may actually naturally decrease among adolescents with asthma as they progress to young adulthood[83]; providers should provide assistance in helping youth with asthma quit.

## Conclusion

J.V. was counseled regarding the potential health risks of his cigarette and marijuana smoking, but he was not interested initially in cutting back or quitting. An initial harm reduction approach was used, ensuring his safety when he was using marijuana, including ensuring he never rode in a car with youth who were using substances. With frequent follow-up and motivational enhancement techniques, J.V. ultimately cut back on his marijuana use and requested assistance in quitting cigarettes. Nicotine replacement therapy (a patch and chewing gum) was prescribed, and he set a quit date. With the close supervision of his mother as well as close clinical follow-up, he was successful in quitting. Nonetheless, he continues to smoke marijuana on weekends with friends, and his provider continues to encourage him to cease marijuana use altogether for his health.

**Box 2**

**Case example 2: type 1 diabetes mellitus**

T.B. is a 16-year-old young woman with T1DM diagnosed at age 7, who reports use of alcohol in social settings on 2 or 3 weekend nights per month. She previously had generally good glycemic control with her hemoglobin (Hgb) A1c between 7.0% and 7.5%, but at her most recent visit, her Hgb A1c was 8.2%. She is on a basal-bolus regimen with insulin glargine administered every night and insulin aspart with meals.

Careful screening by her endocrinologist reveals that T.B. first began drinking alcohol this year with friends. She denies current use of other substances, noting that she does not like the idea of inhaling anything, and although she tried "molly" on a single occasion at a party, she is afraid of getting in trouble with the law and plans to avoid illicit drugs moving forward. She receives excellent grades in school, and this has not changed with her substance use. T.B. would like to attend a competitive college.

She denies drinking alone, reporting that she only ever consumes alcohol in social situations. T.B. never drives while drinking and always ensures a ride from another friend who has a safe plan to get home. She reports "drinking to get drunk" and usually consumes 4 or 5 beers with 1 or 2 occasional shots on a typical night with her friends. Recently, however, she had to be picked up by her parents after she was found vomiting at a house party, and T.B. disclosed shortly after that on another occasion, she blacked out after drinking on an empty stomach.

*Considerations*

- Binge drinking is common among adolescents with T1DM,[9] and alcohol consumption is associated with risk for hypoglycemia.[8,84] Consistent with recommendations from the American Diabetes Association[85] and the American Academy of Pediatrics,[75] clinicians should carefully screen adolescents with T1DM to ascertain their substance use intensity and frequency.

- Hypoglycemia can be delayed by several hours after drinking, which can be particularly hazardous to adolescents who drink and then fall asleep. Compounding this, glucagon for treatment of hypoglycemia may be less effective when youth have been drinking. Clinicians should determine whether youth with T1DM have ever drank to the extent of vomiting or blacking out, which can have hazardous consequences for blood glucose levels.

- In the long term, alcohol and other substance use is associated with poor glycemic control in adolescents with T1DM.[8,18] Clinicians might consider whether an adolescent with poor glycemic control may have an underlying substance use disorder and should consider more carefully monitoring for hyperglycemia among adolescents who use alcohol.

- Misuse of stimulants and other recreational club drugs such as ecstasy may place adolescents with T1DM at excess risk for diabetic ketoacidosis.[18,86,87] When screening for substance use among adolescents with T1DM, clinicians should be certain to ask about use of stimulants and other club drugs.

- Mortality is greatly elevated among youth with T1DM, largely owing to hypoglycemia and ketoacidosis.[88] Psychiatric comorbidity and substance use are associated with this increase in mortality.[89] Clinicians should be aware that the consequences of alcohol and substance use among patients with T1DM can be life-threatening.

## Conclusion

T.B. was initially reluctant to cut back on her drinking, stating that she did not believe she had a drinking problem. As a harm reduction approach, her endocrinologist helped her understand the importance of wearing a medical alert bracelet at all times and counseled her to talk to her friends about the criticality of seeking immediate medical attention if she loses consciousness. Her endocrinologist also helped her understand the criticality of vigilantly checking blood glucose levels around the times of her drinking. T.B. returned for multiple follow-up visits in which she participated in motivational enhancement and increasingly acknowledged the potential risks that alcohol use posed to her ongoing success in school. In her senior year, T.B. continued to drink but in smaller quantities, specifically recognizing the hazards of binge drinking given her T1DM diagnosis.

**Box 3**
**Case example 3: inflammatory bowel disease**

C.Q. is a 17-year-old young man with Crohn disease diagnosed 6 years earlier who currently uses marijuana daily. He has had multiple exacerbations of his IBD that have required long-term hospitalizations for intravenous corticosteroid administration. He has been on methotrexate previously and is currently taking 6-mercaptopurine (6-MP). C.Q. is concurrently being followed for generalized anxiety disorder diagnosed at age 13 years, for which he takes fluoxetine and receives ongoing psychotherapy.

He has smoked marijuana for 3 years and initially smoked only on weekends, but he has now progressed to the point that he smokes daily. When he is not smoking, he notes that his anxiety is worsened. In addition, he feels that his Crohn disease is helped by his marijuana use, and he has even asked his physician for a license for medicinal cannabis, which recently became legal in his state. C.Q. denies any alcohol use, citing its effects on his gastrointestinal tract. He does not use other substances, stating that marijuana is the only drug that he uses because it helps him relax. C.Q. believes marijuana has helped his appetite and attributes a recent improvement in his weight to his ongoing use.

*Considerations*

- Marijuana use is highly prevalent among patients with IBD, with as many as 1 in 3 adolescents reporting past-year use, and 1 in 8 reporting past-month use; nearly one-half report prior binge drinking.[9] The high prevalence of substance use should prompt the clinician to screen all adolescents with IBD, provide brief intervention, and refer to treatment as appropriate.

- Marijuana is legal for medicinal purposes in several jurisdictions in the United States and elsewhere. Studies are mixed as to whether states with medical marijuana laws have observed increases in adolescent marijuana use, but several studies suggest that prevalence of use may indeed be increasing.[46,47,49–51,90,91]

- Substance use (particularly heavy alcohol use) among patients with IBD can exacerbate hepatotoxicity associated with medications such as methotrexate and 6-MP.[28,29] Adolescents with IBD should be counseled regarding the potential excess risk associated with substance use while taking hepatotoxic medications.

- Adolescents who use substances may be less likely to adhere to their IBD medications,[9] possibly placing them at risk for illness exacerbation. Medication adherence should be carefully assessed among adolescents who use substances, and conversely, adolescents with serious or repeat exacerbations should be screened for use.[92–94]

- Gastrointestinal motility is altered among patients who use marijuana.[22,23,55,57,95] It is unclear whether these changes are beneficial; some studies report improvement in Crohn disease outcomes with marijuana use,[22,23,57] but one observational study showed risk for poorer long-term outcomes.[22]

- No data on cannabis for IBD exist for adolescents, and it is unknown what cannabinoid compound, dose, route, or schedule would be ideal. At this time, particularly in the face of known long-term adverse health and neurocognitive risks of marijuana use among adolescents,[58–62] cannabis cannot be recommended for IBD.

## Conclusion

C.Q. so strongly believed that marijuana was helping his IBD that he was not interested in cutting back or quitting at any time, even despite frequent and ongoing visits for motivational enhancement, which he ultimately stopped attending when he turned 18 years old. Before this, however, he was carefully counseled about the potential adverse health and neurocognitive harms of long-term heavy marijuana use[58–62] as well as the lack of available evidence for efficacy of marijuana for IBD. He ultimately chose to enroll in a randomized clinical trial of dronabinol for adults with Crohn disease.

initiating smoking may have precipitated an asthma diagnosis in the first place. Regardless of whether a diagnosis of asthma precedes smoking or vice versa, from the health care provider's perspective, it is critical to recognize that tobacco use has clear deleterious effects on disease management and symptom control.[13] Alcohol use and marijuana use are clearly prevalent among youth with asthma, and youth who smoke cigarettes are themselves even more likely to use other substances.[9,10,14–16]

### Type I Diabetes Mellitus

For adolescents with T1DM, several studies have identified lower prevalence of alcohol and other substance use compared with the general adolescent population,[7,8,17] but a more recent survey highlighted that in one clinic-based sample, more than 1 in 3 adolescents with T1DM reported past-year alcohol use and nearly 1 in 2 reported lifetime binge drinking.[9] In this same study, nearly 1 in 5 adolescents with T1DM reported past-month marijuana use. The lower prevalence of substance use reported in some studies may be due to sampling young adolescents; some data suggest that adolescents with T1DM may have lower prevalence of substance use in their early teen years but have similar prevalence to the general youth population by the end of adolescence.[17] Data from Australia highlight a high prevalence of street drug use among adolescents with T1DM, which is concerning given the appetite-altering effects of many substances with resultant effects on blood glucose levels.[18,19]

### Other Chronic Medical Conditions

Data on substance use among adolescents with other chronic medical conditions are lacking. However, in light of findings from one sample of youth from subspecialty clinics serving adolescents with asthma/cystic fibrosis, T1DM, arthritis, or IBD showing that there may be disease-specific differences in prevalence of alcohol and marijuana use,[9] further studies are merited to understand the epidemiology of substance use across a wide array of chronic medical conditions.

## HOW SUBSTANCES MAY ALTER THE COURSE OF ILLNESS AMONG YOUTH WITH CHRONIC MEDICAL CONDITIONS

Clinically significant harm can result from the use of substances in the setting of a chronic medical condition. Potential mechanisms include the direct physiologic effects of alcohol and drugs, toxic effects, interaction with medications used for chronic disease management, effects resulting from the route of administration of substances, and behavior changes resulting from substance use. **Table 1** reviews these mechanisms and provides some examples documented in the medical literature.

The first of these mechanisms, physiologic or metabolic changes exerted by substances, may involve direct action of the substance at the cellular level and/or indirect effects mediated by the central nervous system (CNS). For example, stimulants act directly on the cardiovascular system by enhancing transmission at sympathetic nerve terminals that innervate myocardium and the peripheral vasculature and also enhance CNS-mediated increases in heart rate, blood pressure, and systemic vascular resistance.[20,21] Although poorly studied, it is probable such physiologic changes acutely place adolescents with chronic hypertension, structural heart disease, or cardiac conduction abnormalities at even higher risk of morbidity or mortality. In addition, a newer body of evidence reveals that cannabinoids such as Δ-9-tetrahydrocannabinol (THC) have a direct effect on cannabinoid receptors in the gastrointestinal tract.[22] Resulting physiologic effects may include decreased intestinal motility, secretion, and

**Table 1**
**Potential mechanisms for changes in symptoms or course of illness as a result of substance use among youth with chronic medical conditions**

| Mechanism | Examples | Reference(s) |
|---|---|---|
| Direct physiologic or metabolic effects of the substance | Cocaine, methamphetamine, and other stimulants with catecholaminergic effects increase blood pressure, potentially worsening control among patients with cardiovascular or renal disease | 96–98 |
| | Among patients with type 1 diabetes, chronic alcohol use worsens glycemic control, whereas acute alcohol consumption is associated with hypoglycemia | 8,18,84 |
| | Stimulants may precipitate ketoacidosis among patients with type I diabetes | 18,86,87 |
| | Marijuana use is associated with alterations in gastrointestinal motility among patients with IBD | 22,23,55,57,95 |
| Toxic effects of the substance on cells and tissues | Alcohol causes direct hepatocellular damage, with implications for patients with pre-existing liver disease; this damage may be further exacerbated by certain medications, such as acetaminophen, methotrexate, 6-MP | 28,29 |
| | Heroin use can cause renal tubular injury and progressive focal segmental glomerular sclerosis, which may further compromise function in patients with chronic kidney disease | 99 |
| Interaction with medications used for disease management | Alcohol delays gastric emptying, potentially affecting first-pass metabolism of some medications required for chronic disease management (eg, propranolol, opioids, benzodiazepines) | 30,33 |
| | Alcohol induces cytochrome P450 2C9, potentially affecting the metabolism of medications using this enzyme (eg, warfarin, phenytoin); THC is also metabolized by cytochrome P450 2C9 (as well as cytochrome P450 3A4), leading to potential medication interactions, particularly with antiepileptic drugs | 33,100–103 |
| | Disulfiram-like reactions (marked by nausea and vomiting) may result from drinking alcohol while taking certain medications (eg, metronidazole, griseofulvin, procarbazine, some cephalosporins) due to inhibition of acetaldehyde dehydrogenase | 33,34 |
| | Alcohol enhances the sedating effect of benzodiazepines, certain antiepileptic drugs, psychotherapeutic agents, and other sedative-hypnotic medications | 30,35 |
| | Drinking alcohol while taking opioids (eg, for chronic pain) enhances respiratory depression and increases risk of overdose | 30,36 |
| Effects related to route of substance administration | Marijuana inhalation is associated with short-term bronchodilation, but in the long term, wheezing, cough, and mucus production among patients with chronic respiratory conditions such as asthma | 37 |
| | Drug injection predisposes to abscesses, endocarditis, and other bacterial and blood-borne infections, which may place users with immunodeficiency at especially high risk | 40–42 |
| Consequences of behaviors resulting from use | Nicotine, alcohol, and marijuana use are associated with worsened medication adherence for chronic medical conditions | 9,11,43,44 |

inflammation, all of which may theoretically be favorable for patients with IBD, although it should be noted that in patients with Crohn disease who use marijuana regularly, long-term outcomes may actually be worse.[23]

The second of these mechanisms is the direct toxic effect of substances on cells and tissues of the body. One of the most thoroughly described examples is the hepatotoxic effect of ethanol.[24] Oxidation of ethanol in the liver produces excess reduced nicotinamide adenine dinucleotide, which inhibits fatty acid oxidation, ultimately leading to hepatic steatosis.[25] Ethanol metabolism in the liver also produces reactive oxygen species, which are directly cytotoxic to hepatocytes.[26,27] These processes are likely deleterious for young people with pre-existing liver disease who drink alcohol, and compounding this, hepatotoxicity may be further exacerbated by medications commonly prescribed for YCMC, such as methotrexate and acetaminophen.[28,29]

The third mechanism is interaction of drugs and alcohol with medications used for chronic disease management. A full review of all possible substance-medication interactions is beyond the scope of this article, but such processes are best understood for alcohol, and ethanol-medication interactions are briefly reviewed here. Ethanol first affects the metabolism of medications by decreasing gastric emptying.[30] This delay in gastric emptying occurs even after one-time consumption of alcohol (ie, it does not require regular alcohol consumption) and alters the normal first-pass metabolism of medications. First-pass metabolism significantly alters plasma levels of propranolol, morphine, meperidine, diazepam, midazolam, lidocaine, and cimetidine. Thus, levels of these medications could be significantly altered among YCMC who ingest alcohol, although extensive studies have not been conducted.[30–32] Alcohol also induces cytochrome P450 2C9, potentially affecting the metabolism of medications metabolized by this enzyme (eg, warfarin, phenytoin).[30] Other interactions of ethanol with medications include disulfiram-like reactions (eg, from metronidazole, griseofulvin, procarbazine, some cephalosporins)[33,34] and enhancement of the depressive effects of certain medications on the CNS and on respiratory drive.[30,35,36]

The fourth mechanism involves complications specific to the route of administration of the substance being used (eg, inhalation, ingestion, injection, or other routes). Smoking marijuana, for example, is associated with increased wheeze, cough, and airway inflammation,[37] which may have critical implications for youth with asthma and for YCMC undergoing surgical procedures requiring general anesthesia with airway intubation.[38,39] Drug injection places users at risk of abscesses and blood-borne bacterial and viral infections, which may have particularly dangerous consequences for youth with immunodeficiency or who are on immunosuppressive medications.[40–42] Similarly, the risk for endocarditis as a result of drug injection could be particularly acute for youth with pre-existing structural or valvular heart disease.[40]

The fourth and final mechanism relates to inferior medication adherence or other disease management among YCMC who use alcohol or drugs. In one recent sample of adolescents with asthma, cystic fibrosis, T1DM, arthritis, or IBD, youth who drank were nearly 80% more likely to report regularly missing medications.[9] Poor medication adherence among young adult heavy drinkers is well described[43] and is further complicated by co-occurring marijuana use.[44] Because adolescence represents a transition period of increasing autonomy and independence, the influence of substance use on self-care and disease management should be critical area for future study.

Although the mechanisms discussed highlight how substances may be harmful to YCMC, there is also the possibility that some substances, or compounds within them, have therapeutic benefits. For no substance is this more passionately debated currently than for marijuana, which in the United States and elsewhere has been legally approved in many jurisdictions for medicinal use.[45–51] Major professional bodies, including the American Academy of Pediatrics, remain opposed to use of marijuana for medicinal purposes outside the usual drug approval regulatory processes (eg, by the US Food and Drug Administration).[48] This opposition is in part in response to the lack of strong empirical evidence that marijuana has medicinal benefits in conditions that manifest during adolescence.

Nonetheless, small observational studies and anecdotal reports have shown that for some young people with intractable epilepsy,[52,53] severe autism,[54] IBD,[23,55] and arthritis,[56] certain cannabinoids present in marijuana may have a beneficial effect. In addition, a recent placebo-controlled trial of 21 adults with Crohn disease showed improvement in symptoms with cannabis use when other therapies had failed.[57] This study did not include adolescents, and it is possible adolescents' pathophysiologic profile may differ and that they are at greater risk for long-term harms of chronic marijuana use.[58–62] Other proposed clinical applications for cannabis include symptomatic management of nausea, poor appetite, and pain, as well as treatment of multiple sclerosis, spinal cord injury, and glaucoma.[63] Nonetheless, owing to its status as an illegal, controlled substance in the United States and elsewhere, high-quality randomized-controlled trials of cannabinoids are lacking. Until careful studies demonstrate the safety, tolerability, efficacy, and proper dosing of cannabinoids for chronic disease, practitioners should continue to exercise caution given the well-established long-term health and adverse neurocognitive effects of marijuana for adolescents and young adults.[58–62]

Finally, in addition to substances affecting the course of chronic medical conditions, certain disease processes can in turn affect the metabolism of drugs of misuse. A commonly cited example is that benzodiazepines require oxidation by the liver for their metabolism and elimination, and therefore, the misuse of benzodiazepines by adolescents with liver disease may be especially hazardous (with the exception of lorazepam, oxazepam, and temazepam, which do not require extensive modification by the liver).[29,64]

## ROUTINE HEALTH CARE AND SCREENING

During adolescent periodic and routine preventive health care visits, screening for drug use including nonmedical use of prescription medications is recommended[65] and should also be conducted at behavioral health visits and specialty clinic visits. Research has shown that the health provider is a trusted source of information that adolescents and their families look to for advice on drug use, even more so than the Internet or social media sources.[66,67]

Preventive messages to YCMC are critical. YCMC may not visit the primary care provider's office often and therefore may not have the opportunity to learn about the risks posed by substance use and nonmedical use of prescription drugs. Similarly, owing to school absences for medical visits, they may be less likely to receive substance use prevention education. Even if they do, universal prevention messages may not apply as readily to YCMC and the additional risks they may have as someone managing a chronic medical condition.

There is much literature on the need for adolescents to have private health conversations with their provider, and when confidentiality is explained at the beginning of the visit, adolescents are often open to disclosing substance use as well as other sensitive information pertaining to mental health and sexual health. Conversely, they are unlikely to disclose this information when their parent or guardian is present.[68,69]

When adolescents and young adults are given private time one-on-one with the provider, they often disclose information on substance use and nonmedical use of prescription medications that can be helpful in optimizing the care and well-being of the adolescents and young adults.

At specialty clinic appointments for chronic disease management, providers may be more likely to focus on illness treatment and less likely to ask about substance use or to inform YCMC of the risks of substance use, particularly as it pertains to their specific condition. Specialty providers may be less likely to realize that YCMC are in need of this information or lack sufficient time to discuss these concerns if disease management concerns prevail.[9]

Routine screening and brief intervention can be obtained effectively either during face-to-face encounters or by using computer- or phone-assisted applications.[70,71] These tools not only screen but also can deliver personalized preventive messages in real time to the adolescent. Some adolescents are even more likely to disclose sensitive information during computerized screening than during face-to-face interview with a provider. This method is beneficial for providers who must manage significant clinical time constraints; once the adolescent is with the provider, the screening information is available to guide the encounter and any needed intervention.

There are readily available, free screening forms that have been validated in this age group. The CRAFFT screen and Screening To Brief Intervention (S2BI) questionnaires are valid and reliable for screening adolescent substance use and are quick to administer in the busy clinical setting.[72–74] Such screens are recommended as a routine component of Screening, Brief Intervention, and Referral to Treatment, which is universally recommended by the American Academy of Pediatrics.[75]

## SUMMARY

Like their peers in the general youth population, YCMC are at risk of experimentation and regular substance use, including nonmedical use of prescription medications. However, given dangerous disease-substance interactions, the stakes for detecting and intervening on substance use are perhaps even higher for YCMC. Given the risk for nonadherence with chronic disease management among substance-using youth, it is incumbent on primary care providers, specialty providers, and behavioral health specialists to be vigilant in asking about substance use and providing brief counseling and referral to formal substance use treatment when appropriate. Doing so is likely not only to prevent the direct harm of alcohol and drug use but also to simultaneously improve chronic disease treatment outcomes.

## REFERENCES

1. Johnston LD, O'Malley PM, Miech RA, et al. Monitoring the future national results on drug use: 2014 overview, key findings on adolescent drug use. Available at: http://www.monitoringthefuture.org/pubs/monographs/mtf-overview2014.pdf. Accessed February 24, 2015.
2. Substance Abuse and Mental Health Services Administration. Results from the 2013 National Survey on Drug Use and Health: summary of national findings, NSDUH Series H-48, HHS Publication No. (SMA) 14–4863. Rockville (MD): Substance Abuse and Mental Health Services Administration; 2014.
3. Johnson NB, Hayes LD, Brown K, et al. CDC national health report: leading causes of morbidity and mortality and associated behavioral risk and protective factors—United States, 2005-2013. MMWR Surveill Summ 2014;63:3–27.

4. Sawyer SM, Drew S, Yeo MS, et al. Adolescents with a chronic condition: challenges living, challenges treating. Lancet 2007;369:1481–9.

5. Van Cleave J, Gortmaker SL, Perrin JM. Dynamics of obesity and chronic health conditions among children and youth. JAMA 2010;303:623–30.

6. Britto MT, Garrett JM, Dugliss MA, et al. Risky behavior in teens with cystic fibrosis or sickle cell disease: a multicenter study. Pediatrics 1998;101: 250–6.

7. Jacobson AM, Hauser ST, Willett JB, et al. Psychological adjustment to IDDM: 10-year follow-up of an onset cohort of child and adolescent patients. Diabetes Care 1997;20:811–8.

8. Glasgow AM, Tynan D, Schwartz R, et al. Alcohol and drug use in teenagers with diabetes mellitus. J Adolesc Health 1991;12:11–4.

9. Weitzman ER, Ziemnik RE, Huang Q, et al. Alcohol and marijuana use and treatment nonadherence among medically vulnerable youth. Pediatrics 2015;136(3): 450–7.

10. Forero R, Bauman A, Young L, et al. Asthma, health behaviors, social adjustment, and psychosomatic symptoms in adolescence. J Asthma 1996;33: 157–64.

11. Precht DH, Keiding L, Madsen M. Smoking patterns among adolescents with asthma attending upper secondary schools: a community-based study. Pediatrics 2003;111:e562–8.

12. Mo F, Robinson C, Choi BC, et al. Analysis of prevalence, triggers, risk factors and the related socio-economic effects of childhood asthma in the Student Lung Health Survey (SLHS) database, Canada 1996. Int J Adolesc Med Health 2003; 15:349–58.

13. Strachan DP, Butland BK, Anderson HR. Incidence and prognosis of asthma and wheezing illness from early childhood to age 33 in a national British cohort. BMJ 1996;312:1195–9.

14. Weekes JC, Cotton S, McGrady ME. Predictors of substance use among black urban adolescents with asthma: a longitudinal assessment. J Natl Med Assoc 2011;103:392–8.

15. Guo S-E, Ratner PA, Johnson JL, et al. Correlates of smoking among adolescents with asthma. J Clin Nurs 2010;19:701–11.

16. Hublet A, De Bacquer D, Boyce W, et al. Smoking in young people with asthma. J Public Health (Oxf) 2007;29:343–9.

17. Martínez-Aguayo A, Araneda JC, Fernandez D, et al. Tobacco, alcohol, and illicit drug use in adolescents with diabetes mellitus. Pediatr Diabetes 2007;8: 265–71.

18. Lee P, Greenfield JR, Gilbert K, et al. Recreational drug use in type 1 diabetes: an invisible accomplice to poor glycaemic control? Intern Med J 2012;42: 198–202.

19. Ng RSH, Darko DA, Hillson RM. Street drug use among young patients with type 1 diabetes in the UK. Diabet Med 2004;21:295–6.

20. Gorelick DA, Baumann MA. The pharmacology of cocaine, amphetamines, and other stimulants. In: Ries RK, Fiellin DA, Miller SC, et al, editors. ASAM Principles of Addiction Medicine. 5th edition. Philadelphia: LWW; 2014.

21. Afonso L, Mohammad T, Thatai D. Crack whips the heart: a review of the cardiovascular toxicity of cocaine. Am J Cardiol 2007;100:1040–3.

22. Izzo AA, Camilleri M. Emerging role of cannabinoids in gastrointestinal and liver diseases: basic and clinical aspects. Gut 2008;57:1140–55.

23. Storr M, Devlin S, Kaplan GG, et al. Cannabis use provides symptom relief in patients with inflammatory bowel disease but is associated with worse disease prognosis in patients with Crohn's disease. Inflamm Bowel Dis 2014;20:472–80.

24. O'Shea RS, Dasarathy S, McCullough AJ. Alcoholic liver disease. Am J Gastroenterol 2010;105:14–32 [quiz: 33].

25. Friedman SL. Mechanisms of hepatic fibrogenesis. Gastroenterology 2008;134: 1655–69.

26. Albano E. Oxidative mechanisms in the pathogenesis of alcoholic liver disease. Mol Aspects Med 2008;29:9–16.

27. Dey A, Cederbaum AI. Alcohol and oxidative liver injury. Hepatology 2006;43: S63–74.

28. Navarro VJ, Senior JR. Drug-related hepatotoxicity. N Engl J Med 2006;354:731–9.

29. Kim JW, Phongsamran PV. Drug-induced liver disease and drug use considerations in liver disease. J Pharm Pract 2009;22(3):278–89.

30. Chan L-N, Anderson GD. Pharmacokinetic and pharmacodynamic drug interactions with ethanol (alcohol). Clin Pharmacokinet 2014;53:1115–36.

31. Pond SM, Tozer TN. First-pass elimination basic concepts and clinical consequences. Clin Pharmacokinet 1984;9:1–25.

32. Parlesak A, Billinger MH-U, Bode C, et al. Gastric alcohol dehydrogenase activity in man: influence of gender, age, alcohol consumption and smoking in a Caucasian population. Alcohol Alcohol 2002;37:388–93.

33. Fraser AG. Pharmacokinetic interactions between alcohol and other drugs. Clin Pharmacokinet 1997;33:79–90.

34. Ren S, Cao Y, Zhang X, et al. Cephalosporin induced disulfiram-like reaction: a retrospective review of 78 cases. Int Surg 2014;99:142–6.

35. Hesse LM, von Moltke LL, Greenblatt DJ. Clinically important drug interactions with zopiclone, zolpidem and zaleplon. CNS Drugs 2003;17:513–32.

36. Fiske WD, Jobes J, Xiang Q, et al. The effects of ethanol on the bioavailability of oxymorphone extended-release tablets and oxymorphone crush-resistant extended-release tablets. J Pain 2012;13:90–9.

37. Tetrault JM, Crothers K, Moore BA, et al. Effects of marijuana smoking on pulmonary function and respiratory complications: a systematic review. Arch Intern Med 2007;167:221–8.

38. Mallat A, Roberson J, Brock-Utne JG. Preoperative marijuana inhalation–an airway concern. Can J Anaesth 1996;43:691–3.

39. Mills PM, Penfold N. Cannabis abuse and anaesthesia. Anaesthesia 2003;58:1125.

40. Gordon RJ, Lowy FD. Bacterial infections in drug users. N Engl J Med 2005;353: 1945–54.

41. Degenhardt L, Hall W. Extent of illicit drug use and dependence, and their contribution to the global burden of disease. Lancet 2012;379:55–70.

42. Lloyd-Smith E, Kerr T, Hogg RS, et al. Prevalence and correlates of abscesses among a cohort of injection drug users. Harm Reduct J 2005;2:24.

43. Grodensky CA, Golin CE, Ochtera RD, et al. Systematic review: effect of alcohol intake on adherence to outpatient medication regimens for chronic diseases. J Stud Alcohol Drugs 2012;73:899–910.

44. Peters EN, Leeman RF, Fucito LM, et al. Co-occurring marijuana use is associated with medication nonadherence and nonplanning impulsivity in young adult heavy drinkers. Addict Behav 2012;37:420–6.

45. D'Souza D, Ranganathan M. Medical marijuana: is the cart before the horse? JAMA 2015;313:2431–2.

46. Choo EK, Benz M, Zaller N, et al. The impact of state medical marijuana legislation on adolescent marijuana use. J Adolesc Health 2014;55(2):160–6.

47. Wall MM, Poh E, Cerda M, et al. Adolescent marijuana use from 2002 to 2008: higher in states with medical marijuana laws, cause still unclear. Ann Epidemiol 2011;21:714–6.

48. Ammerman S, Ryan S, Adelman WP. The impact of marijuana policies on youth: clinical, research, and legal update. Pediatrics 2015;135:584–7.

49. Harper S, Strumpf EC, Kaufman JS. Do medical marijuana laws increase marijuana use? Replication study and extension. Ann Epidemiol 2012;22:207–12.

50. Hasin DS, Wall M, Keyes KM, et al. Medical marijuana laws and adolescent marijuana use in the USA from 1991 to 2014: results from annual, repeated cross-sectional surveys. Lancet Psychiatry 2015;2(7):601–8.

51. Lynne-Landsman SD, Livingston MD, Wagenaar AC. Effects of state medical marijuana laws on adolescent marijuana use. Am J Public Health 2013;103: 1500–6.

52. Vogelstein F. One man's desperate quest to cure his son's epilepsy—with weed. Available at: http://www.wired.com/2015/07/medical-marijuana-epilepsy/. Accessed August 3, 2015.

53. Gonzalez D. For children's seizures, turning to medical marijuana. Available at: http://lens.blogs.nytimes.com/2015/03/26/medical-marijuana-eases-childhood-seizures/. Accessed August 3, 2015.

54. Borchardt D. Desperate parents of autistic children trying cannabis despite lack of studies. Available at: http://www.forbes.com/sites/debraborchardt/2015/06/10/desperate-parents-of-autistic-children-trying-cannabis-despite-lack-of-studies/. Accessed August 3, 2015.

55. Lahat A, Lang A, Ben-Horin S. Impact of cannabis treatment on the quality of life, weight and clinical disease activity in inflammatory bowel disease patients: a pilot prospective study. Digestion 2012;85:1–8.

56. Fitzcharles M-A, Clauw DJ, Ste-Marie PA, et al. The dilemma of medical marijuana use by rheumatology patients. Arthritis Care Res (Hoboken) 2014;66:797–801.

57. Naftali T, Bar-Lev Schleider L, Dotan I, et al. Cannabis induces a clinical response in patients with Crohn's disease: a prospective placebo-controlled study. Clin Gastroenterol Hepatol 2013;11:1276–80.e1.

58. Hall W, Degenhardt L. Adverse health effects of non-medical cannabis use. Lancet 2009;374:1383–91.

59. Meier MH, Caspi A, Ambler A, et al. Persistent cannabis users show neuropsychological decline from childhood to midlife. Proc Natl Acad Sci U S A 2012; 109:E2657–64.

60. Moore TH, Zammit S, Lingford-Hughes A, et al. Cannabis use and risk of psychotic or affective mental health outcomes: a systematic review. Lancet 2007; 370:319–28.

61. Hadland SE, Knight JR, Harris SK. Medical marijuana: review of the science and implications for developmental-behavioral pediatric practice. J Dev Behav Pediatr 2015;36:115–23.

62. Hadland SE, Harris SK. Youth marijuana use: state of the science for the practicing clinician. Curr Opin Pediatr 2014;26:420–7.

63. Amar Ben M. Cannabinoids in medicine: a review of their therapeutic potential. J Ethnopharmacol 2006;105:1–25.

64. Witek MW, Rojas V, Alonso C, et al. Review of benzodiazepine use in children and adolescents. Psychiatr Q 2005;76:283–96.

65. Hagan JF, Shaw JS, Duncan PM. Bright futures: guidelines for health supervision of infants, children, and adolescents, 3rd edition Available at: http://brightfutures.aap.org/3rd_Edition_Guidelines_and_Pocket_Guide.html. Accessed August 3, 2015.

66. Kim SU, Syn SY. Research trends in teens' health information behaviour: a review of the literature. Health Info Libr J 2014;31:4–19.

67. Selkie EM, Benson M, Moreno M. Adolescents' views regarding uses of social networking websites and text messaging for adolescent sexual health education. Am J Health Educ 2011;42:205–12.

68. Britto MT, Tivorsak TL, Slap GB. Adolescents' needs for health care privacy. Pediatrics 2010;126(6):e1469–76.

69. Ford C, English A, Sigman G. Confidential health care for adolescents: position paper for the Society for Adolescent Medicine. J Adolesc Health 2004;35:160–7.

70. Harris SK, Csemy L, Sherritt L, et al. Computer-facilitated substance use screening and brief advice for teens in primary care: an international trial. Pediatrics 2012;129:1072–82.

71. Chisolm DJ, Gardner W, Julian T, et al. Adolescent satisfaction with computer-assisted behavioural risk screening in primary care. Child Adolesc Ment Health 2008;13:163–8.

72. Levy S, Weiss R, Sherritt L, et al. An electronic screen for triaging adolescent substance use by risk levels. JAMA Pediatr 2014;168:822–8.

73. Knight JR, Sherritt L, Shrier LA, et al. Validity of the CRAFFT substance abuse screening test among adolescent clinic patients. Arch Pediatr Adolesc Med 2002;156:607–14.

74. Knight JR, Shrier LA, Bravender TD, et al. A new brief screen for adolescent substance abuse. Arch Pediatr Adolesc Med 1999;153:591–6.

75. Levy SJ, Kokotailo PK. Substance use screening, brief intervention, and referral to treatment for pediatricians. Pediatrics 2011;128:e1330–40.

76. Silverman RA, Boudreaux ED, Woodruff PG, et al. Cigarette smoking among asthmatic adults presenting to 64 emergency departments. Chest 2003;123:1472–9.

77. Leuenberger P, Schwartz J, Ackermann-Liebrich U, et al. Passive smoking exposure in adults and chronic respiratory symptoms (SAPALDIA study). Swiss study on Air Pollution and Lung diseases In Adults, SAPALDIA team. Am J Respir Crit Care Med 1994;150:1222–8.

78. Gilliland FD, Islam T, Berhane K, et al. Regular smoking and asthma incidence in adolescents. Am J Respir Crit Care Med 2006;174:1094–100.

79. Primack BA, Soneji S, Stoolmiller M, et al. Progression to traditional cigarette smoking after electronic cigarette use among US adolescents and young adults. JAMA Pediatr 2015;169(11):1018–23.

80. Leventhal AM, Strong DR, Kirkpatrick MG, et al. Association of electronic cigarette use with initiation of combustible tobacco product smoking in early adolescence. JAMA 2015;314:700.

81. Kalkhoran S, Glantz SA. Modeling the health effects of expanding e-cigarette sales in the United States and United Kingdom: a Monte Carlo Analysis. JAMA Intern Med 2015;175(10):1671–80.

82. Collaco JM, Drummond MB, McGrath-Morrow SA. Electronic cigarette use and exposure in the pediatric population. JAMA Pediatr 2015;169:177–82.

83. Bae J. Influence of asthma on the longitudinal trajectories of cigarette use behaviors from adolescence to adulthood using latent growth curve models. J Prev Med Public Health 2015;48:111–7.

84. Wolpert H, Anderson B, Harris M. Transitions in care: meeting the challenges of type 1 diabetes in young adults. Alexandria (VA): American Diabetes Association; 2009.

85. Peters A, Laffel L. Diabetes care for emerging adults: recommendations for transition from pediatric to adult diabetes care systems: a position statement of the American Diabetes Association, with representation by the American College of Osteopathic Family Physicians, the American Academy of Pediatrics, the American Association of Clinical Endocrinologists, the American Osteopathic Association, the Centers for Disease Control and Prevention, Children with Diabetes, The Endocrine Society, the International Society for Pediatric and Adolescent Diabetes, Juvenile Diabetes Research Foundation International, the National Diabetes Education Program, and the Pediatric Endocrine Society (formerly Lawson Wilkins Pediatric Endocrine Society). Diabetes Care 2011;34:2477–85.

86. Lee P, Greenfield JR, Campbell LV. Managing young people with type 1 diabetes in a "rave" new world: metabolic complications of substance abuse in type 1 diabetes. Diabet Med 2009;26:328–33.

87. Seymour HR, Gilman D, Quin JD. Severe ketoacidosis complicated by "ecstasy" ingestion and prolonged exercise. Diabet Med 1996;13:908–9.

88. Laing SP, Swerdlow AJ, Slater SD, et al. The British Diabetic Association Cohort Study, II: cause-specific mortality in patients with insulin-treated diabetes mellitus. Diabet Med 1999;16:466–71.

89. Laing SP, Jones ME, Swerdlow AJ, et al. Psychosocial and socioeconomic risk factors for premature death in young people with type 1 diabetes. Diabetes Care 2005;28:1618–23.

90. Wen H, Hockenberry JM, Cummings JR. The effect of medical marijuana laws on adolescent and adult use of marijuana, alcohol, and other substances. J Health Econ 2015;42:64–80.

91. Hill K. Medical marijuana does not increase adolescent marijuana use. Lancet Psychiatry 2015;2:572–3.

92. Leung Y, Heyman MB, Mahadevan U. Transitioning the adolescent inflammatory bowel disease patient: guidelines for the adult and pediatric gastroenterologist. Inflamm Bowel Dis 2011;17:2169–73.

93. Lu Y, Markowitz J. Inflammatory bowel disease in adolescents: what problems does it pose? World J Gastroenterol 2011;17:2691–5.

94. Philpott JR. Transitional care in inflammatory bowel disease. Gastroenterol Hepatol (N Y) 2011;7:26–32.

95. Naftali T, Mechulam R, Lev LB, et al. Cannabis for inflammatory bowel disease. Dig Dis 2014;32:468–74.

96. Turner BC, Jenkins E, Kerr D, et al. The effect of evening alcohol consumption on next-morning glucose control in type 1 diabetes. Diabetes Care 2001;24:1888–93.

97. Schwartz BG, Rezkalla S, Kloner RA. Cardiovascular effects of cocaine. Circulation 2010;122:2558–69.

98. Lange RA, Hillis LD. Cardiovascular complications of cocaine use. N Engl J Med 2001;345:351–8.

99. Blowey DL. Nephrotoxicity of over-the-counter analgesics, natural medicines, and illicit drugs. Adolesc Med Clin 2005;16:31–43, x.

100. Joffe HV, Xu R, Johnson FB, et al. Warfarin dosing and cytochrome P450 2C9 polymorphisms. Thromb Haemost 2004;91:1123–8.

101. Lee CR, Goldstein JA, Pieper JA. Cytochrome P450 2C9 polymorphisms: a comprehensive review of the in-vitro and human data. Pharmacogenet Genomics 2002;12:251–63.

102. Stout SM, Cimino NM. Exogenous cannabinoids as substrates, inhibitors, and inducers of human drug metabolizing enzymes: a systematic review. Drug Metab Rev 2014;46:86–95.

103. Patsalos PN, Perucca E. Clinically important drug interactions in epilepsy: general features and interactions between antiepileptic drugs. Lancet Neurol 2003; 2:347–56.

# Objective Testing
## Urine and Other Drug Tests

Scott E. Hadland, MD, MPH[a,b,*], Sharon Levy, MD, MPH[b,c]

### KEYWORDS

- Substance abuse detection • Adolescents • Substance-related disorders • Ethanol
- Street drugs • Urine

### KEY POINTS

- Routine laboratory testing of adolescents, whether in primary care, school, or at home is not recommended, though testing may be useful in several clinical situations.
- Laboratory testing is complex and requires careful attention to specimen collection and interpretation of results.
- As with all laboratory testing, drug testing offers limited information and should always be interpreted in a clinical context.

It is incumbent on clinicians to detect substance use early and intervene to reduce acute risks and to improve the life course trajectory of addiction and its harms. For clinicians working with adolescents, screening for alcohol and drug use is a critical skill that allows for brief intervention and referral to treatment, an approach endorsed by major professional bodies,[1–3] including the American Academy of Pediatrics (AAP).[4] Screening is best conducted using a validated instrument (such as the Screening to Brief Intervention (S2BI) instrument[5]) that can then prompt a discussion between the clinician and adolescent.

At first blush, routine screening of adolescents by testing urine or other bodily fluids might seem like a reasonable strategy for detecting substance use; but this approach

Conflict of Interest Statement: The authors have no conflicts of interest to disclose.

Dr S.E. Hadland is supported by the Division of Adolescent and Young Adult Medicine at Boston Children's Hospital and the Leadership Education in Adolescent Health Training Program T71 MC00009 (MCH/HRSA) and by a National Research Service Award 1T32 HD075727 (NIH/NICHD). Dr S. Levy is supported by 1R01AA021913–01 (NIH/NIAAA).

[a] Division of Adolescent/Young Adult Medicine, Department of Medicine, Boston Children's Hospital, 300 Longwood Avenue, Boston, MA 02115, USA; [b] Department of Pediatrics, Harvard Medical School, 25 Shattuck Street, Boston, MA 02115, USA; [c] Division of Developmental Medicine, Department of Medicine, Boston Children's Hospital, 300 Longwood Avenue, Boston, MA 02115, USA

* Corresponding author. Division of Adolescent/Young Adult Medicine, Department of Medicine, Boston Children's Hospital, 300 Longwood Avenue, Boston, MA 02115.

E-mail address: scott.hadland@childrens.harvard.edu

Child Adolesc Psychiatric Clin N Am 25 (2016) 549–565

http://dx.doi.org/10.1016/j.chc.2016.02.005

childpsych.theclinics.com

is fraught with inaccurate findings and misinterpretation and, worse, leads to mistrust on the part of the adolescent and missed opportunities for nuanced discussions about substance use with a clinician. Abstinence from all substances is recommended throughout adolescence because of the impact of alcohol, marijuana, and other drugs on brain development.[6] Routine drug testing of all adolescents, however, is insensitive for detecting sporadic use and risks obscuring opportunities for counseling and brief interventions that may be better identified by self-report.[7]

Although routine laboratory testing is not recommended for adolescents, there are several indications for which this procedure may provide useful information to supplement a clinical history or to regularly monitor patients in treatment for substance use disorders. Here, the authors review drugs commonly included in testing panels, bodily fluids, and tissues tested, indications for testing, practical concerns, and issues unique to drug testing adolescents as contrasted with its use in adults.

## DRUGS TESTED

Although it is possible to test for use of an individual drug, multiple drugs or classes are usually tested at the same time using a single biological sample.[8] The most commonly used immunoassay (IA) drug test panel includes the Substance Abuse and Mental Health Services Administration-5 (SAMHSA-5), a standard panel established in the 1980s under the Drug-Free Workplace Act. The SAMHSA-5 includes amphetamines, marijuana (tetrahydrocannabinol [THC]), cocaine metabolites, opiates (including heroin, morphine, and codeine but not synthetic opioids, such as oxycodone, hydrocodone, buprenorphine, or methadone), and phencyclidine (PCP).[8,9] Most drug screens available commercially have panels that expand beyond the SAMHSA-5 to also include benzodiazepines, barbiturates, and additional opiates.[8]

Alcohol and drugs vary substantially in their windows of detection, largely owing to their degree of fat solubility. For example, THC and other highly fat-soluble compounds have a very long half-life of elimination and can be detected in urine up to weeks after last use among heavy users. The various windows of detection for several commonly used substances are shown in **Table 1**.[10]

## SOURCES FOR TESTING

There are multiple sources for biological specimens (often referred to as *biological matrices* in the scientific literature): urine, blood, saliva, hair, breath, sweat, and meconium. These various tissues and bodily fluids exhibit different rates and durations of excretion that result in different detection windows for substances, as demonstrated in **Fig. 1**.

When substances are ingested, they are absorbed in the gastrointestinal tract and distributed to tissues of the body.[9] Substances that are injected, inhaled, or snorted bypass gastrointestinal absorption and are delivered immediately to tissues. Because many drugs are lipid soluble, they must undergo metabolism in the liver to render them water soluble, which then allows them to be eliminated in urine. Blood and breath reflect moment-to-moment serum levels of an ingested substance and offer the earliest and shortest windows of detection for substances.[8] Sweat and saliva reflect the presence of a drug within the body several hours later. Urine offers a somewhat longer window of detection for substances, usually varying from 1 day after consumption to several weeks. Hair and meconium offer the longest windows of detection (weeks to months). Advantages and disadvantages of different matrices for drug testing are shown in **Table 2**.

Here the authors review the various biological matrices for drug testing.

**Table 1**
**Windows of detection in urine for various substances**

| Substance | Detection Windows by Drug Test Type | | | |
| --- | --- | --- | --- | --- |
| | Urine | Hair | Oral Fluid | Sweat |
| Alcohol | 10–12 h ETG, up to 48 h | N/A | Up to 24 h | N/A |
| Amphetamines | 2–4 d | Up to 90 d | 1–48 h | 7–14 d |
| Methamphetamine | 2–5 d | Up to 90 d | 1–48 h | 7–14 d |
| Barbiturates | Up to 7 d | Up to 90 d | N/A | N/A |
| Benzodiazepines | Up to 7 d | Up to 90 d | N/A | N/A |
| Cannabis (marijuana) | 1–30 d | Up to 90 d | Up to 24 h | 7–14 d |
| Cocaine | 1–3 d | Up to 90 d | 1–36 h | 7–14 d |
| Codeine (opiate) | 2–4 d | Up to 90 d | 1–36 h | 7–14 d |
| Morphine (opiate) | 2–5 d | Up to 90 d | 1–36 h | 7–14 d |
| Heroin (opiate) | 2–3 d | Up to 90 d | 1–36 h | 7–14 d |
| PCP | 5–6 d | Up to 90 d | N/A | 7–14 d |

Lysergic acid diethylamide, mushrooms, synthetic cannabinoids, and ecstasy (3,4-methylenedioxy-methamphetamine) will not be detected by typical drug testing.

*Abbreviation:* ETG, ethyl glucuronide.

*From* National Center on Substance Abuse and Child Welfare. Drug testing practice guidelines, substance abuse and mental health services administration. 2011. Available at: https://ncsacw.samhsa.gov/files/IA_Drug_Testing_Bench_Card_508.pdf. Accessed October 12, 2015.

## Urine

Of all the matrices, urine is the most commonly used for adolescent drug testing and is the most thoroughly studied.[9,11] However, for adolescent patients, its collection is somewhat invasive because it requires either a sophisticated collection protocol that is not readily available in medical offices or direct observation (eg, by a clinician

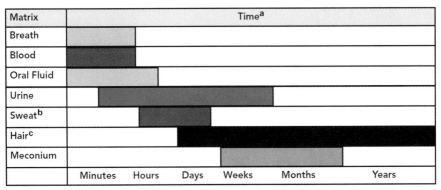

**Fig. 1.** Drug detection times for different biological specimens used in drug testing. [a] Very broad estimates that also depend on the substance, the amount and frequency of the substance taken, and other factors previously listed. [b] As long as the patch is worn, usually 7 days. [c] Seven to 10 days after use to the time passed to grow the length of hair but may be limited to 6 months' hair growth. However, most laboratories analyze the amount of hair equivalent to 3 months of growth. (*From* Substance Abuse and Mental Health Services Administration. Clinical drug testing in primary care. Technical assistance publication [TAP] 32. Rockville (MD): 2012. HHS publication No. [SMA] 12-4668.)

**Table 2**
**Advantages and disadvantages of various matrices (ie, bodily fluids and tissues) used for drug testing**

| Matrix | Advantages | Disadvantages |
|---|---|---|
| Urine | • Available in sufficient quantities<br>• Higher concentrations of parent drugs and/or metabolites than in blood<br>• Availability of POCTs<br>• Well-researched testing techniques | • Short to intermediate window of detection<br>• Easy to adulterate or substitute<br>• May require observed collection<br>• Potential for shy bladder syndrome, cannot produce a specimen |
| Oral fluid | • Noninvasive specimen collection<br>• Easy to collect<br>• Reduced risk of adulteration<br>• Directly observed specimen collection<br>• Parent drug rather than metabolite can be assay target<br>• Able to detect same-day use, in some cases<br>• Availability of POCTs<br>• Detect residual drug in the mouth | • Limited specimen volume<br>• Possibility of contamination from residual drug in mouth that cannot be correlated with blood concentrations<br>• Short window of detection<br>• Requires supervision of patients for 10–30 min before sampling<br>• Salivation reduced by stimulant use<br>• Need for elution solvent to efficiently remove drugs adsorbed to collection device<br>• Potential for cannabinoids in oral fluid to arise from contamination of the oral cavity rather than excretion in saliva from blood |
| Sweat | • Detects recent use (fewer than 24 h with a sweat swipe) or allows for cumulative testing with the sweat patch (worn for up to 7–14 d)<br>• Noninvasive specimen collection<br>• Difficult to adulterate<br>• Requires little training to collect specimen<br>• May be an economical alternative to urine | • Few facilities and limited expertise for testing<br>• Risk of accidental or deliberate removal of the sweat patch collection device<br>• Unknown effects of variable sweat excretion among individuals<br>• Only a single sweat collection patch available so multiple analyses cannot be done if needed (ie, more than one positive initial test)<br>• May be affected by external contaminants<br>• Requires 2 visits, one for patch placement and one for patch removal |
| Blood | • Generally detects recent use<br>• Established laboratory test method | • Expensive, except to detect ethanol<br>• Limited window of detection<br>• Invasive specimen collection (venipuncture)<br>• Risk of infection<br>• Requires training to collect specimen<br>• May not be an option for individual with poor venous access |

*(continued on next page)*

| Table 2 (continued) | | |
|---|---|---|
| Matrix | Advantages | Disadvantages |
| Hair | • Longest window of detection<br>• May be able to detect changes in drug use over time (from 7–10 d after drug use to 3 mo, depending on length of hair tested)<br>• Directly observed specimen collection<br>• Noninvasive specimen collection<br>• 4 tests cover 1 y<br>• Easy storage and transport<br>• Difficult to adulterate or substitute<br>• Readily available sample, depending on length of hair tested | • Cannot detect use within the previous 7–10 d<br>• Difficult to interpret results<br>• Costly and time consuming to prepare specimen for testing<br>• Few laboratories available to perform testing<br>• No POCTs currently available<br>• Difficult to detect low-level use (eg, single-use episode)<br>• May be biased with hair color (dark hair contains more of some basic drugs [cocaine, methamphetamine, opioids] because of enhanced binding to melanin in hair)<br>• Possibility of environmental contamination<br>• Specimen can be removed by shaving |
| Breath | • Well-established method for alcohol testing<br>• Readily available | • Used only for alcohol and other volatiles<br>• Short window of detection<br>• May be difficult to obtain adequate sample, especially with patients who are very intoxicated or uncooperative<br>• Uncommon in clinical setting |
| Meconium | • Can detect maternal drug abuse and fetal or infant exposure<br>• Wide window of drug detection (third trimester of gestation)<br>• Noninvasive collection from diaper<br>• Generally, adequate specimen amount | • Narrow collection window that can be missed, especially in babies with low birth weight<br>• Testing not available in all laboratories<br>• Requires extra steps (weighing and extraction)<br>• Confirmation assays more difficult than for urine |

Abbreviation: POCTs, point-of-care tests.
From Substance Abuse and Mental Health Services Administration. Clinical drug testing in primary care. Technical assistance publication [TAP] 32. Rockville (MD): 2012. HHS publication No. [SMA] 12-4668.

or a parent) to prevent tampering.[7,12] Compounding this, many pediatricians are unfamiliar with proper collection procedures and with the limitations of urine drug screening.[11]

Currently, the most commonly used urine drug testing approach involves automated IA either alone as a point-of-care test or as an initial screen for a 2-step testing procedure.[7,8] Results from IA are qualitative (ie, a drug or its metabolite is denoted either present or absent, without the quantity reported). In the 2-step approach, a screening IA is followed by confirmatory gas chromatography-mass spectrometry (GC-MS). If any substances are positive on the initial IA, a separate quantity of the same sample is then subjected to GC-MS as a confirmatory test for those same substances, with negative results on the IA disregarded. GC-MS provides a quantitative result to help guide the clinician, which can be used to follow serial samples and determine whether the metabolite concentration is increasing or decreasing, which may suggest ongoing use or abstinence, respectively. Even still, caution is warranted as levels may vary with urine concentration, the amount of drug used, and time since last use, thus making an absolute determination regarding whether use is ongoing difficult.

IA is often used as a point-of-care test given its convenience, low cost, and relatively rapid results (although results are often not available quickly enough to guide clinical management in emergent situations).[7] Most home urine drug test kits use IA. Although IA has high sensitivity, it has poorer specificity than GC-MS owing to cross-reactivity, whereby compounds in the biological specimen other than the actual substance or its metabolite bind to the assay and trigger a false-positive result. (For example, PCP assays can turn positive if an individual consumes dextromethorphan, a common component of cough syrup.) Additionally, IA drug tests performed in isolation do not distinguish among drugs within a class (ie, IA cannot distinguish between various amphetamines, barbiturates, benzodiazepines, or opiates).[8] GC-MS is not performed as a point-of-care test and usually must be sent to a laboratory, resulting in a delay.[7] Newer but less widely used technologies include liquid chromatography-mass spectrometry and tandem mass-spectrometry, which can be used to bypass the initial screening IA and identify a larger number of substances and metabolites.[8]

Often, laboratories report the urine creatinine, which helps the clinician correct for the relative concentration or dilution of the urine. Concentration of the urine by the kidneys results in elevated levels of drug metabolites; therefore, urine concentrations of certain drugs and their metabolites are usually divided by the urine creatinine. An example of this is THC, whose excretion in the urine can continue for up to 1 month after most recent use in heavy users[13]; urine samples positive for THC must be carefully interpreted to distinguish ongoing excretion from new use. Urine THC concentration should be divided by the urine creatinine concentration in order to determine whether the creatinine-normalized THC concentration is increasing or decreasing with consecutive urine samples,[14] and these ratios can then be compared with nomograms of THC excretion in order to make a clinical interpretation.[15] Practical issues, such as timing of the urine sample collection, specimen collection techniques, validation of the sample, and result interpretation, are covered later in this article.

### Blood

Drug testing of blood samples is usually only performed in emergency situations; because of the invasiveness of obtaining a blood sample, the need for specially trained phlebotomists, and the expense of blood drug testing, it is rarely performed in primary care settings.[7,9] An additional limitation is that obtaining blood samples requires venipuncture, and locating venous access among injection drug users can be very difficult.[9] Unlike urine samples, blood samples generally detect alcohol and drug compounds themselves rather than their metabolites. Blood testing typically detects substance use that occurred within 2 to 12 hours of the test.[7]

### Oral (Saliva)

Oral fluid testing is less commonly used; but oral samples represent a convenient, promising matrix for many settings. Unlike urine samples, oral samples are not easily tampered with and can be collected with minimal invasion of privacy.[15,16] Oral secretions contain either the original drug compound or its metabolite for approximately 24 to 48 hours after last use.[9,15,16] Importantly, the use of breath sprays, mouthwash, or other oral rinses containing alcohol does not affect drug testing results as long as they are not used within 30 minutes of sample collection.[17] To collect an oral sample, a swab is placed adjacent to the lower gums against the inner cheek and left in place for several minutes before being inserted into a vial for transportation to the laboratory.[9] Point-of-care oral testing is also available in some settings.[18]

### Hair

Hair drug tests have the advantage of detecting substance use days to months or, in some cases, years later.[9,19] Drug metabolites are present in hair as early as 1 week after the most recent use; because metabolites remain trapped in the core of the hair as it grows, hair provides a rough timeline of use over an extended period.[9,20] Hair grows at a rate of approximately 0.5 in per month, and so the standard 1.5-in hair sample obtained close to the root in most drug testing protocols gives information over the past 3-month drug use.[8]

Because of the long period of detection for hair samples, they are useful for detecting chronic substance use, understanding the duration of patients' drug use over the long-term, and indicating periods of abstinence.[20–22] Conversely, hair testing is not helpful in detecting sporadic use when weekly or even monthly drug testing is required as part of a drug treatment plan.[9] Additionally, drug use often must be relatively heavy in order for testing to detect levels in hair. Other limitations of hair testing include that individuals can surreptitiously remove the sample through shaving; that sweat production can cause drug metabolites to travel proximally up the hair shaft, thus, affecting drug test interpretation; and that drugs can be incorporated into hair through simple exposure from second-hand smoke.[23,24] An additional potential consideration is that drug concentrations can be affected by the melanin content of hair, resulting in potentially higher concentrations of certain drugs in dark hair as compared with blond or red hair.[15,25] Bleaching or coloring the hair may also alter concentrations of metabolites.[26]

The hair sample is typically cut from the back of the head using scissors, cutting as close to the scalp as possible to estimate the most recent drug use.[9] For patients who are bald or who have shaved their head, hair can be taken from the armpit, face, or other unshaven part of the body, so long as a sufficiently long enough sample can be taken. No point-of-care hair drug testing currently exists.

### Breath

Breath testing, often referred to colloquially as the "Breathalyzer" test after the original brand name testing device (Smith and Wesson, Springfield, MA), is used exclusively for instantaneous estimation of blood alcohol content.[8] Breath testing provides an accurate measure of the actual blood alcohol content at that moment in time and is more frequently used in law enforcement or in emergency departments than in primary care. The US Department of Transportation (DOT) maintains an active list of approved breath testing devices for the interested reader (https://www.transportation.gov/odapc/approved-evidential-breath-testing-devices).[27]

### Sweat

The US Food and Drug Administration (FDA) has approved a patch for collection of sweat for drug testing that is placed on the skin for 3 to 7 days before being sent to a laboratory for interpretation.[8,9] In Europe, a wipe is also available that is not currently FDA approved because of concerns regarding its accuracy.[9,12] Sweat testing checks for substances and their metabolites in the bloodstream in the hours before and while the patch is applied.[8,9] Currently, sweat testing is only available for the SAMHSA-5.

Patches that pucker or show other evidence of interference when removed have been designed in attempt to reduce tampering.[8]

### Meconium

Meconium is obtained from newborns and used as a measure of maternal substance use in the third trimester.[8,12,28,29] Meconium is present in a newborn's first several stools. Meconium testing is used as a screen in the newborn nursery or neonatal intensive care unit when maternal substance use during pregnancy is suspected and can have critical legal consequences for guardianship of the child.[30] Meconium testing can also inform clinical management of neonatal abstinence syndrome and other newborn withdrawal syndromes.

## INDICATIONS FOR DRUG TESTING

According to the American Society for Addiction Medicine, drug testing should be used "to discourage nonmedical drug use and diversion of controlled substances, to encourage appropriate entry into addiction treatment, to identify early relapse and to improve outcomes of addiction treatment through the use of long-term post-treatment monitoring."[8] Because substance use is often secret, adolescents may not be forthcoming; drug testing may be useful when history is negative in the context of clinical signs and symptoms suggesting substance use.[7] Indications for adolescent drug testing are explored here.

### Emergent Care

Drug tests are commonly used in emergent situations, such as when an adolescent presents with altered mental status.[7,8] Some common clinical scenarios include attempted suicide, motor vehicle injury or other injury in which substance use may have been a contributor, unexplained seizures, syncope, arrhythmia, or toxidromal signs that suggest a particular intoxication or withdrawal pattern.[7] In such cases, consent for the drug screen is inferred; its results may be used to guide clinical management. However, drug testing results are generally not available immediately and cannot be reliably used early in emergent management; therefore, initial decisions, such as whether to provide naloxone for suspected opioid overdose, should be made by the clinician based on presenting signs and symptoms.[7,8] Additionally, because highly sensitive drug testing may detect substances at limits far lower than therapeutic doses, drug screens may identify additional substances that are present but not contributing to the acute intoxication or withdrawal picture and may therefore be misleading.[7] Once patients are stabilized, however, drug testing results may be helpful in determining subsequent management, particularly once confirmatory testing results are available.

### Assessment of Behavioral or Other Mental Health Concerns

In primary care or mental health care settings, substance use by an adolescent may be suspected as underlying or complicating symptoms of depression, anxiety, inattention, hyperactivity, or other broader concerns, such as a school failure or interpersonal difficulties.[7,9] In these situations, voluntary drug testing (ie, drug testing with the assent of the adolescent and the consent of a guardian) may serve as a helpful complement to a careful history. A positive drug screen might indicate substance use that an adolescent previously denied, leading to an opportunity for an honest conversation.[7] However, as highlighted later in the discussion of interpretation of results, there are several limitations in drug testing that might result in a negative result despite clinically significant substance use by an adolescent.

## Substance Use Treatment

Drug testing is performed as a routine component of outpatient adolescent substance use treatment.[7,9] It serves multiple roles, including preventing adverse effects of pharmacotherapy (eg, precipitating opioid withdrawal if a clinician provides naltrexone for alcohol use disorder if that patient were also surreptitiously using opioids) and monitoring for use of illicit substances during treatment and/or adherence with prescribed medications, such as stimulants for comorbid attention-deficit/hyperactivity disorder (ADHD) or buprenorphine for opioid use disorder.[9] In residential substance use treatment, drug testing helps support the drug-free therapeutic environment.[8]

In monitoring for illicit drug use during treatment, testing should be performed at random times, as discussed later, because adolescents are often aware of the short window of detection in urine for many substances and might otherwise simply abstain from use for the several days leading up to a scheduled test.[7,9] Testing should also be performed frequently enough (eg, at least weekly) to detect any use occurring during treatment.[8] A positive drug screen should never serve as grounds for termination from the substance use treatment program but rather should prompt a careful conversation between the adolescent and clinician to reconsider the current treatment plan[7,8]; multiple positive drug tests may indicate the need for a higher level of care, for example.[8]

Contingency management, which relies on incentives to encourage ongoing abstinence for adolescents with a substance use disorder, often uses drug testing for monitoring.[31] Adolescents who attend their scheduled visits and/or have negative urine drug tests are provided monetary prizes or other rewards to reinforce their treatment plan adherence.[9,31,32] In many settings, the value of prizes increases incrementally with each successive attended visit or negative drug screen, which further improves the efficacy of treatment.[31,33,34]

## Other Settings

Several other potential settings for adolescent drug testing exist. The DOT federally mandates workplace drug testing for private-sector transportation workers, and many of the current standards for workplace testing have emerged from these regulations.[9] For example, the SAMHSA-5 urine drug screen was codified in the late 1980s for DOT workplace testing. Some adolescents and young adults may find themselves seeking or maintaining employment in settings where drug screening is routine.[7] Drug screens from nonfederal employers can and often do expand their drug testing panels to include substances in addition to those on the SAMHSA-5.[9] Many policies regarding when, where, and how employers can test their employees are set by states; a full review is beyond the scope of this article; but a complete, up-to-date listing of relevant policies is available at a cost from the Drug and Alcohol Testing Industry Association (DATIA), an independent industry organization.[35]

Some jurisdictions have proposed drug screening in school. However, this approach is opposed by the AAP because of insufficient evidence that it discourages adolescent drug use, difficulty in correctly interpreting results, and potential adverse consequences, such as disciplinary action, decreased participation in sports and other school activities, breaches of confidentiality, and increased use of substances not included in the drug testing panel used.[36] Similarly, although home urine drug tests are commercially available for purchase from, for example, drugstores and online marketplaces, use of these over-the-counter home tests by parents without the guidance of a clinician is not recommended because of the complexities in interpreting results.[7]

(Use of over-the-counter drug screens is distinguished from formal drug screens collected at home under the guidance of a clinician to be sent to an approved laboratory, which is frequently recommended as part of drug treatment.) Youths involved in the criminal justice system are typically routinely drug tested, and the specifics of this practice vary from state to state.[8]

## PRACTICAL CONCERNS IN ADOLESCENT DRUG TESTING
### Adolescent Assent/Parental Consent and Confidentiality

Once a practitioner thinks that drug testing (usually urine) would be helpful clinically, he or she should have a careful discussion with both the adolescent and parent regarding the potential benefits (ie, supporting reducing substance use) and the limitations of testing.[7] Any questions should be addressed; then the clinician should communicate to the adolescent the recommendation for drug testing, emphasizing the potential benefits (confirming a history of no recent substance use, improving trust with parents, and so forth). Assent should always be obtained from the adolescent, and permission to share results of any drug tests with his or her parent should be sought.

In addition to the usual privacy provisions dictated by the Health Insurance Portability and Accountability Act of 1996 (HIPAA), programs providing substance use diagnosis, treatment, or referral for treatment are subject to stricter confidentiality requirements under federal regulations.[9] These regulations are contained in Volume 42 of the Code of Federal Regulations, Part 2, often referred to by practitioners as Part 2 provisions. Whereas under HIPAA, personal health information can be disclosed among an adolescent's providers without written consent if done as part of routine clinical care, Part 2 requires written permission from adolescent patients for any disclosure. As always, if emergent clinical care for the adolescent is required, consent is implied and written permission need not be obtained. Many readers of this article are unlikely to be affected by Part 2 regulations.

The age at which an adolescent can independently seek, consent for, and receive substance use treatment services varies from state to state.[37] In some cases, a minor's emotional, social, and cognitive maturity is considered in addition to chronologic age. Moreover, whether an adolescent's parent must, by law, be notified once the adolescent has consented for treatment varies across states. Readers are encouraged to seek out regulations in their own states; the National District Attorneys Association compiles a list of relevant state laws and regulations that providers can review.[38]

### Test Selection and Timing

The clinician should also carefully consider what tests should be included in a drug screen. The SAMHSA-5, though widely available, notably misses several commonly used substances, including alcohol, opioids and synthetic cannabinoids, among other drugs and their metabolites[39]; clinicians should ensure that the laboratory they work with is able to broadly test for these commonly used substances. The SAMHSA-5 also tests for certain substances that are not commonly used in many places in the United States. An example is PCP, which is included in the SAMHSA-5 despite very low prevalence of use in most settings. In fact, where prevalence is low, a positive PCP screen is likely to be false, having been triggered by cross-reactivity with another compound (eg, dextromethorphan, a component of many cough syrups, is often implicated; even though technically a false positive, such a result may indicate misuse of cold medications).[40]

For adolescents who use marijuana, metabolites are detected in the urine for longer than other substances owing to the fat solubility of cannabinoids. For intermittent users, metabolites can be detected in the urine for up to 1 week after last use; for daily users, they can be detected for up to 1 month.[13] For adolescents who drink alcohol, urine ethyl glucuronide and ethyl sulfate are helpful tests with a window of detection of several days. Liver tests, such as aspartate aminotransferase, alanine aminotransferase, and gamma-glutamyl transferase are also somewhat sensitive to alcohol use but have poor specificity, thus, limiting their use.[41–43] Carbohydrate-deficient transferrin is a more specific marker for ongoing heavy alcohol use but requires drinking in excess of 40 g/d of ethanol for several weeks (approximately 3 standard drinks per day) and may not accurately detect intermittent heavy drinking.

Random drug testing is preferred to scheduled drug testing.[8] Because the window of detection for most substances varies between 1 to 3 days, adolescents who hope to evade detection on a drug test simply need to abstain from substance use for several days beforehand (though a longer period of abstinence is required for marijuana, as highlighted earlier). Random testing entails notifying the adolescent (or preferably, the adolescent's parent or guardian) of an immediate testing time. Carefully counseling the adolescent and his or her family beforehand about the expectation to immediately complete random drug tests as part of the treatment plan is essential. Random tests should occasionally be done on consecutive days to avoid drug use immediately after testing.

### Specimen Collection

Proper specimen collection procedures are critical for ensuring an adequate urine sample for drug testing. The Internet provides advice on a host of mechanisms for defeating urine drug tests that range from simple to sophisticated. A survey of practicing pediatricians found that, although most have ordered urine drug tests for an adolescent patient, most often these tests are collected without supervision, making it relatively easy for an adolescent to defeat a test.[11]

The most easily accomplished methods for tampering with a urine sample are adding water or other fluids or substituting a previously collected sample. Simple specimen validity checks (described later) can identify most samples that have been adulterated. Nonetheless, supervised sample collection is recommended to discourage tampering and increase the utility of testing.

The DOT describes 2 adequate methods for collecting a urine sample for drug testing.[12] For most routine workplace testing with adults, a collection protocol is used that does not involve direct observation. In this protocol, urine samples are collected in a private bathroom without running water, soap, or other liquids and with toilet water stained blue. No outer clothing, bags, or brief cases are permitted in the bathroom. The sample is checked for temperature immediately after it is produced. Although effective, this protocol is expensive to implement and monitor. Some commercial laboratories may offer this service, though it must be ordered separately and adds significant expense to the cost of a test, which may not be covered by insurance.

An alternative acceptable collection method requires direct observation of the specimen as it is being produced. This method is more invasive, though is simpler and does not require a specialized bathroom. This alternate collection protocol is often not practical in a clinical office.

For adolescents receiving treatment of substance use problems or disorders, urine specimens can be collected at home under the supervision of a parent or guardian. First morning specimens are recommended because the bladder is reliably full and urine is most concentrated. Random, unannounced tests are difficult to prepare for; repeated testing over several weeks is likely to detect ongoing use. A series of negative drug tests over several weeks provide strong support for a report of abstinence. Thus, home urine collection may be a reasonable mechanism for monitoring an adolescent that is receiving treatment of a substance use disorder.

Although urine specimens may be collected at home, it is recommended that all urine drug tests be coordinated with a medical professional and only ordered in the context of an appropriate clinical indication. As noted earlier, the AAP recommends against suspicionless drug testing, whether at home, school, medical offices, or in other settings, because these tests provide little useful clinical information and may cause tension between an adolescent and parents, school administrators, physicians, or other adults. Furthermore, the AAP discourages physicians from recommending drug tests for home use interpreted by families because they rely on relatively nonspecific and insensitive enzyme-linked panels and may generate false-positive and false-negative results. (Again, this is distinguished from home collection of drug tests to be sent to a laboratory for formal interpretation under the guidance of a clinician in a substance use treatment program, which is commonly indicated.)

### Specimen Validation

Regardless of collection procedures, validity checks are recommended for all urine specimens. The DOT recommends checking temperature, creatinine, and specific gravity on every urine sample.[12] Temperature is checked immediately after voiding. Urine specimen cups with temperature strips that fluoresce between 90°F and 100°F facilitate temperature validation. Urine creatinine and specific gravity can be ordered together with a drug test panel. Many commercial laboratories also offer adulterant panels that can detect many substances added to a test in vitro.

Creatinine is a product of muscle metabolism that can be used as a marker of urine concentration. According to the DOT's guidelines, urine samples with a random creatinine between 2 and 20 mg/mL should be considered dilute; a specimen with a creatinine less than 2 mg/mL should be considered substituted (ie, not urine) or artificially diluted (ie, water has been added).[12] Because adolescence is the period in life during which muscle mass is greatest, this creatinine range may need to be adjusted for larger teens. For example, a specimen with a creatinine between 20 and 50 mg/mL may be considered dilute if the specific gravity is also low.

A dilute specimen suggests that a teen has recently consumed a large volume of fluid. This may occur incidentally or intentionally in attempt to drive the concentration of a drug or metabolite to less than the detection level of the test. It is not possible to distinguish between these possibilities based on the results of a urine test alone, and clinical correlation is advised whenever interpreting negative drug test. Repeat drug testing may be warranted using first morning specimens if possible. A dilute urine sample can still be positive, although in such cases it is possible to miss other substances present in lower concentrations. For example, a urine specimen may be positive for marijuana but too dilute to identify low levels of cocaine.

### Interpretation of Results

As with all laboratory tests, urine drug tests can yield false-positive and false-negative results. Unlike most other laboratory results, however, results of urine drug tests can be accurate and still yield misleading information; in other words a test can yield a true negative result in the context of ongoing psychoactive substance use (eg, if the test was performed outside the window of detection of the drug that the adolescent was using) or a true positive result in the context of no use of psychoactive substances (eg, if the test detects substances found in food such as poppy seeds, which can trigger an opioid screen, or in a patient's prescribed medications, such as stimulants for ADHD, which can trigger an amphetamine screen). Urine drug tests may also yield ambiguous results if a test is too dilute for interpretation or does not match a patient's stated history. Because of their differing properties, different interpretation strategies are required for IA screening tests as compared with confirmatory GC-MS tests.

### Interpretation of immunoassay tests

Enzyme-linked IA tests are relatively quick, inexpensive, and easy to perform and, as such, are often used by laboratories as a first-line screen. This testing format identifies drugs or metabolites above a certain threshold concentration in the urine. Typically the threshold concentration is set high enough to limit detection of low levels of drugs or metabolites that may be found in foods. For example, poppy seeds contain very low levels of morphine that can be detected by sensitive tests; but under usual circumstances concentrations of morphine in the blood and urine from consuming typical amounts of poppy seeds will be well under the detection threshold.

IA is nonspecific and cross-reactions can occur. As an example, quinolone antibiotics can cross-react with an opioid panel yielding a false-positive test result. To eliminate this type of error, IA tests should be confirmed with a more definitive chromatographic test (eg, GC-MS), particularly if a test result is unexpected and does not correlate with a patient's history.

### Interpretation of confirmatory chromatography tests

Chromatographic tests generally take longer to perform and are more labor intensive and more expensive than IA, though newer technologies may address these issues. Chromatographic tests are specific and are not susceptible to cross-reactions; thus, false-positive results are rare. However, chromatographic tests can detect prescribed medications (such as stimulants used for ADHD treatment); it is impossible to distinguish whether a patient used the medication as prescribed or misused it by using more than prescribed or using an alternate route of administration (eg, crushing and snorting pills).

### Interpretation of negative tests

Whether IA or chromatographic testing is preformed, special consideration should be given to the interpretation of negative tests. A drug test will be negative despite ongoing drug use in 4 different circumstances:

- The window of detection has passed. The window of detection for most substances is 2 to 3 days, and drug use will not be detected after this period. One notable exception is heavy, chronic use of cannabis, which can result in prolonged excretion for up to 4 weeks,[14] complicating interpretation during this period.
- The patient has used a substance not detected by the testing panel. Athough nearly any substance can be tested for in urine, standard test panels are limited to commonly used substances. For example, synthetic cannabinoids are not detected by standard tests for cannabis and should be ordered separately if use is suspected. Inhalants are excreted by the lungs and cannot be detected in a urine specimen.
- The concentration of the substance is less than the detection limit of the test. This circumstance is uncommon with chromatographic tests, which are typically very sensitive, but may occur with IA tests, which have a set cutoff threshold typically designed to eliminate false positives from cross-reaction or trace amounts of a

drug or metabolite that may be found in food products. Intentional urine dilution may result in a falsely negative test.

- The specimen has been substituted or adulterated. Distinct from most instances of laboratory medicine, patients may be motivated to falsify test results by substituting or adulterating specimens. Proper specimen collection techniques (see earlier discussion), use of temperature testing, and adulterant panels can minimize opportunities for interfering with testing in this way.

### Presenting drug test results to adolescents

Reviewing positive urine drug test results presents the simultaneous challenges of sharing relevant information while maintaining a therapeutic alliance with an adolescent patient and his or her family. Before ordering a drug test, a discussion of how results will be reported and to whom can help maximize the utility of drug testing.

In most instances it is useful to have a private conversation with the adolescent to clarify interpretation of the drug test result. Simply sharing that the drug test yielded an unexpected result without revealing specific details may set the stage for an honest conversation about substance use; at times, patients will reveal use of substances that were not detected by the test. If patients give a history that is consistent with the drug test results, then the conversation can move on to a discussion of next steps, which could include changes to the treatment plan. Sharing drug test results together with a plan may facilitate a positive conversation. For example, a clinician may report to parents that their son has recently used marijuana and has now agreed to speak with a counselor about anxiety and marijuana use.

When a drug test result is dilute or otherwise ambiguous, a clinical interview may be helpful. Starting with a simple statement about an unexpected test result without revealing all of the details can serve as an open-ended way of beginning the conversation. If a patient does not report substance use, then the clinician can review methods for reducing the chance of a dilute specimen by providing a first morning urine if possible or, if not, limiting water intake in the hour before giving a sample. Repeat testing may be useful.

During a clinical interview an adolescent may offer an explanation that is consistent with the observed drug test results, such as a new prescription medication or supervised use of cold medication. This history can be confirmed with a parent, and the drug test can be interpreted as negative (ie, consistent with a history of no illicit substance use).

In some instances an adolescent's history may be inconsistent with observed drug test results. As with all laboratory testing, drug test results provide limited information and clinical correlation is always advised. A single positive drug test may be spurious and can be treated that way if patients otherwise seem to be doing well and adhering to the treatment plan. In these cases, repeat urine testing is recommended; a second occurrence of a positive drug test is unlikely to be another false-positive result. In this case, the clinician may recommend modifications to the treatment plan.

### SUMMARY

Drug testing, when carefully collected and thoughtfully interpreted, offers a critical adjunct to clinical care and substance use treatment. However, because test results can be misleading if not interpreted in the correct clinical context, clinicians should always conduct a careful interview with adolescent patients to understand what testing is likely to show and then use testing to validate or refute their expectations. Because of the ease with which samples can be tampered, providers should also carefully reflect on their own collection protocols and sample validation procedures to ensure optimal accuracy.

**REFERENCES**

1. Moyer VA. Screening and behavioral counseling interventions in primary care to reduce alcohol misuse: U.S. preventive services task force recommendation statement. Ann Intern Med 2013;159:210–8.
2. National Institute on Alcohol Abuse and Alcoholism. Alcohol screening and brief intervention for youth: a practitioner's guide. Bethesda (MD): National Institutes of Health; 2011.
3. Higgins-Biddle J, Hungerford D, Cates-Wessel K. Screening and brief interventions (SBI) for unhealthy alcohol use: a step-by-step implementation guide for trauma centers. Atlanta (GA): Centers for Disease Control and Prevention; 2009.
4. Levy SJ, Kokotailo PK. Substance use screening, brief intervention, and referral to treatment for pediatricians. Pediatrics 2011;128:e1330–40.
5. Levy S. Effects of marijuana policy on children and adolescents. JAMA Pediatr 2013;167:600–2.
6. Hagan JF, Shaw JS, Duncan PM. Bright futures: guidelines for health supervision of infants, children, and adolescents, 3rd edition Available at: http://brightfutures. aap.org/3rd_Edition_Guidelines_and_Pocket_Guide.html. Accessed October 12, 2015.
7. Levy S, Siqueira LM, Ammerman SD, et al. Testing for drugs of abuse in children and adolescents. Pediatrics 2014;133:e1798–807.
8. American Society for Addiction Medicine. Drug testing: a white paper of the American Society of Addiction Medicine (ASAM). Chevy Chase (MD): American Society of Addiction Medicine; 2013.
9. Substance Abuse and Mental Health Services Administration. Clinical drug testing in primary care. Technical assistance publication (TAP) 32. Rockville (MD): Substance Abuse and Mental Health Services Administration; 2012. HHS publication No. (SMA) 12–4668.
10. National Center on Substance Abuse and Child Welfare/Substance Abuse and Mental Health Services Administration. Drug testing practice guidelines. Available at: https://ncsacw.samhsa.gov/files/IA_Drug_Testing_Bench_Card_508.pdf. Accessed October 10, 2015.
11. Levy S, Harris SK, Sherritt L, et al. Drug testing of adolescents in ambulatory medicine: physician practices and knowledge. Arch Pediatr Adolesc Med 2006;160:146–50.
12. Jones RK, Shinar D, Walsh JM. Detection and measurement of drugs. State Knowl. Drug-impaired driving. NHTSA Rep. DOT HS 809 642. Washington, DC: US National Highway Traffic Safety Administration; 2003.
13. Grotenhermen F. Pharmacokinetics and pharmacodynamics of cannabinoids. Clin Pharmacokinet 2003;42:327–60.
14. Schwilke EW, Gullberg RG, Darwin WD, et al. Differentiating new cannabis use from residual urinary cannabinoid excretion in chronic, daily cannabis users. Addiction 2011;106:499–506.
15. Cone EJ. New developments in biological measures of drug prevalence. In: Harrison L, Hughes A, editors. The validity of self-reported drug use: improving the accuracy of survey estimates. Bethesda (MD): National Institute on Drug Abuse; 1997. p. 108–29.
16. Dams R, Choo RE, Lambert WE, et al. Oral fluid as an alternative matrix to monitor opiate and cocaine use in substance-abuse treatment patients. Drug Alcohol Depend 2007;87:258–67.

17. Bosker WM, Huestis MA. Oral fluid testing for drugs of abuse. Clin Chem 2009; 55:1910–31.

18. Drummer OH. Drug testing in oral fluid. Clin Biochem Rev 2006;27:147–59.

19. Boumba V, Ziavrou K, Vougiouklakis T. Hair as a biological indicator of drug use, drug abuse or chronic exposure to environmental toxicants. Int J Toxicol 2006;25: 143–63.

20. Dolan K, Rouen D, Kimber J. An overview of the use of urine, hair, sweat and saliva to detect drug use. Drug Alcohol Rev 2004;23:213–7.

21. Warner E, Lorch E. Laboratory diagnosis. In: Ries RK, Fiellin DA, Miller SC, et al, editors. SAM Principles of Addiction Medicine. 5th edition. Philadelphia: American Society of Addiction Medicine; 2014.

22. Pragst F, Balikova MA. State of the art in hair analysis for detection of drug and alcohol abuse. Clin Chim Acta 2006;370:17–49.

23. Henderson GL, Harkey MR, Zhou C, et al. Incorporation of isotopically labeled cocaine and metabolites into human hair: 1. Dose-response relationships. J Anal Toxicol 1996;20:1–12.

24. Ropero-Miller JD, Huestis MA, Stout PR. Cocaine analytes in human hair: evaluation of concentration ratios in different cocaine sources, drug-user populations and surface-contaminated specimens. J Anal Toxicol 2012;36:390–8.

25. Dasgupta A. Handbook of drug monitoring methods: therapeutics and drugs of abuse. Totowa (NJ): Springer; 2008.

26. Pötsch L, Skopp G, Moeller MR. Influence of pigmentation on the codeine content of hair fibers in Guinea pigs. J Forensic Sci 1997;42:1095–8.

27. US Department of Transporation. Approved evidential breath testing devices. Available at: https://www.transportation.gov/odapc/approved-evidential-breath-testing-devices. Accessed October 4, 2015.

28. Concheiro M, Jones HE, Johnson RE, et al. Maternal buprenorphine dose, placenta buprenorphine, and metabolite concentrations and neonatal outcomes. Ther Drug Monit 2010;32:206–15.

29. Gray T, Huestis M. Bioanalytical procedures for monitoring in utero drug exposure. Anal Bioanal Chem 2007;388:1455–65.

30. Hudak ML, Tan RC. Neonatal drug withdrawal. Pediatrics 2012;129:e540–60.

31. Stanger C, Budney AJ. Contingency management approaches for adolescent substance use disorders. Child Adolesc Psychiatr Clin N Am 2010;19:547–62.

32. Hartzler B, Lash SJ, Roll JM. Contingency management in substance abuse treatment: a structured review of the evidence for its transportability. Drug Alcohol Depend 2012;122:1–10.

33. Shearer J, Tie H, Byford S. Economic evaluations of contingency management in illicit drug misuse programmes: a systematic review. Drug Alcohol Rev 2015;34:289–98.

34. Dennis M, Godley SH, Diamond G, et al. The Cannabis Youth Treatment (CYT) study: main findings from two randomized trials. J Subst Abuse Treat 2004;27:197–213.

35. Drug & Alcohol Testing Industry Association. Ultimate guide to state drug testing laws. Available at: http://www.datia.org/publications/ultimate-guide-to-state-drug-testing-laws.html. Accessed October 12, 2015.

36. Levy S, Schizer M. Adolescent drug testing policies in schools. Pediatrics 2015; 135:782–3.

37. Center for Substance Abuse Treatment. Chapter 8—Legal and ethical issues. Substance abuse and mental health administration. Rockville (MD): Substance Abuse and Mental Health Services Administration; 1999.

38. National District Attorneys Association. Minor consent to medical treatment laws. Available at: http://www.ndaa.org/pdf/Minor Consent to Medical Treatment (2). pdf. Accessed September 25, 2015.

39. Johnston LD, O'Malley PM, Miech RA, et al. Monitoring the future national survey results on drug use: 1975-2014, Overview, key findings on adolescent drug use. Ann Arbor (MI): Institute for Social Research. The University of Michigan; 2015.

40. Rengarajan A, Mullins ME. How often do false-positive phencyclidine urine screens occur with use of common medications? Clin Toxicol 2013;51:493–6.

41. Nanau RM, Neuman MG. Biomolecules and biomarkers used in diagnosis of alcohol drinking and in monitoring therapeutic interventions. Biomolecules 2015;5:1339–85.

42. Warner E. Laboratory diagnosis. Principles of Addiction Medicine. 3rd edition. Chevy Chase (MD): American Society of Addiction Medicine; 2003. p. 337–48.

43. Center for Substance Abuse Treatment. The role of biomarkers in the treatment of alcohol use disorders. Rockville (MD): Substance Abuse and Mental Health Services Administration; 2006.

# Index

*Note:* Page numbers of article titles are in **boldface** type.

Child Adolesc Psychiatric Clin N Am 25 (2016) 567–577
http://dx.doi.org/10.1016/S1056-4993(16)30048-7
1056-4993/16/$ – see front matter

childpsych.theclinics.com

# *Moving?*

## *Make sure your subscription moves with you!*

To notify us of your new address, find your **Clinics Account Number** (located on your mailing label above your name), and contact customer service at:

**Email: journalscustomerservice-usa@elsevier.com**

**800-654-2452** (subscribers in the U.S. & Canada)
**314-447-8871** (subscribers outside of the U.S. & Canada)

**Fax number: 314-447-8029**

**Elsevier Health Sciences Division**
**Subscription Customer Service**
**3251 Riverport Lane**
**Maryland Heights, MO 63043**

*To ensure uninterrupted delivery of your subscription, please notify us at least 4 weeks in advance of move.